The Age of the Inquiry

Inquiries in health and social care attract public interest, wide coverage in the media and are influential in shaping policy and service provision. *The Age of the Inquiry* examines inquiries across a range of services: into child protection tragedies, mental health homicides, abuse in learning disability services and in residential and nursing care for older people. Leading writers in the field have been brought together to analyse some of the key inquiries of the 1990s and the beginning of the twenty-first century.

The contributors discuss a wide range of inquiries in terms of their processes, findings and applications. Readers will find new and original accounts of high profile inquiries such as the Climbié Inquiry, as well as being introduced to inquiries that are less familiar. The value of inquiries is hotly debated and their positive and negative impacts are highlighted. The book also includes accounts from professionals who have chaired inquiries, those who have been subjected to their scrutiny, and from parents whose son died in a mental health tragedy which was the subject of an inquiry. Proposals for the future form and conduct of inquiries are included, and a number of the contributors use their personal experiences of participating in inquiries to inform their suggestions.

Nicky Stanley is Professor of Social Work at the University of Central Lancashire and Director of the MA in Social Work Programme. She undertakes research and has published extensively in the fields of child protection, mental health and interprofessional work.

Jill Manthorpe is Professor of Social Work at King's College London where she is Co-Director of the Social Care Workforce Research Unit. She is currently researching in the areas of workforce planning, dementia, adult protection and risk, where her work is widely published.

The Age of the Inquiry

Learning and blaming in health and social care

Edited by Nicky Stanley and Jill Manthorpe

Routledge
Taylor & Francis Group

LONDON AND NEW YORK

First published 2004
by Routledge
11 New Fetter Lane, London EC4P 4EE

Simultaneously published in the USA and Canada
by Routledge
29 West 35th Street, New York, NY 10001

Routledge is an imprint of the Taylor & Francis Group

© 2004 Nicky Stanley and Jill Manthorpe

Typeset in Garamond and Gill by BC Typesetting Ltd, Bristol
Printed and bound in Great Britain by
MPG Books Ltd, Bodmin, Cornwall

British Library Cataloguing in Publication Data
A catalogue record for this book is available from the British Library

Library of Congress Cataloging in Publication Data
A catalog record for this book has been requested

ISBN 0–415–28315–9 (hbk)
ISBN 0–415–28316–7 (pbk)

The Age of the Inquiry

Learning and blaming in health and social care

Edited by Nicky Stanley and Jill Manthorpe

Routledge
Taylor & Francis Group

LONDON AND NEW YORK

First published 2004
by Routledge
11 New Fetter Lane, London EC4P 4EE

Simultaneously published in the USA and Canada
by Routledge
29 West 35th Street, New York, NY 10001

Routledge is an imprint of the Taylor & Francis Group

© 2004 Nicky Stanley and Jill Manthorpe

Typeset in Garamond and Gill by BC Typesetting Ltd, Bristol
Printed and bound in Great Britain by
MPG Books Ltd, Bodmin, Cornwall

British Library Cataloguing in Publication Data
A catalogue record for this book is available from the British Library

Library of Congress Cataloging in Publication Data
A catalog record for this book has been requested

ISBN 0–415–28315–9 (hbk)
ISBN 0–415–28316–7 (pbk)

Contents

Tables and boxes

Tables

Boxes

Contributors

Paul Cambridge is a Senior Lecturer in Learning Disability at the Tizard Centre, University of Kent at Canterbury.

Roger Clough is Emeritis Professor of Social Work at the University of Lancaster and a former Chief Inspector with Cumbria Social Services. He now undertakes research through the Eskrigge Social Research consultancy.

Alan Corbett is Head of Therapy at CARI (Children at Risk in Ireland). Prior to this he was Director of Respond, an organisation that provides a range of services to victims and perpetrators of sexual abuse who have learning disabilities.

Brian Corby is Professor of Social Work Studies at the University of Central Lancashire.

Sylvia Duncan is a Consultant Clinical Psychologist at the Baker and Duncan Family Consultancy.

Audrey and **Paul Edwards** are the parents of Christopher whose mild mental illness led him to cause a breach of the peace for which he was remanded to prison for three days. Within nine hours of entering prison he was beaten to death by his cell mate who had schizophrenia. When not discharging her parental responsibilities, Audrey was a Court Reporter and Paul was the Chief Executive of social housing authorities in the UK and Australia.

Rachel Fyson is a Research Fellow at The Ann Craft Trust, an organisation that works to prevent the abuse of people with learning disabilities.

Deborah Kitson is Director of The Ann Craft Trust.

Jill Manthorpe is Professor of Social Work at King's College London and Co-Director of the Social Care Workforce Research Unit. She is Chair of the Hull and East Riding Adult Protection Committee.

Andrew McCulloch is Chief Executive of the Mental Health Foundation. His experience of inquiries includes sitting as a panel member, giving evidence and acting as secretary to an inquiry.

Pete Melia was Senior Clinical Nurse and Clinical Manager for the Personality Disorder Services at Ashworth Hospital from 1997 to 2001. He is currently employed as a Nurse Consultant in Forensic Mental Health at the Hutton Centre Regional Secure Unit in Middlesbrough. He is a Visiting Lecturer at Teesside University.

Eileen Munro is a Reader in Social Policy at the London School of Economics.

Camilla Parker is an independent legal consultant specialising in mental health law and policy and human rights.

Bridget Penhale is a Senior Lecturer in Gerontology at the University of Sheffield.

Herschel Prins is External Professor at the University of Loughborough, Visiting Professor at Nottingham Trent University and Hon. Visiting Fellow, Scarman Centre, Leicester University.

Peter Reder is now retired, he was previously Consultant Child and Adolescent Psychiatrist at the West London Mental Health Trust.

Dave Sheppard is a partner in the Institute of Mental Health Law and an independent consultant and trainer on mental health law and practice. He has been a social work member of three independent inquiries following homicide.

Nicky Stanley is Professor of Social Work at the University of Central Lancashire.

The inquiry as Janus

Nicky Stanley and Jill Manthorpe

Inquiry reports in health and social care have been issuing in a seemingly con-tinuous stream since the early 1990s in the UK. This flow has been dominated by some major, eye-catching features. Public attention has focused on inquiries into homicides committed by users of mental health services and those addressing the deaths of children known to statutory services. This book also covers inquiries into the care of people with learning disabilities and older people. These groups may attract less public interest and fewer head-lines but are similarly vulnerable. Indeed, one of the major achievements of the inquiries has been to bring detailed accounts of the experiences of some of the most stigmatised and socially excluded groups to the forefront of public awareness. The Climbié Inquiry (Laming 2003), for instance, paints a picture of the housing and financial difficulties experienced by families from abroad living in London, the Longcare Inquiry (Buckinghamshire County Council 1998) provides a vivid account of the squalor and petty depredations of institutional life, and the 'care' of older people with dementia is revealed to be brutish in Beech House and Rowan Ward.

The inquiries also convey the experiences of those who are most reliant on health and welfare services. The reports tell the stories of individuals who spend long periods engaged in complex transactions with professionals, who live with constant professional intrusions into their personal or family lives, or who live in institutions where their time and activities are structured by others. The interactions between those who use services and those who provide them are recorded at a level of detail rarely available to those who are not themselves employed by these services. The accounts provided by inquiry reports show recipients of services in a variety of roles: they may make repeated requests for help or support, they may seek to evade statutory scrutiny, and they may attempt to exploit or abuse services and professionals. Similarly, professionals are depicted as failing to respond to the needs of vulnerable people, actively pursuing those who need help, and abusing or exploiting those who rely on them for protection.

In order to maintain a focus upon those who are socially excluded and reliant on services, this book concentrates on inquiries which have involved social care and health organisations. This has resulted in the omission of some of the major inquiries of the last decade: the Bristol Royal Infirmary Inquiry (Kennedy 2001), the Alder Hey Hospital Inquiry (Redfern *et al.* 2001) and the Shipman Inquiry (Smith 2002, 2003). These inquiries, alongside those discussed in this book, have had a significant impact on public perceptions of professional expertise and authority. However, as they have focused primarily on health services, they record the experiences of a much wider group of people who are using universal services available to the broad population.

This book is devoted to inquiries into health and social care services in England and Wales published since 1990: it is the period since then that we have designated the 'age of the inquiry'. This approach excludes some of the key inquiries into child deaths which took place in the 1980s, but these have been fully discussed elsewhere (Stevenson 1989; Corby 2002). Although inquiries into individual child deaths went 'underground' in the 1990s with Part 8 Reviews (generally internal to local statutory services) replacing formal inquiries, some high profile inquiries (e.g. Bridge Child Care Consultancy Service 1995; Newham Area Child Protection Committee 2002; Norfolk Health Authority 2002) have emerged – these are discussed more fully in Chapter 4. The period has also seen a number of inquiries into abuse in children's homes (Stanley 1999) and, in Chapter 6, Brian Corby analyses the process and impact of the largest of these inquiries: the North Wales Tribunal. The 1990s saw an explosion in the number of mental health inquiries into homicide following the guidance issued by the NHS Executive in 1994 stating that, 'in cases of homicide it will always be necessary to hold an inquiry' (Department of Health 1994). The sheer quantity of these inquiries and the attendant cost implications are evident in Chapter 9 which provides a comprehensive list of all those published since 1985. Inquiries involving the care of older people or people with learning disabilities have been fewer in number but still attract considerable public interest as the report into Rowan Ward (Commission for Health Improvement 2003) demonstrates (see Chapter 12).

The interest evoked by inquiries is not only attributable to their content, the form is also relevant. The inquiry report tells a story. It is a narrative account replete with human drama and action. Every inquiry report has its heroes, villains and victims but, for the reader, the outcome of their interactions is known at the outset. The dramatic tension of the story told by the inquiry report resides in the judgement delivered by the inquiry team. The reader is invited to identify with the lofty perspective of the inquiry panel and to pass judgement upon the actions of the protagonists with the benefit of hindsight. This is essentially a moral judgement about whether professionals have done the job expected of them and whether they have adequately protected those they were charged to protect. Parton (1985) borrowed the term 'moral panic' from the work of Cohen (1973) to describe the response to child care inquiries of the 1970s and 1980s. While the use of the term 'panic' has provoked some criticism (Merrick 1996), the focus on the moral nature of the tale told by the inquiry team is justified. However, the inquiry team and the reader of the report examine events from the high vantage point that is hindsight. Hindsight suggests causal associations which may not have existed between omissions of care and tragic events (Stanley and Manthorpe 2001) and some of the more reflective inquiry reports acknowledge the distinction between hindsight vision and the viewpoint available at the time to professionals under scrutiny.

As a means of balancing the 'omniscient' stance of the inquiry team and the reader of the inquiry report, Part I of this book is devoted to commentaries that are self-avowedly partial and offer alternative perspectives. Herschel Prins' chapter presents the views of a number of those who have chaired inquiries and provides an insight into the processes of managing and co-ordinating the work of the inquiry team. The second chapter, by Paul and Audrey Edwards, is a personal account of the inquiry process from the viewpoint of family members who sought to participate in the process as equal partners in inquiry. The difficulties they encountered in their attempts to do so illuminate the extent to which the inquiry process has been captured and controlled by the legal profession. Finally, in this first part, Pete Melia's chapter offers a picture of the process of inquiry from the perspectives of patients and staff at Ashworth Hospital. This account explores the immediate impact of an inquiry on those who are being inquired into and highlights the potential of inquiries for blaming individuals and holding them to account.

The following four parts of the book cover inquiries into child care services, mental health homicides, the care of people with learning disabilities and the care of older people. The inquiries discussed include both those examining individual cases and those which address large-scale institutional abuse. While the triggers for these two types of inquiries may differ considerably, both forms of inquiry explore the interface between professional practice that is simply poor and that which can be labelled as neglectful or abusive. We have argued elsewhere (Manthorpe and Stanley 1999) that responses to institutional abuse need to distinguish between the actions and responsibilities of individual staff and organisational failings. This also applies to inquiries which examine individual deaths and harm, and this distinction between individual and organisational accountability emerged as an explicit theme of the Climbié Inquiry (Laming 2003).

There is considerable debate as to whether inquiries should continue in their present form (Grounds 1997; Reder and Duncan 1998; Eldergill 1999) and the establishment of the National Patient Safety Agency (Department of Health 2001) indicates some commitment to reform of the current system. In addition to considering the impact of inquiries on policy and practice, this book offers a number of different evaluations of both the process and the form of inquiries. We consider that the strength of the inquiry format lies in its capacity to position itself on the boundary between past events and future developments. Like Janus, god of the new year, it can look both backwards and forwards and some of the inquiry reports that have had the most impact are those that acknowledge this dual vision and use the evidence of past events to inform planning for the future.

The depth of the backwards gaze of inquiries varies. Some reports, like the Blom-Cooper *et al.* (1996) inquiry into the case of Jason Mitchell, explore the early experiences of perpetrators of homicide or abuse in depth. Others confine themselves to perusing the history of contact with statutory services. Exposing an individual's developmental history at length can serve to make abuse or violence in later life more explicable and perhaps less horrific for readers. However, there are some rarely acknowledged questions concerning the rights of those who are the subject of inquiry reports to privacy in relation to information that might be considered to be outside the events which constitute the proper focus of an inquiry. Consent for publication of such material is not always sought.

The breadth and scope of the inquiry's forward gaze is usually determined by the level at which an inquiry is commissioned and pitched. Inquiries such as the North Wales Tribunal and the Victoria Climbié Inquiry are instigated by central government, absorb considerable resources and attract national media attention. They are, by their very nature, required to comment on the national rather than local picture. Other inquiries may reflect the interests of the Chair in addressing broad policy issues or legislative reform. Blom-Cooper *et al.*'s (1995) inquiry into the case of Andrew Robinson, which argued the case for a new Mental Health Act, is a good example of this. The following section considers why some inquiries assume pre-eminence.

Inquiries of note

Many of the inquiries discussed in this book will be familiar to almost all readers – others have had little exposure. This book discusses the 'iconic' inquiries but we hope that it also provides exploration of some of those inquiries that are more submerged. In Chapter 8, for example, some rarely considered mental health inquiries involving female perpetrators are discussed. In considering why certain inquiries receive attention, both at the time of publication and in the longer term, six key factors can be identified to explain why certain inquiries achieve 'iconic' status. Not all inquiries of note are characterised by all these factors but one or a combination of factors appears significant in shaping the level of the social reaction.

- Inquiries assume pre-eminence when the event or series of events involve multiple 'victims'. A number of victims make for a wide group of affected individuals, families and citizens. The sheer quantity of individuals affected by Beech House (see Chapter 10), the North Wales Inquiry (see Chapter 6) and in Longcare (see Chapter 12) demands a high profile inquiry which can function as a means for addressing the enormity or scale of the 'crime' or event.

- Related to this 'quantitative' approach, the identity of 'victims' seems to contribute to the impetus to have an inquiry – particularly if those harmed are children or vulnerable. Heightened vulnerability, among children for example, is integral to presumed 'innocence', and evokes empathy from the public. This gives the voice of relatives, such as Victoria Climbié's parents, a poignant authority and capacity for testimony, since the vulnerability of those affected may make it difficult for their own voices to be heard (see Manthorpe 1999). However, Paul and Audrey Edwards' account in Chapter 2 shows that some relatives may struggle to be listened to and to receive a response. Victims who are perceived as 'ordinary citizens' also provoke public concern. The random and arbitrary nature of events dramatises the risks faced by 'ordinary' innocent members of the public whose sense of safety is consequently undermined. This public sense of insecurity helps account for the high level of interest in those inquiries which the Clunis Inquiry (Ritchie *et al.* 1994) exemplified. This anxiety was developed and sustained by the campaigning work of Jayne Zito, Jonathan Zito's widow, who established the Zito Trust to work for improvements in mental health services and legislation.

  Those inquiries where the voice of those affected by events is less easy to portray as 'defenceless', tread a difficult path in portraying individuals as victims, as Melia's discussion of Ashworth Hospital patients' experience of the Fallon Inquiry demonstrates in Chapter 3. Individuals who are socially excluded do not always evoke public sympathy, but individual presumptions of innocence can override possible antipathy to social groups, such as looked after children or adults with learning disabilities. Hence, inquiries such as the North Wales Tribunal attract public interest although judgemental debates continue about the victims' integrity (see, for example, Webster 1998).

- A further reason for some inquiries to resonate with the public is that they focus on events which are atypical and 'horrific'. As the distressing events catalogued by the Victoria Climbié Inquiry (see Munro, Chapter 4) demonstrate, it is not simply that a child died but that her suffering was perceived to be long-term, deliberate and caused by neglect or cruelty. The collision of the horrific with the 'innocent' or 'ordinary' status of the victim provokes high emotional responses from the public.

- Inquiries usually involve retrospective analysis of events which have unfolded over time and thus opportunities are seen to have existed for intervention by professionals charged with the protection of vulnerable individuals. Key inquiries not only pose the question 'what happened?' but 'how could such events continue?' and 'why did no one act?'

Chronologies can serve to expose long series of professional interventions which, with the benefit of hindsight, assume the status of missed opportunities. Inquiries that assume pre-eminence carry the promise that fault-finding or blame is possible and that the inquiry will be able to deliver clear answers and allocate responsibility.

- Our reading of large numbers of inquiries also suggests that there are factors to consider which are less predictable in determining whether an inquiry comes to be an emblem of what is wrong with health or social care. These relate to the timing of inquiry process and publications: for example, Fyson and her colleagues in Chapter 10 discuss the way in which the Longcare Inquiry locked in to debates about criminal justice and court procedures. Inquiries may chime with debates and policy initiatives, and may be picked up as examples of the need for reform. In relation to community mental health, the inquiries that have had a particular impact have fed into receptive policy debates, as McCulloch and Parker observe in Chapter 7.

- Finally, 'iconic' inquiries are generally accessible and this enables their findings and, in some cases, the evidence (see Corby in Chapter 6) to be considered afresh. Accessibility can be a matter of publication in a form that endures. We have ourselves found it very difficult to access some inquiries and hope that Chapter 9 assists in providing readers with sources. But accessibility is also a matter of style and comprehensiveness: some inquiries are much easier to read than others. There have been a number of valuable commentaries published (Peay 1996; Butler and Drakeford 2003). These have enabled the inquiries' messages to be circulated more widely but have inevitably tended to highlight some inquiries and ignore others.

The media and the message

The media clearly play a key role in magnifying the profile of some inquiries. The six factors discussed above influence the priorities of the media but, more importantly, mediate the interaction between the media and the development of policy and practice. It would be naive to see this impact as unidirectional. The media are not homogeneous and any influence on inquiries may represent, to varying degrees, critiques of government, distrust in professionals, political standpoints and public expressions of sympathy, outrage or disbelief. Moreover, much media reporting is not by journalists but includes viewpoints and commentary from welfare 'insiders', such as academics, senior managers or policy commentators. The notion that the media represent external scrutiny of welfare is diluted by the complex movements of comment, information and expertise.

At times, inquiries are instigated by media exposure and the function of the media as the last resort for the whistleblower is recognised in legislation (Public Interest Disclosure Act 1998). During the 1990s, however, the thresholds for inquiries were formalised and, in Chapter 5, Reder and Duncan outline the route whereby child death inquiries have been moved from a seemingly haphazard response to events to a formulaic process of decisions about the shape and scale of an inquiry. In our view, the 1990s will stand out as the decade when inquiries in British welfare emerged, alongside audit and inspection regimes, as a dominant means whereby social and health care services were scrutinised. The media's role in attracting public interest has fuelled decisions to hold individual inquiries (Butler and Drakeford 2003), but the media have also contributed to the view that inquiries have been too numerous, too expensive and insufficiently effective in changing systems or addressing practice. Doubts concerning the continued value of inquiries are reinforced when it appears easy for some authors to use others' reports as if they represent their own findings or reflections. Chapter 12 draws attention to the word-for-word repetition in the North Lakeland Trust (North Lakeland Healthcare 2000) inquiry report of a passage from the Beech House Inquiry Report (Camden and Islington Community Health Services NHS Trust 1999).

During the 1990s, access to inquiries was revolutionised by electronic media. The Climbié Inquiry Report was not the first to be available on-line (the *Case Review in Respect of PM*, Manby *et al.* 1998, probably has that dubious honour), but evidence was posted on its web site on a day-to-day basis. This stands in contrast to many previous inquiries where the final report presented the key findings and the detailed processes of hearing and examining evidence were either summarised for the reader or remained hidden. Similarly, some reports were easily accessible to a wide readership while others were hard to obtain. Although the increase in accessibility signalled by the Climbié Inquiry provides, on the face of it, a process that is open and more transparent in permitting other inferences to be drawn from the evidence, the volume of material is potentially disempowering as it becomes indigestible and overwhelming. Synopses and analyses of inquiries have been welcomed to assist in making the material manageable (for example, Reith 1998; Parker and McCulloch 1999; and Sinclair and Bullock 2002). All summaries, of course, provide an interpretation of the original material and some are explicitly designed to raise issues or to make connections that appear to have been underlooked, for example, the role of alcohol and drug misuse in mental health homicides (Ward and Applin 1998).

Images also play a key part in imprinting people or events on the minds of public and professionals alike and many readers will retain strong impressions of the much-used pictures of Christopher Clunis (the perpetrator of the homicide of Jonathan Zito) and the photograph of Victoria Climbié screened on television and published in the press. Both photographs convey the ethnicity of the subject of inquiry but, while photographs of Victoria communicate a sense of a childhood that has been lost, those of Clunis emphasise his size and race. Media images of black perpetrators of mental health homicides have fed the 'big, black and dangerous' stereotype which has contributed to the noted tendency for high levels of control and coercion to be employed with black users of mental health services (Fernando *et al.* 1998).

Not only does the media impact on the decision to hold an inquiry and on the public response to its findings, it is increasingly playing a role in the process of inquiry itself. Inquiry witnesses can appear conscious of the ways in which their evidence may be picked up and interpreted by the media. Media reporting may influence witnesses' willingness to appear before inquiries as well as shaping the nature of their evidence.

The relationship between the media and inquiries can be characterised as dynamic, and more recent inquiries, such as the Climbié Inquiry, have shown an awareness of this interactive relationship and a readiness to use and exploit the potential of the media.

This book draws largely on the inquiry reports themselves as primary sources. As documents, however, they relate to a variety of readerships and perhaps the key role of the media lies in the identification of matters germane to its readership. The media will continue to emphasise the human drama and 'bad news' aspects of inquiries since, as Anderson (1997) notes, these contribute to news value. If inquiries continue to be more publicly accessible then the media's role in distilling findings will be further needed. Ironically, greater accessibility can make interpretation more significant while underplaying its mechanisms.

Using inquiries

The effort, time, expense, together with professional and personal involvement invested in inquiries, make it important that their aftermath is used positively to inform policy, practice and learning. There is mixed evidence on the use made of inquiries, not surprisingly, since, as Reder and Duncan (1996) have noted, inquiries have various or multiple purposes. The chapters contained in this volume indicate the layers of influence potentially addressed by inquiries: at policy, service delivery and educational levels. In policy terms, inquiries provide impetus for reform or throw fresh light on complex issues. Butler and Drakeford (2003: 6) characterise the relationship between inquiries, policy and scandal as symbiotic and argue that inquiries can both disrupt or accelerate policy drives. In Chapter 3, Melia identifies the negative contribution of the Fallon Inquiry to national debate on the treatment of personality disorder. The Climbié Inquiry was the impetus behind the Green Paper, *Every Child Matters* (Chief Secretary to the Treasury 2003) on child protection, but some of the policy issues identified by the report, such as the recruitment and retention of child care social workers and the effectiveness of Area Child Protection Committees (ACPCs), were already under discussion. Within adult services, the impact of inquiries is less easy to discern, with *No Secrets* (Department of Health 2000a) making little reference to inquiries and more to issues around standards of care. Developments in adult protection with increased multi-agency working and agreed policy and procedures may lead to local inquiries in order to promote service improvements through analysis of critical incidents or adverse events. Agreement over the form of such inquiries and their thresholds is being developed, often modelled on child protection reviews (Manthorpe 2003). Campaigns in adult protection have drawn on the examples of poor practice provided by inquiries such as Longcare and Beech House. However, in contrast, Fyson and her colleagues (Chapter 10) consider that the influence of inquiries has been limited in learning disability policy. Inquiries seem to have provided contributory evidence, and evidence that is of high standing, rather than anecdotal, that reform is required.

It is more difficult to establish how inquiries impact on local policy and practice. As Prins notes in Chapter 1, inquiry teams rarely have the opportunity to monitor the implementation of their recommendations. Sinclair and Bullock's (2002) review observes that the task of conducting a serious case review is so demanding that there may be little energy or enthusiasm for translating recommendations into practice. However, in Chapter 11, Cambridge provides some concrete proposals as to how inquiries can be made more relevant and easily translatable into practice.

In reading recent inquiry reports, the shadow of previous inquiries becomes discernible in the actions of the protagonists. In relation to practice, the influence of inquiries weighs heavily on front-line workers and their managers. Health and social care professionals are too often depicted as motivated by the need to be seen to follow guidelines or procedure rather than the needs of the service user. The reports show them passing on responsibility to other professionals or closing cases, so relinquishing their responsibility for messy and demanding problems that cannot easily be made sense of or resolved. In the Climbié Inquiry, the social work practice in the London Borough of Haringey was described by a union representative who was also a social worker as 'conveyor belt social work'. The phrase conveys the sense that cases need to be kept moving, to be passed on through the system as fast as possible to ensure that no one gets stuck with responsibility for what might happen. Likewise, the inquiry team reporting on the case of Kenneth Grey (Mishcon *et al.* 1995: 7) comments that:

> this case reminded us of a sprint relay race where Kenneth Grey was the baton passed from hand to hand, and as he was passed on to the next runner in the race, so the previous runner handed over responsibility for him . . .

In a climate where care professionals are exposed to high levels of personal criticism and hostility in the media, the fear of being held responsible for a tragedy increases. Practice which seeks to avoid personal exposure to blame by moving cases on fails to engage in any depth with the needs of those who use services. 'Conveyor belt' practice may also be attributed to limited resources and high demands on health and social care practitioners, but the 'blame culture' fostered by inquiries has played a significant role here.

In the area of teaching and professional development, inquiries are used for several purposes. Inquiries are documents with which students and practitioners can engage, identifying both with the position of the practitioners but also with the interests of those who are subject to harm. The narrative approach can prove effective for students since it portrays the 'real' world of practice with its resource constraints, movements of personnel, difficulties in communication and general realignment of services, policies and imperatives. We need to be cautious, however, in using inquiries uncritically. They emphasise events that are unusual and may promote anxiety and conservatism. They may fuel stereotyping and concerns about violence, and they may instil a fear that other professionals will be unreceptive or incompetent. Most importantly, they relate to what went wrong, and although good practice is mentioned, this often becomes buried. In some areas of policy and practice, for instance, the field of interprofessional communication and collaboration, inquiries appear to have pushed research studies to one side and are being interpreted and used as hard evidence. The extent to which the accounts provided by inquiry reports are representative of broad standards of professional practice remains open to question. A shift in emphasis is discernible in the National Patient Safety Agency's (Department of Health 2001) approach to risk management which incorporates analysis of 'near misses' into the evidence base of everyday practice. The development of such processes within health services could usefully be transferred to the context of social care.

Finally, in considering the value of inquiries, the needs of family members and others must be acknowledged. The predominance of the legal inquisitorial mode of inquiries has had the effect of disempowering those whose interests the process should serve. As Paul and Audrey Edwards note in Chapter 2, family members may be admitted to the process but allowed no power in relation to it. Consent to publish information is not always sought from perpetrators or others, such as Ashworth's patients, who are allocated a status resembling that of the criminal in the dock in the inquiry process. Sinclair and Bullock (2002) likewise highlight the failure to involve family members in serious case reviews of child deaths. In Chapter 1, Prins comments on how rarely mental health inquiries are used to inform the future care of service users who commit homicides. The process needs to be more participatory and less wedded to the development and delivery of a moral verdict. The Climbié Inquiry made a significant move towards a more participatory approach with its 'second phase' consisting of expert seminars. The Commission for Health Improvement made progress in this direction by appointing Vicky Farnsworth, a self-advocate with learning disabilities, to its inquiry team into services at Bedfordshire and Luton NHS Trust (Batty 2003). This opening up of inquiries is to be welcomed; developing the process further could enhance their value. More movement in this direction might also serve to extend the benefits of inquiries to a wider group.

The future of inquiries

The inquiries of the 1990s and the early years of the twenty-first century have been harnessed to the managerialist and modernising agenda dominating British health and social services in this period. Their messages have been both framed and interpreted as a call for greater accountability. This is particularly apparent in relation to the Climbié Inquiry which, rather than rejecting the 'blame culture', adopted a broad paintbrush to spread blame widely through the echelons of both health and social care agencies. The Green Paper *Every Child Matters* (Chief Secretary to the Treasury 2003) published in response to this inquiry included a chapter headed 'Accountability and Integration' which argued the need for a lead person to be identified at all levels of policy making and practice in children's services. However, what is not clear is the mechanism by which increased accountability improves the quality of services. Improved clarity concerning who should do what may make it easier to identify what has gone wrong and who is to blame but does not necessarily guarantee a better service. Indeed, we have argued in this chapter that the 'blame culture' which has been fostered and fed by inquiries has led to defensive practice with health and social care professionals failing to engage with the real needs of service users because they are too heavily focused on adhering to procedure and are anxious about assuming responsibility in the absence of authority and resources.

It is high time that inquiries were unyoked from the process of allocating blame and allowed to focus on the learning that can be gleaned from their dual vision. The Department of Health's publication, *An Organisation with a Memory* (2000b), announced a new approach to learning from errors, adverse events and near misses in the NHS. The implementation plan (Department of Health 2001: 40) for this strategy identified the development of a 'blame-free culture' in which mistakes and negligence can be reported without fear of retribution as key to the success of this initiative. *An Organisation with a Memory*, for example, identified suicides by hanging from bed or shower rails committed by mental health in-patients as an area where risks could be reduced and the new system of reporting adverse events could be particularly effective. However, it is not currently clear whether the new approach is also to apply to mental health homicides.

In our view, the costs of continuing to hold full-scale inquiries into individual mental health homicides have begun to outweigh the benefits. Inquiries have ceased to yield new messages at the national level, but still have much to say about local services and local performance and we consider that the local interagency reviews into child deaths, now known as serious case reviews, offer a useful model for reviewing mental health homicides or serious events in other services in a manner that is non-adversarial and time-limited. This model of review could be still more open and participative so that service users and family members could contribute to the process. A sense of control and ownership of a review into homicide might serve to reduce families' needs to 'discover who is to blame'. Individual professionals may well be poorly trained, incompetent, negligent and make mistakes. Such practices need to be singled out and remedied if services and professionals are to command trust and respect. However, identifying and addressing poor or abusive practice needs to be undertaken constructively, in a manner that discriminates. Blame is too often experienced by those working in health and social care as a sledgehammer which fails to acknowledge the capacity for human error under the stress that emanates from the nature of the work and a lack of resources.

However, reviews into child deaths also have something to learn from the world of inquiries into homicide. *The Confidential Inquiry into Homicides and Suicides by Mentally Ill People* (Boyd 1996; Appleby *et al.* 1999, 2001) has been extremely successful in its work of collating and extrapolating common themes from mental health homicides and suicides. One particularly useful aspect of the Confidential Inquiry's work has been the presentation of statistics relating to homicides committed by users of mental health services alongside those occurring in the wider population (see Appleby *et al.* 2001). Child care services might also benefit from an approach which located child deaths that occur as a result of abuse or neglect in the context of national statistics on child deaths, including road traffic casualties and other forms of accidental death. Such an approach would reframe the task of safeguarding children's lives as a broad social responsibility, not just a task for professionals.

Currently, overviews of inquiries involving children are not readily accessible. Although central government receives copies, commentators have noted difficulties in obtaining details of all serious case reviews for a particular period. A number of key studies (Reder and Duncan 1999; Sinclair and Bullock 2002) have had to utilise samples whose representativeness is open to question. The establishment of a national body, equivalent to the Confidential Inquiry, which received and logged anonymised reports of all serious case reviews would, in our view, be a useful development. We are less convinced of the need for a three-tier structure for reviews, such as Reder and Duncan's (1998) proposal for introducing an additional regional body to undertake reviews: this appears to introduce a new layer to what is already an expensive and complex process. The government's formal response to the Climbié Inquiry, *Keeping Children Safe* (Department of Health *et al.* 2003: 118–20), proposes replacing the current system for local reviews with a similar structure: local screening groups would scrutinise all unexpected child deaths and identify those which required a serious case review. Serious case reviews would be undertaken by an independent team. A national overview of serious case reviews is also promised. While this might move to a distance some of the resource demands which serious case reviews place on services, these independent review teams would need to be constituted in such a way that they could allow families to contribute to their work. They would also need to be empowered to check that recommendations for local change were implemented. Alternatively, this role might be undertaken by the new integrated inspection services headed by Ofsted (Chief Secretary to the Treasury 2003).

In the case of inquiries involving the institutional abuse of children, older people or people with learning disabilities, we believe that abuse on a large scale by those formally entrusted with the case of vulnerable people does require a full-scale independent inquiry. Nevertheless such inquiries need to be constructed in such a way as to allow service users and their families to participate in and have some ownership of the process. In Chapter 13, Clough and Manthorpe consider the arguments for allowing inspectorates to assume the functions of inquiries and suggest that the new Commission for Social Care Inspection should address the interface between inspection and inquiries.

Other chapters in this book offer different views on the value and future of inquiries. Our aim in bringing inquiries into different services together in a single volume has been to promote the learning that inquiries can offer. Reflecting on the lessons of inquiries across user groups illuminates the extent to which their messages are transferable and may also suggest new applications for their findings. Here, we have indicated that not only can messages be applied across different fields, inquiries into health and social might also benefit from careful consideration of the form and process of inquiries across user groups. At the time of writing, the future of inquiries is under deliberation. Seismic shifts in the structure of services at the levels of central and local government make change imminent although its direction is unclear. We hope that this book contributes to the critical debate around the role of inquiries and increases the opportunities to use their lessons constructively.

References

Anderson, A. (1997) *Media, Culture and the Environment*, London: University College London Press.

Appleby, L., Shaw, J., Amos, T. and McDonnell, R. (1999) *Safer Services: National Confidential Inquiry into Suicide and Homicide by People with Mental Illness*, London: Department of Health.

Appleby, L., Shaw, J., Sherratt, J., Amos, T., Robinson, J. and McDonnell, R. (2001) *Safety First: Five Year Report of the Confidential Inquiry into Suicide and Homicide by People with Mental Illness*, London: Department of Health.

Batty, D. (2003) 'The voice of experience', *The Guardian*, 16 April.

Blom-Cooper, L., Hally, H. and Murphy, E. (1995) *The Falling Shadow: One Patient's Mental Health Care 1978–1993*, London: Duckworth.

Blom-Cooper, L., Grounds, A., Guinan, P., Parker, A. and Taylor, M. (1996) *The Case of Jason Mitchell: Report of the Independent Panel of Inquiry*, London: Duckworth.

Boyd, W. (Chair) (1996) *Report of the Confidential Inquiry into Homicides and Suicides by Mentally Ill People*, London: Royal College of Psychiatrists.

Bridge Child Care Consultancy Service (1995) *Paul: Death Through Neglect*, London: The Bridge Child Care Consultancy Service.

Buckinghamshire County Council (1998) *Independent Longcare Inquiry*, Buckingham: Buckinghamshire County Council.

Butler, I. and Drakeford, M. (2003) *Social Policy, Social Welfare and Scandal: How British Public Policy is Made*, London: Palgrave.

Camden and Islington Community Health Services NHS Trust (1999) *Beech House Inquiry: Report of the Internal Inquiry Relating to the Mistreatment of Patients Residing at Beech House, St. Pancras Hospital During the Period March 1993–April 1996.* London: Camden and Islington Community Health Services NHS Trust.

Chief Secretary to the Treasury (2003) *Every Child Matters*, London: The Stationery Office. Cm 5860.

Cohen, S. (1973) *Folk Devils and Moral Panics*, London: Paladin.

Commission for Health Improvement (2003) *Investigation into Matters Arising from Care on Rowan Ward, Manchester Health and Social Care Trust*, London: Commission for Health Improvement.

Corby, B. (2002) 'Interprofessional cooperation and inter-agency coordination', in K. Wilson and A. James (eds) *The Child Protection Handbook*, second edition, London: Ballière Tindall.

Department of Health (1994) *NHS Executive Guidance on the Discharge of Mentally Disordered People and Their Continuing Care in the Community*, (HSG(94)27/LASSL(94)4) London: HMSO.

Department of Health (2000a) *No Secrets: Guidance on Developing and Implementing Multi-Agency Policies and Procedures to Protect Vulnerable Adults from Abuse*, London: Department of Health.

Department of Health (2000b) *An Organisation with a Memory*, London: Department of Health.

Department of Health (2001) *Building a Safer NHS for Patients: Implementing an Organisation with a Memory*, London: Department of Health.

Department of Health (2003) *Every Child Matters*, London: The Stationery Office. Cm 5860.

Department of Health, Home Office, Department for Education and Skills (2003) *Keeping Children Safe: The Government's Response to the Victoria Climbié Inquiry Report and Joint Inspectors' Report Safeguarding Children*, London: Department of Health. Cmnd. 5861.

Eldergill, A. (1999) 'Reforming inquiries following homicides', *Journal of Mental Health Law*, October: 111–36.

Fernando, S., Ndegwa, D. and Wilson, M. (1998) *Forensic Psychiatry, Race and Culture*, London: Routledge.

Grounds, A. (1997) 'Commentary on the inquiries: Who needs them?', *Psychiatric Bulletin*, 21: 135–55.

Kennedy, I. (2001) *Inquiry into the Management and Case of Children Receiving Complex Heart Surgery at the Bristol Royal Infirmary*, Norwich: The Stationery Office.

Laming, H. (2003) *The Victoria Climbié Inquiry: Report of an Inquiry by Lord Laming*, London: The Stationery Office.

Manby, M., Evans, I. and Hall, S. (1998) *Case Review in Respect of PM. Born 15th September 1993, Died 6th December 1997. Report of an Independent Review Panel for North East Lincolnshire Area Child Protection Committee*, Grimsby: North East Lincolnshire ACPC.

Manthorpe, J. (1999) 'Users' perceptions: Searching for the views of users with learning disabilities', in N. Stanley, J. Manthorpe and B. Penhale (eds) *Institutional Abuse: Perspectives Across the Life Course*, London: Routledge.

Manthorpe, J. (2003) 'Informing local inquiries: developing local reviews in adult protection', *Journal of Adult Protection*, 5(4): 18–25.

Manthorpe, J. and Stanley, N. (1999) 'Conclusion: Shifting the focus from "bad apples" to users' rights', in N. Stanley, J. Manthorpe and B. Penhale (eds) *Institutional Abuse: Perspectives Across the Life Course*, London: Routledge.

Merrick, D. (1996) *Social Work and Child Abuse*, London: Routledge.

Mishcon, J., Dick, D., Welch, N., Sheehan, A. and Mackay, J. (1995) *The Grey Report: Report of the Independent Inquiry Team into the Care and Treatment of Kenneth Grey to East London and the City Health Authority*, London: East London and City Health Authority.

Newham Area Child Protection Committee (2002) *Ainlee. Part 8 Review*, Newham: ACPC.

Norfolk Health Authority (2002) *Summary Report of the Independent Health Review*, Norwich: Norfolk Health Authority.

North Lakeland Healthcare (2000) *External Review Report*, NHSE: Carlisle North Lakeland Healthcare and North Cumbria Health Authority.

Parker, C. and McCulloch, A. (1999) *Key Issues from Homicide Inquiries*, London: Mind.

Parton, N. (1985) *The Politics of Child Abuse*, Basingstoke: Macmillan.

Peay, J. (ed.) (1996) *Inquiries After Homicide*, London: Duckworth.

Reder, P. and Duncan, S. (1996) 'Reflections on child abuse inquiries', in J. Peay (ed.) *Inquiries After Homicide*, London: Duckworth.

Reder, P. and Duncan, S. (1998) 'A proposed system for reviewing child abuse deaths', *Child Abuse Review*, 7(4): 280–6.

Reder, P. and Duncan, S. (1999) *Lost Innocents*, Routledge: London.

Redfern, M., Keeling, J.W. and Powell, E. (2001) *The Royal Liverpool Children's Inquiry: Summary and Recommendations*, www.rlcinquiry.org.uk/download/sum.pdf

Reith, M. (1998) *Community Care Tragedies: A Practice Guide to Mental Health Inquiries*, Birmingham: Venture Press.

Ritchie, J., Q.C., Dick, D. and Lingham, R. (1994) *The Report of the Inquiry into the Care and Treatment of Christopher Clunis*, London: HMSO.

Sinclair, R. and Bullock, R. (2002) *Learning from Past Experience – A Review of Serious Case Reviews*, London: Department of Health.

Smith, J. (2002) *First Report: Death Disguised*, London: The Stationery Office.

Smith, J. (2003) *Second Report: The Police Investigation of March 1998*, London: The Stationery Office. Cmnd. 5853.

Stanley, N. (1999) 'The institutional abuse of children: An overview of policy and practice', in N. Stanley, J. Manthorpe and B. Penhale (eds) *Institutional Abuse: Perspectives Across the Life Course*, London: Routledge.

Stanley, N. and Manthorpe, J. (2001) 'Reading mental health inquiries: Messages for social work', *Journal of Social Work*, 1(1): 77–99.

Stevenson, O. (1989) 'Multidisciplinary Work in Child Protection', in O. Stevenson (ed.) *Child Abuse: Public Policy and Professional Practice*, Hemel Hempstead: Harvester Wheatsheaf.

Ward, M. and Applin, C. (1998) *The Unlearned Lesson: The Role of Alcohol and Drug Misuse in Inquiries*, London: Wynne Howard Publishing.

Webster, R. (1998) *The Great Children's Home Panic*, Chichester: Wiley.

Part I

Participating in inquiries

Chapter 1

Mental health inquiries – 'Cui Bono?'[1]

Herschel Prins

Introduction

This chapter concerns itself with mental health inquiries, mainly those into homicides committed by persons known to the mental health services both in the NHS and related agencies such as social services, probation and prisons. My own experience embraces chairmanship of three rather different mental health inquiries; first, that into the death of Orville Blackwood at Broadmoor Hospital (Prins *et al.* 1993); second, that into the absconsion from day leave of a medium-secure unit offender-patient during a visit to a zoo and theme park (Prins *et al.* 1997); third, that into a homicide committed by a patient known to the mental health services (Prins *et al.* 1998). Although these inquiries were somewhat different in nature they all involved a common theme – the assessment and management of risk. In the Blackwood case, the risk of dangerous behaviour was somewhat *over-emphasised* (a rather unusual finding), in the Holland and Patel Inquiries the risks of future problematic behaviour were *under-estimated* (for a detailed presentation and discussion of these three cases see Prins 1999, Chapter 4). Each threw up problems relating to chairmanship. However, my views deriving from these experiences could well be seen as highly idiosyncratic; in order to offset this probability I addressed a letter of inquiry to thirteen persons who had chaired mental health inquiries, almost exclusively those into homicides. Following reminders, nine chairmen/women replied to my letter and I am most grateful to them for their assistance. Anonymity was guaranteed so that their views have been expressed in composite fashion later in this chapter. My choice of respondents was based largely on those I could contact comparatively easily. Because of this, the sample cannot be regarded as strongly representative; for this reason, the views I have collated should therefore be regarded with a degree of caution. Before proceeding to an analysis of my respondents' views, it may be useful to provide a degree of context-setting.

Inquiries have a long and honourable history. Social problems requiring subsequent legislative action have nearly always been investigated by inquiries. For example, the Gowers Commission into Capital Punishment provided the spur for the introduction of the Homicide Act of 1957 with its provision for Diminished Responsibility. Two inquiries of forensic-psychiatric importance were the inquiry into the circumstances under which Graham Young was released from Broadmoor only to kill by means of poison within a few months of such release (Aarvold *et al.* 1973), and the wide-ranging review of the law and practice relating to mentally abnormal offenders under the chairmanship of Lord Butler of Saffron Walden that followed it (Home Office and DHSS 1975). Today, the tradition of inquiries seems well entrenched. Whenever 'ill' befalls, there are calls for an inquiry – whether these 'ills' consist of disasters at sea, in the air or on land, the mass murder of children, defaulting doctors, their murder of their patients or the alleged illicit activities of our democratic representatives. The social and political climate in which the urge to seek redress takes place is very important in relation to criminal justice and psychiatry (particularly forensic-psychiatry). Concerns about public protection have become central to much criminal justice and forensic-psychiatric thinking and practice. Such concerns were very well summed up by Faulkner, a former senior civil servant with extensive Home Office experience. He stated:

> The 1990s have been characterized by an 'exclusive' view of society which distinguishes between the 'deserving majority' which needs to be protected from the undeserving, feckless minority, who must be excluded and, in many cases incarcerated.

Faulkner identified:

> an ideological battle taking place between the exclusionists who dominated the last Parliament's programme of criminal punishments, demonization of children, hostility to single parents and refugees, and [the] inclusionists who are talking increasingly of citizenship and civic responsibility.
>
> (Faulkner 1997: 26)

The constitution of inquiries

Inquiries take many forms. Peay has provided a useful summary of their infinite variety – from full-scale public Tribunals of Inquiry to fairly informal investigations (see also Walshe 2002). She categorises them as follows:

- Statutory Tribunals and Inquiries.
- Statutory Inquiries.
- Tribunals of Inquiry.
- Non-statutory Inquiries.

- Inquiries after Homicides. (Peay 1996a: 12–18), these *can* be invested with statutory powers by the Secretary of State under Section 125 of the Mental Health Act 1983.

Membership will of course vary according to the inquiry's remit. However, some surprising formats have appeared in the past. The so-called 'Profumo' affair, which one would have thought might have called for a full-scale 'public inquiry' was in the hands of a single judge – the late Lord Denning; he conducted his investigation in private and has been said to have acted as 'detective, solicitor, counsel and judge' (Royal Commission on Tribunals of Inquiry, Chairman Salmon, L.J. 1966, Cmnd. 3121 at p. 44. Quoted in Peay 1996a: 14). Most mental health inquiries will have at least three to four members representing, for example, the disciplines of psychiatry, social services, nursing and the law. Occasionally, there have been five or six member panels (as in the Jason Mitchell Inquiry, Blom-Cooper *et al.* 1996).

At the outset of an inquiry a decision will need to be reached as to whether the inquiry will be held in private or in public, a dichotomy which fails to embrace any sense of a mid-way position. Sir Cecil Clothier QC, who has extensive experience of inquiries in various forms, provides thoughtful comments on this aspect:

> It is thus a fundamentally important decision to be made at the outset of any inquiry whether to hold it entirely in public, entirely in private, or partly in each. *Whatever decision is made about this, it will not satisfy everyone.* [Emphasis added.] The media will always be in favour of a public inquiry, piously exclaiming that the sole purpose is to inform an anxious readership. But of course a public inquiry affords exciting copy and often ready-made headlines, sometimes for months on end.
>
> (Clothier 1996: 51)

He continues:

> A tiresome cliché has been invented, namely a 'full public inquiry', as if there was some sort of half-baked inquiry which might suffice on occasion . . . they are hoping that someone or other close to the events in question, whom they often believe they have already identified, will have to appear publicly to be suitably chastised.
>
> (Clothier 1996: 51)

In our inquiry into Orville Blackwood's death at Broadmoor Special Hospital we were placed under some pressure:

> . . . by both the POA and Orville Blackwood's family to conduct a public inquiry, to let all parties have the right to hear oral evidence put before us

and to cross-examine witnesses. We resisted those pressures. We were under pressure to concentrate on particular issues and to reach particular conclusions, and we were very aware of the public expectations that were raised (or diminished) by the establishment of this Inquiry.

(Prins *et al.* 1993: 3)

At the time we were conducting our inquiry at Broadmoor, my colleague and friend Sir Louis Blom-Cooper QC was conducting his wide-ranging inquiry into complaints about patient ill-treatment at Ashworth Hospital. Although the two inquiries had *some* aspects in common, there were major differences. For example, our inquiry was concerned specifically with policy and procedures within Broadmoor Hospital. 'Our criticisms, where we had them [were] aimed more at practice and custom than at individuals' (p. 3) (but the media sometimes erroneously linked the two). Sir Louis is an advocate of public inquiries and, indeed, has much experience of them. However, he has acknowledged that expense is an important factor since public inquiries involve substantial legal representation for all parties concerned; such representation may also lengthen the proceedings considerably (arguments for and against public inquiries were cogently set out in Blom-Cooper 1993 and 1999). The extent of his considerable experience in this field is described in some detail by Feldman (1999).

Of course, the decision whether or not to hold an inquiry in public or in private is a matter for the sponsoring body and *not* the inquiry team. It is my impression that a non-lawyer asked to chair a public inquiry would be reluctant to do so unless counsel to the inquiry had been appointed or a lawyer had been appointed to act as adviser/secretary to the inquiry panel. I would have been very reluctant to hold the Blackwood Inquiry in public without considerable legal advice and support.

Most homicide inquiries have been held in private – wisely in my view. In public inquiries, the proceedings tend inevitably to operate on an adversarial as opposed to an inquisitorial basis. Decisions to hold them in private or in public seem somewhat arbitrary. For example, the inquiry into the care and treatment of Christopher Clunis chose to sit in private, as did the inquiry into the death of the young volunteer, Jonathan Newby (Davies *et al.* 1995). The inquiries into the Robinson and Mitchell cases were held in public (Blom-Cooper *et al.* 1995, 1996). I can find no evidence that either of these latter inquiries would have been hampered in any way had they been held in private. There are good reasons for believing that private hearings allow witnesses to give sensitive and often emotive evidence and to feel less constrained and stressed. At a conference on the future of inquiries, the Responsible Medical Officer in the Mitchell case gave a moving account of the impact of the inquiry on himself and his family; for him it was clearly a traumatic experience, for even if no blame attaches, professionals are likely to feel, perhaps quite irrationally, that they may be to blame. In some way this is more likely to be the case if the hearings are in the full glare of public scrutiny. It may well be that future inquiries will tend to be held in public as a result of the implementation of the Human Rights Act, 1998, and the recent ruling of the European Court that the Edwards/Linford inquiry should have been held in public (case of Paul and Audrey Edwards v. the United Kingdom application no. 46477/99, 14 March 2002, see Chapter 3 in this volume).

Some feel that fairness also demands that the perpetrator of the homicide (who at the time of the inquiry will have been convicted and sentenced) should be asked to consent to all the personal documentation of their case being made available to the inquiry team; in a number of instances this has been done and consent obtained. An opposing view is that in such 'public interest' cases, consent is not required, the view being that difficulties would arise if consent was withheld. The Mitchell and the Ms B (Blom-Cooper *et al.* 1996 and the Dimond *et al.* 1997) inquiry teams suggested that central government should give clearer direction in this matter; namely that disclosure in the public interest should be seen to include disclosure to an inquiry.

Homicide inquiries

Inquiries into serious incidents are not new phenomena in the UK, and there have been numerous inquiries into the care (more frequently lack of care) of the mentally ill and people with mental illness or learning disabilities in institutions (Stanley *et al.* 1999). The focus of such inquiries has changed over the past decade or so to an examination of apparent defects in care in community settings. An important policy development has taken place, namely the introduction of the *National Confidential Inquiry into Homicides and Suicides by Mentally Ill People* (Appleby *et al.* 1997). This was set up under the aegis of the Department of Health and with the co-operation of the Royal College of Psychiatrists, the objectives being to inquire into, and collect overall data on, homicides and suicides committed by people under the care of, or recently discharged into, the community by mental health services. A number of recommendations have emerged from the reports of this inquiry; these have included the need for improved assessment techniques, better contact with patients, better communication between professionals and better liaison between psychiatric professionals and those in close contact with the family carers of patients. The inquiry, now re-named *The National Confidential Inquiry into Suicide and Homicide by People with Mental Illness*, is currently located at the University of Manchester. It is important to note that this inquiry is not concerned with investigating individual cases (see Appleby *et al.* 1997). For a very useful discussion of common themes in individual cases see Reith (1998) and also Prins (1998).

It is important to remember that a number of homicide inquiries pre-dated the central government requirement to hold them from 1994 onwards (Department of Health, NHS Executive 1994). Reference has already been made to the inquiry into the homicides committed by Graham Young (Aarvold *et al.* 1973 discussed by Bowden 1996) and the cases of Simcox in the 1960s and Illiffe (see Prins 1999). Later significant cases were those of Sharon Campbell, who stabbed to death her former social worker, Isabel Schwarz (Spokes *et al.* 1988) and Carol Barratt, a young woman who stabbed to death an 11-year-old girl in a shopping mall following detention under Section 2 of the Mental Health Act 1983. A Mental Health Review Tribunal had ruled firmly against discharge but the Responsible Medical Officer (RMO) discharged her following representations by the patient's mother (Unwin *et al.* 1991). Kim Kirkman was a patient with a long history of psychiatric secure hospital care; he killed a neighbour, but committed suicide before he could come to trial. The inquiry held into his case concluded that there was no way in which Kirkman's homicidal behaviour could have been predicted, but the team did recommend that in future more use might be made by practitioners of actuarial devices and research findings (Dick *et al.* 1991). Michael Buchanan beat to death a complete stranger (a retired police officer) in an underground car park. Buchanan had a long history of both residential child care and psychiatric treatment (Heginbotham *et al.* 1994). Andrew Robinson's and Jason Mitchell's cases were the subject of public inquiries, both chaired by Sir Louis Blom-Cooper and, amongst other matters, both revealed serious deficiencies in risk assessment and management (Blom-Cooper *et al.* 1995, 1996). Finally, the case of Christopher Clunis, probably the best known of all homicide inquiries, has served very much as a pattern to be followed in all the subsequent homicide inquiries mandated by the government instruction of 1994 (Ritchie *et al.* 1994). With a succession of such high profile cases (though minute in relation to the numbers of homicides committed annually overall) and the activities of intruders such as Michael Fagin in Royal Palaces, and Ben Silcock's intrusion into the lions' enclosure at London Zoo, it is not altogether surprising that the politicians decided that more formal procedures should be established for reviewing such cases. However, central government direction was doubtless fuelled by media 'hype'.

Governmental preoccupation is with those who have a history of involvement with mental health services. Although homicides and other serious instances of violence against the person will be the subject of internal inquiries into those known to other services (such as probation or social services), there is no mandate for an independent external inquiry in such cases, though there is nothing to prevent a health authority setting up an independent inquiry into a non-fatal case concerning a patient known to the psychiatric services. This occurred in the case of Benjamin Rathbone who pleaded guilty to the attempted murder of a passenger at Loughborough station by pushing him on to the railway track. Rathbone was subsequently made the subject of a Hospital Order with Restrictions under Sections 37/41 of the Mental Health Act 1983 (Mackay *et al.* 2001).

Emerging themes

From the analysis I carried out of a number of homicide and associated inquiries (Prins 1999) and those enumerated by Reith (1998), it is possible to discern eight emerging themes, as follows:

1 There is still a long way to go towards encouraging mental health and criminal justice professionals to take a broad view of an individual's social functioning in relation to their illness. This may arise, in part, because of the tendency for medical practitioners to play a dominant role in the practice of psychiatry. To some extent this is understandable, given that in cases governed by the current mental health legislation the RMO (Responsible Medical Officer) is held responsible in law for acts of negligence or omission (see also Reith 1998, Chapter 4).

2 The importance of matching past behaviour to present behaviour has often been overlooked. More needs to be done in encouraging workers to compile careful chronologies of patients' lives.

3 Linked with point 2 is the need for the maintenance of adequate records and the development of common systems of recording. For the most part, mental health and criminal justice services have their separate systems of record-keeping.

4 Too little attention is paid to the importance of vulnerability in the assessment and management of risk; that is, of not placing patients and offenders back into situations which may promote the commission of further disastrous actions, and the completion of what the late Doctor Murray Cox (1979: 310) called 'unfinished business'.

5 There is a compelling need to develop more sensitivity to issues of race, culture and gender differences. Most racism in institutions, be they opened or closed, operates at a subliminal level (see Macpherson 1999).

6 Workers need to develop robust approaches to dealing with offenders and offender-patients. Concern for civil liberties has sometimes obscured the need to place public protection at the forefront. A more searching, questioning stance is needed.

7 Levels and modes of communication between professionals still leave a lot to be desired. Top-down approaches to care and management are still too prevalent; sharing of information is still not as good as it might be and some workers are often defensive, taking comfort from the fact that 'knowledge is power'. There is too much of a tendency to hide behind confidentiality as a defence to information sharing, as is the tendency to 'go it alone'.

8   Finally, the roles played by, and support for, family and other close carers have not been adequately addressed – sometimes with tragic consequences.

Current guidance and practice

As already noted, current guidance is laid down by the Department of Health NHS Executive (*Guidance on the Discharge of Mentally Disordered People and Their Care in the Community*. HSG/94/27, 1994). The essential elements of the Departmental instructions are as follows:

In cases of homicide, it will always be necessary for the District Health Authority (now Strategic Health Authority) *to hold an independent inquiry.* The only exception is where the victim is a child; here separate regulations apply. In establishing an independent inquiry, the following points should normally be taken into account:

The remit of the inquiry

This should encompass at least:

- the care and treatment the patient was receiving at the time of the incident;
- the suitability of the care in view of the patient's history and assessed health and social care needs;
- the extent to which that care corresponded with statutory obligations;
- the exercise of professional judgement;
- the adequacy of the care plan and its monitoring by the responsible worker.

Composition of the inquiry panel

Consideration should be given to appointing as chair an independent person (who need not be a lawyer). Other members should include a psychiatrist, and if appropriate, a senior representative from social services and/or a senior nurse and/or a senior health service manager. An undertaking, given at the start of the process, to publish the report will enhance the credibility of the inquiry. In exceptional cases, it may not be desirable for the final report to be made public. In these circumstances, an undertaking should be given at the outset that the main findings will be made available to interested parties.

Scope of inquiry

Most inquiries have followed the general guidelines outlined above, and most set out in some detail the procedures the panel proposes to adopt. They give, for example, a detailed statement of the inquiry's remit, the manner in which witnesses will be asked to give oral and/or written evidence, and arrangements for representation and opportunities for witnesses to respond to any criticisms which might be levelled at them. Since central government guidance does not set boundaries as to the extent of an inquiry's remit, inquiry panels have been left to settle this matter for themselves. A number of panels have commented on the need for firmer guidance, since its absence can lead to difficulties. For example, in the inquiry I chaired into the care and management of Sanjay Kumar Patel (Prins *et al.* 1998), both the social services and the education departments were unhappy that we had extended our remit to cover their services to Sanjay Patel in his childhood and adolescence (Sanjay was aged 19 when he committed the homicide – the killing of a vagrant, Patrick Cullen, in the centre of Leicester). We set out our reasoning in this matter in the following terms:

> It was borne in upon the panel during the course of this inquiry how difficult it was to draw fine dividing lines between the functions of the various agencies involved. In this case, there are a number of areas where inter-agency overlap is unavoidable. This may be particularly relevant for this type of inquiry when it involves the mental health of children and adolescents whose needs are also addressed by other legislation and when young people are in transition between services for children and adolescents and those for adults. . . . The panel has sought to identify the quality of care given to Sanjay Patel by the various agencies and the level of collaboration and co-operation that there was between them. When undertaking this inquiry, the panel had in mind the importance of seeking out, not only the key events in this tragic event so that lessons can be learned from them, but *to highlight these for the information of all those who will have responsibilities for {his} care and management in the future.* [Emphasis added.]
>
> (Prins *et al.* 1998: 3; see also Dimond *et al.* 1997: 36, para 3)

So far as I am aware, few, if any, other inquiry reports have stressed the matters I have placed in emphasis; some may consider that this goes beyond the panel's remit. My colleagues and I chose, we think for good reason, to think otherwise.

Publication and distribution of reports

Both these matters require some degree of rationalisation. For example, some reports are published in good quality glossy format by the commissioning authority (such as a health authority, either alone, or in conjunction with a social service, probation, police or prison authority); and some are published as Command papers by authority of Parliament and printed by the Stationery Office. One or two inquiry reports have been published commercially as books (two notable examples being the reports into the Robinson and Mitchell cases, Blom-Cooper *et al.* 1995, 1996). Such general publications will ensure a wide and more accessible readership.

However, ensuring such a wide readership may encourage an inquiry team to stray beyond their original remit and make much wider recommendations than the task required. Such tendencies are not new; Grounds (1997) observed that similar wide-ranging recommendations were being made into cases of alleged psychiatric-hospital-patient abuse in the late 1960s. Occasionally, reports are published in-house in cyclostyled paper covers; these seem to do less than justice to the matters being investigated and to the work involved in doing so. Failure, for whatever reason, to print enough copies or to reprint them – as was the case in our inquiry into Orville Blackwood's death in Broadmoor (Prins *et al.* 1993) meant that at both time of publication and subsequently, legitimate enquirers were denied access.

There is also the question of dissemination of inquiry reports. They appear in sequential fashion and many of them make very similar recommendations. Following such action as the authorities choose to take at local level, the report is then most likely shelved. As Reith urged: 'The information that is already available needs to be made more accessible by a central body such as the Department of Health so that the available information [e.g. in cumulative inquiry reports] is properly disseminated' (Reith 1998: 17). Crichton and Sheppard (1996: 71) addressed the issue in sharper terms:

> If the current rash of inquiry reports are not widely read and do not influence practice, then they risk being as nationally relevant as a private stamp collection . . . if they are dismissed before they are read and fail to engender a debate of the issues, then a valuable opportunity for improving national practice will be lost.

Finally, some inquiry teams sign the report (usually at the front); others do not. There seems little justification for signatures appearing on the printed copies; if signatures are deemed necessary, then they can be appended to the top copy.

Purpose of inquiries – 'Cui Bono'?

Blom-Cooper has stated that the purpose of inquiries is 'to examine the truth . . . what happened . . . how did it happen, and who if anyone was responsible, culpably or otherwise, for it having happened?' (Blom-Cooper 1993: 20). So far so good, but are there not problems in such a definition of purpose and are there not, indeed, other purposes, explicit or implicit? The search for truth is admirable, but is it as readily ascertainable as might be inferred from Sir Louis' remarks? All of us who work in this field agree that it is very easy to be wise after the event, and that 'hindsight-bias' may lead one to draw facile or quite erroneous conclusions. Coonan *et al.* (1998: 3) put the problem in very balanced context. They stated:

> The essential requirement is that the Inquiry should be fair and just; to be seen to be fair and just, and at the same time provide answers to the fundamental questions: 'How?' and 'Why?' the death occurred. A balance must be struck between the competing demands of the inquisitorial nature of the Inquiry and the requirement to provide some degree of protection to individuals whose credibility and competence is strongly impugned. Serious allegations had been made against specific individuals at the outset. Provided the correct balance is struck, the requirements of seeking the truth, making recommendations, and at the same time identifying individual failure, where appropriate, is both reconcilable and achievable.

As far as I am aware, no homicide inquiry report has stated categorically that omissions or failures in practice could be shown *conclusively* to have caused the homicidal event. The best that can be said is that such failures *may* have been contributory factors. This has led some to question the desirability of such complex, costly and time-consuming procedures. However, it has to be stressed that inquiries into homicides are needed not just to inquire into practices and offer necessary criticism; they are also needed for the purposes of public catharsis, most notably to help the families of the deceased (and in some cases of the perpetrator) to cope with their grief (see also Walshe 2002). Grounds (1997: 134) suggested that 'Families have two over-riding concerns; first, that they should know what happened, even if the process of learning is an ordeal; secondly, [that] what happened to them should not happen to others in the future' (see also Chapter 3 in this volume).

Lingham and Murphy (1996: 22) also put the matter very succinctly:

> Although professionals in the mental health field are understandably reluctant to expose their working practices to public scrutiny, they should recognize that inquiries do not serve only to prevent recurrences of tragic events. They provide explanations for victims, bereaved relatives and for families of mentally ill people who may feel guilty as well as let down by health and social services. The special audit process should be thorough and objective if professionals and managers are to learn from the conclusions.

Lingham and Murphy (1996: 22) also recognised the stress under which witnesses may labour: 'We have both witnessed nervous staff dry up with anxiety, giving their evidence in an uncharacteristically incoherent fashion under hostile cross-examination'.

In a later paper, Lingham (1997) provided helpful advice to witnesses on how they can prepare themselves for what must inevitably be an ordeal.

Time for change

A number of authorities have expressed the view that changes are required in the present system of inquiries. Eastman advocated: 'That the main purpose of inquiries should be pursued separately. This implies that inquiries should investigate only causal explanation and should always be explicitly precluded from expressing a judgement about *professional culpability*' (Eastman 1996: 1070 [emphasis added]. He suggested that judgements about the latter should always be made either through the professional's governing body or through the civil courts.

A further deficiency in the present system must be mentioned. Currently, each inquiry is a single event; the team carry out their mandated tasks and present their report. It is then left to the authorities being reviewed to accept or reject whatever recommendations are made, and to act upon them as they see fit. Very rarely is a panel asked to revisit to ensure that its recommendations have been implemented. Indeed, there seems to be some reluctance to accept such offers, as we found in our inquiry into Orville Blackwood's death in Broadmoor (Prins *et al.* 1993).

The possibilities of loss of useful information through the absence of an effective channel of dissemination was referred to earlier. What direction then should future policy and practice take? In 1999 I recommended the following:

- Mandatory homicide inquiries should either cease or, if they are not abandoned entirely, there should be some clear time limit set on how long ago the perpetrator was in contact with the mental health services. At present, this appears to be limitless and is left to the discretion of individual panels to determine. This is unsatisfactory.
- In the event of formal inquiries being abandoned, there should be set in place more effective systems of monitoring and audit, notably in respect of risk assessment and management (see Eastman 1996). There should be a requirement to report all homicide cases, perhaps to the Department of Health. This (or some other body) would then decide if an independent external inquiry was required.
- Such residual cases should then become the responsibility of a central body (such as the Mental Health Act Commission) who could maintain a register of possible inquiry team members and also act as an inquiry secretariat.

(Prins 1999)

After much debate a new procedure seems to have now been agreed. In future it would appear that independent inquiries into homicides are likely to come under the umbrella of the recently established *National Patient Safety Agency*. This agency serves as an independent body to collect information about clinical errors by health service staff (NHS Federation 2001).

The respondents

The preceding part of this chapter covered matters of particular concern to those who chair mental health inquiries of one kind or another, in particular, homicide inquiries. As stated in the introduction, I considered that a purely personal view might well be somewhat idiosyncratic. For this reason I addressed a number of questions to my thirteen respondents, one of whom preferred to talk around the issues in an extended interview. Almost all of them had undertaken more than one inquiry into mental health or other matters such as child care. One of my respondents had undertaken four into mental health and two into child abuse. Two had undertaken three and, in addition, one had also been a member of mental health inquiry teams on several other occasions, including internal panels of inquiry. Thus, all of my respondents can be said to be persons of considerable experience and reputation. To the best of my knowledge (professional status was not asked for) all, save one, had legal backgrounds and two were Queen's Counsel. The replies of my respondents have been compressed to present composite answers. This is because of my promise of anonymity and non-attribution.

The questions I put to my respondents are summarised under the following headings:

1   Manner of appointment to chair the inquiry.
2   Extent to which chairman/woman had any 'say' in the selection of team colleagues.
3   Provision of support services.
4   Degree of 'lobbying' by interested parties.
5   Public or private debate.
6   Problems relating to possible conflict of interest between parties.
7   Management of 'hearings'.
8   Access to documentation.
9   Problems in drafting final report.
10 Arrangements for promulgation, publication and dissemination of findings. Feedback from appointing authority and any requests for return to undertake 'follow-up'.

Manner of appointment to chair the inquiry

For the majority of my respondents the request to chair the inquiry came 'out of the blue'. One respondent had extensive experience of clinical negligence cases; another was already 'known' to the Department of Health; one or two had experience in chairing 'internal' inquiries so their competence was already 'tested'. In one instance, the respondent had agreed to take on the task on the recommendation of a colleague who had been approached first, but was unable to undertake it. The 'out of the blue' approach was usually by an initial telephone call. One of my respondents had chaired two previous homicide inquiries and turned down a request to undertake a third, not wishing to be 'type-cast'. Only rarely did the request seem to come through the recommendation of a body such as the Mental Health Act Commission. In my own case, my appointment to chair the Blackwood Inquiry was somewhat unusual as another person had been identified for this role but this choice was apparently not considered sufficiently 'independent'. Overall, appointments appear to be rather a matter of chance.

Extent to which chairman/chairwoman had any 'say' in the appointment of panel colleagues

In general, chairmen/women did not have any direct 'say' in the appointment of panel colleagues, though in one or two instances names 'were run past' them and if, for any valid reason, they were not deemed suitable their views would have been taken into account. One or two of my respondents thought that chairmen/women should be consulted and have a right to veto appointments. In general, chairmen/women were very satisfied indeed with the contributions made by their fellow panel members.

Support services

Generally speaking, support services were considered to be very good. In one or two instances they were regarded as 'exceptional' and greatly facilitated the work of the inquiry. In my experience of chairing three inquiries, support was excellent and the final reports owed much to the quality of administrative help we received.

Degree of lobbying by interested parties

Occasional lobbying did occur; for example, requests to hold the inquiry in public rather than in private. In one or two instances, attempts were made to proffer witnesses of an authority's choosing rather than those identified by the inquiry panel. One respondent considered that there had been less lobbying than they had expected. Overall my impression is that lobbying was not a problem. When it arose, it was dealt with effectively (and judicially) by the inquiry panel.

Public or private inquiries

A small minority of respondents favoured public inquiries (but did recognise the problems of expensive and more lengthy hearings). One or two favoured them if the matters being investigated raised issues of serious national concern or notoriety. The majority of respondents favoured inquiries in private, largely on the grounds of them being less intimidatory, litigious and better able to deal with sensitive clinical issues. However, a number of them stressed the need for the findings of inquiries held in private to be made public. Two respondents thought that there might be a trend for more inquiries to be held in public as a result of the implementation of the Human Rights Act 1998.

Problems relating to possible conflicts of interests and the achievement of 'fairness' to all parties

The stresses involved for witnesses in inquiries, whether in private or in public, were noted sympathetically by my respondents. One or two noted the problems involved in reconciling relatives' understandable desire to apportion 'blame' and the need to be fair to witnesses. There was a reported need to ensure a proper factual basis for any criticisms that might be made. Occasionally, there was a need to 'rein in' a colleague adopting either too hard or too sympathetic an approach to a professional witness. Chairmen and women had to operate a delicate balancing act.

Management of hearings

No major problems were identified. Occasionally, witnesses needed to be given a sense of direction to lessen any tendency to ramble or be inconsistent, or to stop the grinding of 'axes'. Emphasis was placed upon the need for the chair to put witnesses at their ease and to facilitate the proceedings generally. Some respondents adopted the practice of asking the relevant panel member to begin the questioning of a witness from their own discipline.

Access to documentation

Several of my respondents would have welcomed clearer government guidance on the compulsory disclosure of documents. Problems had arisen on several occasions when patients or medical advisers refused access to their medical records. A statement concerning what might constitute public interest 'over-ride' would have been welcomed. In one or two instances, problems involved in accessing medical records led to serious delays in the panel's work. This apart, the respondents did not seem to have had difficulty in accessing other medical and allied records. However, comment was made on the poor quality of record-keeping in some cases and an over-abundance of records in others, which took many hours to assimilate and put into comprehensible order!

Problems in drafting the final report

There seemed to be a broad consensus of opinion that drafting the final report could present considerable logistical problems. The difficulties of drafting 'by committee' were alluded to by more than one respondent; it was considered more helpful if the chairman/woman took the initiative in constructing a first draft to be subsequently worked over and amended by the rest of the panel. Occasionally, the sponsoring authority requested changes at the drafting stage. In some cases panels had agreed to these if they were considered justified. In others, requests for change were resisted by the panel. One respondent referred to the dangers of individual panel members wishing to ride personal 'hobby-horses' – a tendency which needed to be resisted firmly. An essential requisite seemed to be that parties likely to be criticised should be informed of any potential criticisms in advance and given the opportunity to comment on them. Sometimes, modifications were made if these concerned matters of fact, but matters of opinion would remain unchanged if the panel considered these had been substantiated by their investigators.

Promulgation, publication and dissemination of findings. Feedback and requests for follow-up by panel

Respondents identified some problems concerning the 'launch' of their report. For example, insufficient publicity being given to the 'launch'; in some cases the panel members were not invited to attend such events. From some of the replies it appeared that, in a few instances, the sponsoring authority did not wish for too much publicity. Hardly ever was there any feedback to panels from sponsoring authorities. Requests to return to see to what extent the panel's recommendations had been acted upon were very rare indeed. Only two of my respondents had been asked to revisit in this way. In one instance the offer was accepted, in the other it was declined on the basis that an independent assessor would be a more appropriate choice. This was acted upon by the sponsoring authority and the panel subsequently informed of the findings. One respondent considered that re-visiting was not appropriate and that the relevant authorities should be trusted to implement any recommendations. Two respondents referred to undue delay in the promulgation of their reports.

Other observations

Respondents were asked to make any additional observations on matters not covered in my questions. One respondent referred to what could best be described as the serendipitous nature of panel membership. Normally, panel members seemed to work well, but where this might not be the case, serious problems could arise. The need to make proper allowance for the time required for an adequate inquiry was stressed. One or two respondents had reservations as to the impact their reports and recommendations would have on future practice. Another respondent considered that there needed to be some degree of control exercised over the number of inquiries taking place. Some respondents raised the important question of venue. While accommodation does not seem to have been a problem in most instances, venue is of course a rather different matter. In most inquiries it is usual to hold the formal panel hearings in, for example, a hotel and arrange for 'site' visits as appropriate. For example, in our inquiry into Orville Blackwood's death, we held most of our 'hearings' at a London hotel. However, we paid several site visits to the unit at which Orville had been detained and also interviewed a number of patients there. We also, at my insistence, visited the local general hospital to which Orville's body had been taken. This was in order to inspect the 'viewing' arrangements for relatives. For various reasons these had been very unsatisfactory and caused Orville's relatives considerable distress. Had we not visited for ourselves, we would not have been able to assess the level of trauma caused to the family. Choice of venue can be a complex matter as, for example, in the current Saville Inquiry into the events of 'Bloody Sunday' in Northern Ireland. In this instance the issue of whether soldiers/witnesses should travel to the province to give their evidence has proved problematic.

Conclusion

Respondents appeared to recognise the inherent tensions involved in balancing the views and feelings of the victims' relatives on the one hand, against those of the professionals involved on the other. Most seemed satisfied with the arrangements for support services and accommodation. Lobbying by interested parties did not seem particularly problematic, and possible conflicts of interest seemed capable of resolution. Most respondents favoured inquiries being held in private, but acknowledged the need for public hearings in certain cases where the public interest or notoriety were of paramount importance. They seemed keenly aware of their role in securing 'fair play' in the conduct of hearings and managing them with an appropriate mixture of informality and 'judicial' restraint. Problems were encountered with access to documentation; more specific guidance from government would have been welcomed here. Drafting the final report was occasionally problematic if sponsoring authorities wished for deletions or amendments. Allowing witnesses to suggest modifications to their factual evidence seemed a helpful device in this respect and panel chairmen and women seemed able to separate this from opinion. It was very rare for panels to be asked to return to the authority to examine to what extent their recommendations had been acted upon; and it was also rare to find the provision of feedback to panels. A repeated word of caution is necessary concerning the responses I obtained. The sample is a very small one; for this reason it would be unwise to over-generalise any conclusions. Had I chosen to survey a larger number of those who had chaired mental health inquiries the results might have been different.

In respect of homicide inquiries in particular, Petch and Bradley (1997: 182) make an apposite observation:

> It has not yet been established why psychiatric patients kill others. . . . However, many inquiries and their reports imply there is something the psychiatric services can do to prevent this happening. The implication is that if a gold standard of care was provided, psychiatric patients would either not kill other people or would do so less frequently. This is far from certain, but if there are things which services can do to reduce the likelihood of homicides by psychiatric patients, the lessons must be learned.

Finally, Peay asks the questions: 'Do . . . "Inquiries After Homicide" explain, expose, expiate or merely excoriate?' (Peay 1996a: 11). I leave readers of this chapter to make up their own minds on this matter.

Acknowledgements

I am most grateful to those respondents who so kindly gave of their time and patience to assist me and for whom I have taken pains to ensure anonymity. My sincere thanks also to Mrs Janet Kirkwood, for yet again making sense of my 'scrawled-over' drafts and producing such excellent finished copy.

Note

1 Who stands to benefit?

References

Aarvold, Sir Carl, Hill, Sir Denis and Newton, G.P. (1973) *Report of the Review of Procedures into the Discharge of Psychiatric Patients Subject to Special Restrictions* (Cmnd. 5191), London: HMSO.
Appleby, L., Shaw, J. and Amos, T. (1997) 'National Confidential Inquiry into Suicide and Homicide by People with Mental Illness', *British Journal of Psychiatry*, 170: 101–2.

Blom-Cooper, L. (1993) 'Public inquiries', in M. Freeman and B. Hepple (eds) *Current Legal Problems*, Oxford: Oxford University Press.

Blom-Cooper, L. (1999) 'Public inquiries in mental health (with particular reference to the Blackwood case at Broadmoor and the patient complaints of Ashworth Hospital)', in D. Webb and R. Harris (eds) *Mentally Disordered Offenders: Managing People Nobody Owns*, London: Routledge.

Blom-Cooper, L., Hally, H. and Murphy, E. (1995) *The Falling Shadow: One Patient's Mental Health Care (1978–1993)*, London: Duckworth.

Blom-Cooper, L., Grounds, A., Guinan, P., Parker, A. and Taylor, M. (1996) *The Case of Jason Mitchell. Report of the Independent Panel of Inquiry*, London: Duckworth.

Bowden, P. (1996) 'Graham Young (1947–1990) 'The St. Albans poisoner: His life and times', *Criminal Behaviour and Mental Health*, Supplement: 17–24.

Clothier, C. (1996) 'Ruminations on Inquiries', in J. Peay (ed.) *Inquiries After Homicide*, London: Duckworth.

Commission for Health Improvement (2003) *Investigation into Matters Arising from Care on Rowan Ward, Manchester Health and Social Care Trust*, London: Commission for Health Improvement.

Coonan, K., Bluglass, R., Halliday, G., Jenkins, M. and Kelly, O. (1998) *Report into the Care and Treatment of Christopher Edwards and Richard Linford*, Chelmsford: North-East Essex Health Authority, Essex County Council, H.M. Prison Service and Essex Police.

Cox, M. (1979) 'Dynamic psychotherapy with sex offenders', in I. Rosen (ed.) *Sexual Deviation* (2nd edn), Oxford: Oxford University Press.

Crichton, J.H.M. and Sheppard, D. (1996) 'Psychiatric inquiries: Learning the lessons', in J. Peay (ed.) *Inquiries After Homicide*, London: Duckworth.

Davies, N., Lingham, R., Prior, C. and Sims, A. (1995) *Report of the Inquiry into the Circumstances Leading to the Death of Jonathan Newby (a Volunteer Worker) on 9 October, 1993*, Oxford: Oxford Health Authority.

Department of Health, NHS Executive (1994) *Guidance on the Discharge of Mentally Disordered People and Their Care in the Community*, HSG/94/27: London: HMSO.

Dick, D., Shuttleworth, B. and Charlton, J. (1991) *Report of the Panel of Inquiry Appointed by the West Midlands Regional Health Authority, South Birmingham Health Authority and the Special Hospitals Service Authority to Investigate the case of Kim Kirkman*, Birmingham: West Midlands Health Authority.

Dimond, B., Bowden, P., Sallah, D., Holden, R. and Lingham, R. (1997) *Summary of the Report into the Care and Treatment of Ms. B*, Bristol: Avon Health Authority.

Eastman, N. (1996) 'Inquiry into Homicides by Psychiatric Patients: Systematic Audit Should Replace Mandatory Inquiries', *British Medical Journal*, 313: 1069–71.

Faulkner, D. (1997) Interview with J. O'Sullivan, *The Independent*, 12 March, p. 5.

Feldman, D. (1999) 'The life and work of Sir Louis Blom-Cooper', in G. Drewry and C. Blake (eds) *Law and The Spirit of Inquiry: Essays in Honour of Sir Louis Blom-Cooper*, The Hague: London: Boston: Kluwer Law International.

Grounds, A. (1997) 'Commentary on the inquiries: Who needs them?', *Psychiatric Bulletin*, 21: 133–4.

Heginbotham, C., Carr, J., Hale, R., Walsh, T. and Warrant, C. (1994) *Report of The Independent Panel of Inquiry Examining the Care of Michael Buchanan*, Brent Park, London: North West London Mental Health Trust.

Home Office and Department of Health and Social Security (1975) *Report of the Committee of Inquiry on Mentally Abnormal Offenders*, Cmnd. 6244. Butler Committee, London: HMSO.

Lingham, R. and Murphy, E. (1996) 'Mental health inquiries', *Health Service Journal*, 31 October: 22–3.

Lingham, R. (1997) 'Inquiries: on the Spot', *Community Care*, September 4–10: 30.

Mackay, R., Badger, G., Damle, A. and Long, R. (2001) *Report of the Independent Inquiry into the Care and Treatment of Benjamin Rathbone*, Leicester: Leicestershire Health Authority.

MacPherson, W. (1999) *The Stephen Lawrence Inquiry* (Advisers Cook, T., Santamu, J., and Stone, R.), Cmnd. 4262 (I) and (II), Vols 1 and 2, London: The Stationery Office.

NHS Federation (2001) *Briefing*, Issue 49, May.

Peay, J. (1996a) 'Themes and Questions: The Inquiry in Context', in J. Peay (ed.) *Inquiries After Homicide*, London: Duckworth.

Peay, J. (ed.) (1996b) *Inquiries After Homicide*, London: Duckworth.

Petch, E. and Bradley, C. (1997) 'Learning the lessons from homicide inquiries: Adding insult to injury', *Journal of Forensic Psychiatry*, 8: 161–84.

Prins, H. (1998) 'Inquiries after homicide in England and Wales', *Medicine, Science and the Law*, 38: 211–20.

Prins, H. (1999) *Will They Do It Again? Risk Assessment in Criminal Justice and Psychiatry*, London: Routledge.

Prins, H., Backer-Holst, T., Francis, E. and Keitch, I. (1993) *Report of the Committee of Inquiry into the Death in Broadmoor Hospital of Orville Blackwood and a Review of the Deaths of Two Other Afro-Caribbean Patients: Big, Black and Dangerous?*, London: Special Hospitals Service Authority.

Prins, H., Marshall, A. and Day, K. (1997) *Report of the Independent Panel of Inquiry into the Circumstances Surrounding the Absconsion of Mr. Holland from the Care of the Horizon NHS Trust on 19 August, 1996*, Harperbury, Hertfordshire: Horizon NHS Trust.

Prins, H., Ashman, M., Steele, G. and Swann, M. (1998) *Report of the Independent Panel of Inquiry into the Care and Treatment of Sanjay Kumar Patel*, Leicester: Leicester Health Authority.

Reith, M. (1998) *Community Care Tragedies: A Practice Guide to Mental Health Inquiries*, Birmingham: Venture Press (BASW).

Ritchie, J., Q.C., Dick, D. and Lingham, R. (1994) *The Report of the Inquiry into the Care and Treatment of Christopher Clunis*, London: HMSO.

Spokes, J.C., Pare, M. and Royle, G. (1988) *Report of the Committee of Inquiry into the After-Care of Miss Sharon Campbell* (Cmnd. 440), London: HMSO.

Stanley, N., Manthorpe, J. and Penhale, B. (eds) (1999) *Institutional Abuse: Perspectives Across the Life Course*, London: Routledge.

Unwin, C., Morgan, D.H. and Smith, B.D.M. (1991) *Regional Fact Finding Committee of Inquiry into the Administration, Care, Treatment and Discharge of Carol Barratt*, Sheffield: Trent Regional Health Authority.

Walshe, K. (2002) *Inquiries: Learning from Failure in the NHS*, Manchester: Manchester Centre For Health Care Management: University of Manchester.

Ward, M. and Applin, C. (1998) *The Unlearned Lesson: The Role of Alcohol and Drug Misuse in Inquiries*, London: Wynne Howard Publishing.

Chapter 2

The family's perspective

Paul and Audrey Edwards

Introduction

In 1994 we were a long-established couple, married for 33 years with two children. Family life had always been important to us. Audrey had not worked during the children's formative years so that she could be there for them as their mother. We took family holidays together and birthdays and Christmas were the highpoints of the year marked by the presentation of gifts and a celebratory meal. Both the children were by then in their twenties and had left home to make their own way in the world but that had only changed the way the family operated: it had not changed its basic unity.

Family life did not prevent us participating in the broader community, for each of us made a contribution through voluntary work and employment. Successful experience of living together in the family was, we believed, a sound basis for working together in the community. We assumed and expected the structures of society, expressed in the law and the major public institutions, to reinforce and support these basic family values. This chapter describes how a family tragedy arising from the onset of mental illness demonstrated to us that, in a crisis, the law was indifferent to our needs and that public institutions placed a higher priority on their own self-protection than on responsibility to members of the community they were supposed to serve. The inquiry process did not meet the needs of our family. We went on to fight for eight years and eventually, with the help of others, secured a decision from the European Court of Human Rights which, if implemented, will ensure families will have the rights we always thought they were entitled to in natural justice (Edwards 2002).

Christopher's story

Our son Christopher was very gentle and caring and also extremely intelligent and hardworking which earned him an honours degree in Economics with Japanese. Following graduation in 1985, he went to Japan to develop his

Japanese language skills and stayed there for nearly two years before returning to England, where he looked for a management trainee position.

Unfortunately he had no success, partly because of the then depressed state of the UK economy and partly because his natural diffidence and reserve prevented him from demonstrating his other excellent qualities in an interview. He became depressed by his experience and in retrospect it is clear he was now showing the first signs of mental illness. We arranged for him to attend a personal development course and following that he obtained a position with a branch of the world-wide Mars organisation. While he enjoyed the social contacts he did not settle to the work and gave it up after ten months towards the end of 1988.

He was clearly under some internal stress which came to a head when he began to pester the Anglican vicar of the area where he was living for immediate confirmation into the Church of England. The pestering of the vicar brought matters to a crisis because one day while the vicar was away the curate called in the police. Christopher appeared in court in 1991 but the matter was not pursued. However, it was now clear to us he needed professional help so we arranged for him to see a psychiatrist privately which led in due course to referral to the NHS and its alleged community care programme.

It was recognised by the private and NHS psychiatrists that Christopher was on the verge of a severe mental illness and needed both medication and specialist assistance, but Christopher – like many people with mental health problems – did not acknowledge he was mentally ill and would not seek treatment. As he was an adult, the NHS would not impose treatment on Christopher; nor would it work through us, his parents and carers, as that would infringe on his independence and right to confidentiality. So the NHS contacts led to nothing and we were his *de facto* carers, without professional guidance, for the next four years.

Over time we made some progress through a lot of loving care, patience, and persistence but this was not sufficient to prevent Christopher one day behaving foolishly and causing a breach of the peace for which he was arrested and brought to court on 28 November 1994. We told the police and court officers of his history of mental illness and his need for the drug Stelazine. Christopher was not, however, sent to hospital but remanded to Chelmsford Prison for three days for psychiatric assessment. Paul spoke to the probation officer at the prison giving her the details of Christopher's mental health history and assumed he would be placed in the prison health care centre.

On the same day Richard Linford appeared before magistrates in another court on charges of criminal assault and criminal damage. He too was remanded to Chelmsford Prison where he was placed in the same cell as Christopher and within nine hours of entering prison he had beaten and kicked Christopher to death very early in the morning of 29 November.

Seeking the truth

On the day of the tragedy we did not know the details of what happened. We knew only Christopher's medical history, and the facts of his arrest and court appearances; we knew nothing at all of Richard's history. Our immediate reaction was to seek a full disclosure of all of the facts surrounding the death of our son. It was, as we have observed in others bereaved by a major tragedy, a desire for knowledge for its own sake not for vengeance or as the basis for legal action. We also assumed that all the public agencies involved would share our wish that all the known facts relating to the tragedy be established and placed on the public record. There had been a major failure in the care of a vulnerable young man and surely, we thought, the public agencies would want to know and share the details with us and the community so that what went wrong could be identified as a basis for corrective action for the future to ensure such a failure could never be repeated.

Our assumption about the public agencies was soon proven to be invalid. They disclosed very little information in response to our written requests and some of the key information they gave us later turned out to be untrue. They did not want to meet us; we did not see a policeman concerned with the case for ten days and then only in response to our specific request and we did not see anyone from the prison until five months after the tragedy and then only on the specific order of the Director General whom we had seen the previous week.

Nor were the official legal processes of any value to us as a source of information about what happened. There was an inquest, but because a trial was imminent its sole function was to authorise the release of Christopher's body some four months after the tragedy. The trial itself was equally unsatisfactory. Listed as a plea and directions hearing – a formal legal process which we might well have not attended – it turned into a full-blown trial on the day. Because Richard Linford pleaded guilty due to diminished responsibility, the trial focused primarily on his mental health. The only witness was a psychiatrist from Rampton Special Hospital who confirmed that Richard was seriously mentally ill and there was a bed for him at Rampton. There was no jury; no witnesses as to the facts of what happened and no opportunity, therefore, for any questioning of those who were involved. The trial was completed within about 40 minutes and when we emerged we were little wiser than we had been on the day of the tragedy. The only new information we gained was that Christopher's ear was missing and Richard's mouth had been bloodstained.

The official legal processes of the state had been fully carried out but the situation we were in was totally unacceptable, both intellectually and emotionally. The Judge had acknowledged that the fact the two young men had been placed in the same cell was a scandal but said it was not one for his court to consider. Surely we – the family of a loved son beaten to death while in the care of the state – had a right to know what had happened, what went wrong and why. Moreover, if the facts were not established and laid on the public record how could we or the community have any confidence that the lessons of the tragedy would be learned and corrective action taken?

We campaigned for a public inquiry through the local media, through the churches, through our MP and even sought the assistance of the Australian government as we all had dual British/Australian citizenship. By chance we discovered there was an NHS guideline stating there should be an independent inquiry in cases where a person receiving treatment from the mental health services was involved in a homicide. We drew this to the attention of our MP who commented 'well spotted' and in due course a public inquiry was announced. The Health Authority in advising us said it had been their intention from the outset that there should be such an inquiry. We found this hard to believe for if this had been their intention surely they would have told us at the outset – we had been making enough noise about it. Nonetheless, we were euphoric. We anticipated an independent public inquiry by authoritative and experienced figures from a range of relevant disciplines and felt confident that now all our questions would be answered.

In fact, a lot of new information came into our possession before the Inquiry was more than a few weeks old. The Crown Prosecution Service had told us after the trial that we could now apply to the Chief Constable for release of the relevant papers to us, though it was entirely at his discretion. We applied and our request was rejected but a few weeks later we obtained informally from another source copies of all the statements taken by the police at the time of the tragedy. The story those documents revealed was shocking and on key issues contradicted previous advice we had been given by both the Prison Service and Essex Police. Although we had not been aware at the time, it was clear that Christopher's behaviour in the court cells had been bizarre. Information about his mental instability had been passed to the prison staff who in turn had asked the court whether the warrant could be changed to require hospital reports, but this was refused. Christopher's disturbed condition was apparent to prison officers when he arrived. He was processed separately from other prisoners and then put in a cell on his own as the escorting officer said 'for his own protection'.

We already knew from local contacts that Richard Linford had been known and feared by neighbours in the small town in which he lived. The statements made it clear that he had a long history of severe mental disorder associated with violence and had more than once been held in psychiatric facilities both sectioned and as a voluntary patient. He was well known to the police for his behaviour and had previously been an inmate in both Norwich and Chelmsford Prisons. Five weeks prior to his appearance at Chelmsford Magistrates Court on 28 November 1994, Richard had been the subject of a case conference involving all the agencies responsible for his welfare. At that conference his GP stated that he was the most intimidating patient she had ever had and that he could murder someone; the specialist psychiatric services, which had previously had him in their care, said staff were frightened of him; while the police inspector present wrote a note to a colleague saying he had been put under pressure to find a way of getting Richard into prison and he was surprised that medical professionals thought that this was either appropriate or practical.

Richard was recognised by the magistrates to be a serious potential risk to others and they remanded him to prison. The police officers delivering him to prison warned the prison officers about the trouble he had been causing earlier in the day and believed prison officers recognised him from his previous stay in the prison. He too was processed separately from other prisoners and put in a cell on his own because, as the escorting prison officer said, 'he was not fit to go in with other inmates'. Even so, later on the same evening of 28 November 1994 he was transferred into the same cell as Christopher and very early in the morning of the following day he beat and kicked Christopher to death. When prison officers realised there was trouble in the cell, six officers gathered outside and looked through the door aperture to see Christopher lying on the floor and Richard standing bloodstained. They could see that Christopher had been assaulted but did not immediately enter the cell; instead they went off to don riot gear and returned later to enter the cell discovering that Christopher was by then dead.

The Inquiry process

Having access to these papers allowed us to frame our questions to the Inquiry on a basis of knowledge. What we wanted from the Inquiry was that their report should disclose the facts on the public record and draw the appropriate conclusions about what changes in policy and practice must be made and identify who should be held responsible.

The Inquiry was formally sponsored by the North Essex Health Authority; Essex County Council and the Prison Service and its establishment was announced on 24 July 1995. The Inquiry Panel was chaired by a QC and comprised a Professor of Forensic Psychiatry; a retired Director of Social Services; a retired Commissioner of the City of London Police and a retired Prison Governor. We asked whether we could recommend terms of reference and when the answer was in the affirmative we made our suggestions and were later told our points had been taken up in the approved version. We then worked intensively for several weeks preparing a submission which summarised what we knew and identified the questions we wanted the Inquiry to answer. We handed over our submission at the beginning of October as requested and were somewhat surprised to discover that a number of the public agencies had not met this deadline. Surely, we thought, with all their experience, staff resources and access to documentation they should have been able to do it at least as quickly as ourselves. Were they taking it seriously?

Our initial euphoria at the announcement of the Inquiry was further diminished when we received a letter advising that, on the representation of one of the public agencies involved, the secretariat function initially carried out by the Essex County Council Legal Department had been transferred to a local firm of solicitors. We expressed our concern that if one of the public agencies involved had sufficient influence to succeed in achieving a change in secretariat the independence of the Inquiry was somewhat compromised which could impact on its readiness to make critical judgements on the performance of the public agencies. We felt also it would have been appropriate to at least consult our views before any such change was made.

We had no knowledge of the local firm of solicitors involved but later, when we discovered it also acted as an estate agents, which was the public face it presented to the community, we expressed our doubts. The solicitors/ estate agents practice was based in Chelmsford which was also the base of the Essex County Council, Essex Police, Chelmsford Prison and the NHS psychiatric unit where Richard Linford had last been treated. Most of the staff of these agents were likely to live in the area. Knowing that estate agencies depend primarily on attracting commissions to sell properties we were concerned that the readiness of the solicitors to press witnesses hard could be influenced by an unwillingness to attract an adverse image among the staff of the public agencies involved who were an important part of its estate agents' client base. We urged that the questioning of witnesses be undertaken by an independent out-of-town barrister but our representations to this effect were rejected.

We believed that the Inquiry should be held in public so that the community was made aware of the facts and we wrote to both the sponsoring agencies and to the Chairman of the Inquiry. The agencies responded that this decision was for the Chairman, who wrote and told us there would be a first phase of the Inquiry during which statements would be gathered from witnesses. At the end of that phase the panel would identify those witnesses from whom it wished to hear oral evidence and looked forward to hearing our evidence at that stage. In addition they would then consider our application for a public hearing, noting that other interested parties might wish to be heard on this issue at the same time. Until that point is reached, the Chairman stated, it would be premature to make any decision in principle.

The next step was an invitation to what was called a Directions Hearing for the Inquiry. We did not know what this involved and wrote to the secretariat asking for advice on what a Directions Hearing entailed and whether we would be able to participate in any way. We did not receive a reply and so on the Friday before the Monday hearing, Paul rang the secretariat and was given an agenda over the phone. This was, we assumed, the meeting at which we would have to make our case to the Inquiry Panel for the hearings to be conducted in public. When we arrived for the hearing in a committee room of the Essex County Council we found the atmosphere intimidating. All the public agencies involved were present accompanied by their solicitors and in some cases their barristers as well; the trade unions and professional bodies of the various staffs under query were also present. We felt strangers in a throng of professionals who knew the rules about Inquiries while we certainly did not. However, the issues were so important to us that we were not prepared to be inhibited by the environment of the committee room.

To our astonishment the whole panel did not come forward on the platform; only one person appeared who announced himself as the Chairman; the other panel members were not present and he stated he would deal with all matters himself. We were shattered when he announced the panel had already decided hearings would be in private so, despite what we had been told earlier, neither we nor any other party would have the opportunity to argue their case before the panel. We made our protest but to no avail and we also sought confirmation that the Inquiry would address the question of whether the public agencies had sought to cover up their failings during their dealings with us following the tragedy but again to no avail. Recognising our dissatisfaction, the Chairman said he would have some good news for us before the end of the session but the good news never emerged. At the end of the meeting we sought clarification from the solicitor providing the secretariat but he was no wiser than we were.

We pressed for clarification of this good news several times but without success. Eventually, some months later we were told that it was a decision that the firm of solicitors would be the secretariat for the whole period of the Inquiry, not just for the setting-up phase. We had not been informed that the appointment of this firm of solicitors had a probationary period and, in view of our reservations about this appointment, this explanation was risible.

We maintained a dialogue with the Inquiry secretariat and gradually built up a number of issues of process on which we sought clarification or assurance. The secretariat faithfully recorded these and referred them to the Chairman who astonished us by advising through the secretariat that he had noted them but did not intend to respond to them. Reluctantly we concluded that we needed to employ a solicitor to represent us in our dealings with the Inquiry. Part of our reluctance was due to the costs involved. When we had discovered at the Directions Hearing that all of the agencies had employed professional legal support we requested that we should receive funding for legal advice to protect our interests in the Inquiry, which we regarded as natural justice. It was inequitable, we argued, that the public agencies whose performances were under examination should have the use of public funds (to which we were contributing through taxes) to protect their interests while we, the bereaved family, were dependent on our own resources. Our plea for financial assistance was rejected but we went ahead and appointed our own lawyers. At a later stage, after further requests, the commissioning agencies did agree to reimburse our legal costs.

The next step was our first meeting with the Inquiry Panel. We had requested and it had been agreed that, prior to meeting with the panel to discuss issues relating to Christopher, we would have a meeting with the Chairman to discuss our outstanding queries and concerns about the Inquiry process. We were introduced into the Inquiry Room where Paul was directed to a witness table. He sat at one side of an open square; on the right hand of the square sat the Inquiry members like a row of judges; opposite Paul were the court reporters; and on the left flank facing the Inquiry Panel sat the secretariat lawyers and our barrister. In front of each of them was a screen on which the text of what was being said was transcribed instantaneously by one of the court reporters. It added to the very formal and controlled environment of the hearing.

Audrey and our daughter Clare were placed some distance away. The Chairman then shattered us by making it clear that he intended to proceed from the outset with the full Inquiry hearing to be followed by the discussion of administrative arrangements. This was contrary to the agreed arrangements, which Audrey had confirmed with the secretariat, that the meeting to discuss our concerns and questions about the process would come first. We were so shocked by this announcement, overawed by the very formal layout of the session with no opportunity to consult with each other and taken aback by the fact that our barrister raised no objection, that we went along with the tide of events. Our barrister took Paul through his initial statement to the police and this was followed by questioning by the secretariat and then by the panel members. The questioning related to our recollection of facts about Christopher's personal history; what had happened when we met him after arrest in the police station and events in the courtroom. By this point, various police and court officials had given evidence to the Inquiry some of which was in conflict with our statements. The tone of some of the questioning by the secretariat was quite aggressive as is indicated by our daughter Clare's comment to her mother at one stage: 'is Dad on trial here?' Paul's evidence was followed by Audrey's and then Clare's. It was a profoundly depressing experience. The euphoria we had felt at the announcement of the Inquiry was totally dissipated; we no longer had confidence that the Inquiry was committed to revealing and publishing all the relevant facts or drawing appropriate conclusions from them.

There had been a tea-break at the end of Paul's evidence during which the Chairman asked to see our barrister privately and, at the end of Clare's evidence, the Chairman said he would now have a private meeting at which our barrister stated we were not needed. Assuming some technical legal issue was to be discussed, we accepted this arrangement. When eventually he returned, it transpired this had been the meeting to discuss the procedural issues about which we had been concerned. Our barrister had not deemed it appropriate for us to be present nor had he raised all the issues we had wanted but had apparently spent the time discussing submissions on legal issues the Chairman might refer to him. We were furious and terminated our barrister's appointment.

We had two further meetings with the Inquiry: the first of which was a relatively low key occasion dealing primarily with aspects of Christopher's mental illness. The final meeting was a different kind of occasion altogether. We had prepared a paper summarising our dissatisfaction with the Inquiry process and the way we had been treated and sent it first to the Department of Health, under whose rules the Inquiry had been established, and we had received an invitation to discuss it with a senior bureaucrat. Following this we discussed it with the three sponsoring agencies and, at their suggestion, it was sent to the Inquiry team and it was arranged that we should discuss it with them. We attended this encounter in a totally different manner to the first. We were not prepared to be overawed by the very formal court-like layout of the meeting room and the Inquiry Panel members had not, in our view, earned the respectful deference we had shown on the first occasion. We were polite, therefore, but quite firm in spelling out our criticisms of the way in which we had been treated and of the way in which the Inquiry was being conducted. Later we even received, what appeared to us, a rather reluctant form of apology from the Chairman. However, while the air had been cleared, it did not appear to us that there were any fundamental changes in the way the Inquiry was conducted.

Our last meeting with the Inquiry Panel was in November 1996, but it was to be a long time before their report was published. We noted from the minutes of some of the public authorities involved, which were available in the local library, that they were becoming concerned at the time taken by the Inquiry and its cost – eventually taking three years and costing approximately £1 million. We had some further conflicts with the Inquiry and the commissioning agencies before the publication date in June 1998. We had pressed that the Inquiry should examine and report on the way we had been treated by the agencies after the tragedy and that, if they were to do this and fulfil the first words of their terms of reference 'To investigate the death of Christopher Edwards in Chelmsford Prison', it was essential they interview the police superintendent and inspector in charge of the investigation. To be fair to the Inquiry they did raise this matter with the Essex Police who refused to allow those officers to appear. It also became clear that the focus of the Inquiry was shifting. For a long time, correspondence from the Inquiry secretariat came under the heading 'Investigation into the death of Christopher Edwards', but suddenly that disappeared and when the report came out it was headed 'Report into the Care and Treatment of Christopher Edwards and Richard Linford' (Coonan et al. 1998), which was an entirely different focus to that indicated by the first words of the terms of reference.

The Inquiry Report

We tried hard to obtain agreement for us to see the report in its draft stage so that we could make comments which could be taken into account in preparing the final version. We knew this opportunity was being made available to each of the public agencies under examination and in our view we, as the victim's family, should have the same opportunity. Our request was, however, denied. What we were offered was the opportunity to read the final report (Coonan *et al.* 1998) on the premises of the Health Authority three days before it was published. We duly turned up at their office on 10 June 1998 and were not greatly impressed by the Inquiry Report. Its 324 pages length with 11 appendices and 85 recommendations reflected, we thought, a wish to justify the three years taken and £1 million spent, rather than a fundamental analysis of the tragedy and the issues raised by it. There was very little in it that we did not already know but we did discover for the first time that when Richard Linford had previously been in Norwich Prison his 'voices' had told him to kill his cellmate and that, when later in Chelmsford Prison, his mental condition had been so disturbed he had to be transferred to Runwell Psychiatric Hospital. We also learned that two prison officers, one of whom passed the cell just before the tragedy was discovered, had refused to give evidence to the Inquiry. The most shocking piece of new information was that it appeared almost certain that the cell alarm system had been rendered ineffective by a prison officer to prevent prisoners disturbing the peace during the night.

The Inquiry Report was published on 15 June 1998. We accepted that the Inquiry had produced a reasonable summary of events but considered it had failed to place those events in the context of major national policy issues, such as the imprisonment of the mentally ill and compared unfavourably with the Lawrence case inquiry which had clearly placed its subject matter in the context of racism within the police. It had also failed to deal properly with evidence that we had been seriously misled by both the Prison Service and Essex Police. Indeed, the conclusion on this issue was self-contradictory, claiming at one point it was due to a mutual misunderstanding of an internal report but acknowledging elsewhere that that report had not been completed until 16 December 1994, while we had produced documentary evidence containing the misleading statement dated 9 December 1994.

Some of the comments in the report were, in our view, very questionable. After listing several criticisms of one of the psychiatrists, including that he consistently downplayed the risks; failed to communicate his decisions; delayed meetings when he knew Richard Linford was a management problem; failing to exercise authority in chairing meetings and had no perception of urgency when there was a need for action, the Inquiry team still felt able to conclude that he was a conscientious and caring psychiatrist!

We were also surprised to read in the report that we were quoted as saying the responses to our queries by the NHS authorities were open, detailed and prompt, so we referred back to our submission in which we had actually said that the responses by the NHS authorities were considerably more detailed, open and prompt *than those of the Prison Service and the Police.* Nor did it address conflicts between the evidence of two senior prison officers and that of the duty governor to whom they reported. The two officers stated Christopher's behaviour had been strange, that they had twice tried to get the warrant changed so he could be sent for hospital reports and that he had been put in a holding cell to be processed separately from other prisoners. The duty governor stated that Christopher appeared calm and there was nothing unusual in his demeanour or behaviour and that he was not aware of the possibility of mental illness in respect of either of the two men.

These examples, and others, undermined confidence in the findings and recommendations of the report. We did, in fact, prepare a comprehensive analysis setting out our detailed criticisms of both the Inquiry Report and its process which, we believed, had also been defective in that it took too long, cost an excessive amount; and had been insensitive to the victim's family. We submitted this assessment to the commissioning agencies and they in turn, with our agreement, passed it on to the Inquiry Panel members. We never received any feedback. Our overall impression of the Inquiry Report was of a bland acceptance of the inevitability of such tragedies and an unwillingness to hold anyone to account for failure. It was, we thought, a damage control exercise on behalf of the agencies with punches pulled, rather than a root and branch analysis of all aspects of the tragedy with appropriate conclusions drawn to ensure appropriate change.

Our relationship with the Inquiry would have been much improved if there had been a greater degree of diplomacy, sensitivity and transparency but, even if these qualities had been present, there still would have been a fundamental difference. Our solicitor told us that it had been indicated to him by the barrister that the Inquiry regarded us as witnesses to certain facts about Christopher, in the same way as prison officers, police, and medical staff were regarded as witnesses to other facts. That is certainly how we were treated and helps explain why there was strong resistance to our efforts to be more positively involved. We could not accept the role which the Inquiry wanted us to assume. After Christopher, we were the people most severely harmed by the tragedy and we were convinced we had a right to be involved as more than mere witnesses to certain facts.

Going beyond the Inquiry

As the Inquiry Report was so unsatisfactory we initiated formal representations through the official complaints processes of each of the agencies involved. Neither the Prison Service Ombudsman nor the Chief Inspector of Prisons was authorised to investigate our complaint about the Prison Service so we had to go to the Parliamentary Ombudsman. He 'found fully justified the complaint by Mr and Mrs Edwards that the Prison Service had misled them as to some of the circumstances which had led to the death in custody of their son', and that 'the effect had been to maintain a false impression concerning the possible extent of the Prison Service's culpability regarding the death'. The Police Complaints Authority upheld 15 of our complaints against Essex Police relating to failures in the way they dealt with both Christopher and Richard before the tragedy, in the investigation process and in the way they liaised with us.

The NHS rejected our complaints against two of the psychiatrists involved but the General Medical Council (GMC) 'were concerned at the standard of the doctors' practice', and expressed their concern in writing to both doctors. Amazingly the NHS was not aware of the GMC ruling on two of its senior professional employees until we brought it to its attention.

The key element of our complaint to the Essex Magistracy Court's Committee was that although, as the Inquiry Report stated, 'the Bench expressed its concern about Christopher Edwards' personal safety in prison' (subsequently confirmed to us personally by one of the magistrates), no such message had been conveyed to the Prison. The Committee, however, advised us that contrary to the Inquiry Report, it had 'concluded that it is beyond doubt that the Bench did not express any concerns about your son's safety in open court or otherwise and that the Bench did not ask the legal advisor to convey any message to the prison'.

The Health and Safety Executive did issue 'An Improvement Notice for Crown Employees' to Chelmsford Prison and in February 2000 told us it was preparing a guidance note for inspectors on issues to address in prison environments, of which they would send us a copy. In December 2003 we were told by the Health and Safety Executive that the 'initial intention to revise internal guidance had in large part been overtaken by more strategic work'.

Our experience with the agencies and the Inquiry has led us to question whether confidence can be placed in agencies of the state to handle such issues. Their perspective was one of institutional self-preservation rather than promoting the community interest. Our belief in the need for recognition of the harm which had been suffered by the victim and his family and in the need to have the full truth placed on the public record as a basis for healing and reconciliation, coupled with a wish to involve the whole community, were an instinctive reaching out for what we later learned was called restorative justice. In autumn 2003 we eventually met with the prison officers who had been involved with Christopher during his time in prison and this proved beneficial to all concerned.

Restorative justice initiatives of various kinds came to occupy a great deal of our time and energy but we had one last legal battle to fight. We remained dissatisfied with the outcome of the official processes for addressing our complaints and approached the civil rights organisation Liberty, which agreed that a case could be made to the European Court of Human Rights that our rights under the Human Rights Convention had been breached. It took some three years but eventually, on 14 March 2002, the court ruled unanimously in our favour on all our major representations.

The Court ruled that Richard's condition had been known well enough to establish he was a real and serious risk to any cellmate, but there had been a failure to bring this to the attention of the Prison Service. There had been various failings in the treatment of Christopher and Richard, including a too brief and cursory screening examination on arrival at the prison. There had therefore been a breach of the state's obligation to protect Christopher's life.

The Court also ruled that our right to an effective investigation into Christopher's death had been violated. It noted that there had been no inquest and the trial had not involved any investigation of witnesses. The multi-agency inquiry had not been an effective investigation because it had no power to compel witnesses to attend and had been held in private, while we had not been represented and were unable to question witnesses. In its comments, the Court pointed out that we had to wait until publication of the final version of the multi-agency inquiry report to discover the substance of the evidence about what had occurred and that, given our close and personal concern, we could not be regarded as having been involved in the procedure to the extent necessary to safeguard our interests. Finally, the Court judged that the established legal processes did not provide a means of determining our claim that the authorities failed to protect our son's right to life nor any means of securing an award of compensation for the harm we had suffered.

This judgement (Application 46477/99) has been hailed in a variety of quarters as a landmark judgement which should be of considerable benefit to families affected by tragedies and who wish to have the assurance of a thorough, independent and objective investigation in which their interests are properly protected (Edwards 2002).

The future of inquiries

We assume therefore that the UK government is now revising the rules and procedures for future public inquiries, taking into account the European Court judgement and comments on the deficiencies in the process we were required to accept. Even before the conclusion of the multi-agency inquiry, we had reached some conclusions about the essential requirements for a successful inquiry and had presented them at a conference on Deaths of Offenders organised by the ISTD (now The Centre for Crime and Justice Studies) at Brunel University in 1997. Our presentation was included in the published papers (Edwards and Edwards 1998). This built upon our review of our experience with the multi-agency inquiry which we presented to the Department of Health, the commissioning agencies and then the Inquiry Panel in the second half of 1996. These recommendations were framed particularly in the context of inquiries into homicides involving a person who had been diagnosed as mentally ill. We believe, however, that they are relevant to all similar inquiries and that they would be at least a useful starting point in considering how to establish a protocol for future inquiries which complies with the ECHR ruling. These recommendations with one later amendment are set out below:

(a)   families of victims should be told as soon as possible that an inquiry will be held even though its formal initiation will need to be deferred until completion of legal action;

(b)   inquiries should be required to prepare and make available to interested parties a strategic plan and timetable for the conduct of the Inquiry;

(c)   the victim's family should be:
  (i)   consulted on the terms of reference, inquiry membership, secretarial arrangements and any changes thereto;
  (ii)   given every opportunity to identify the questions they want raised and the information they believe should be made available to the inquiry; and informed whether their representations have been accepted and, if not, why not;
  (iii)   given a full explanation of procedures and what they can expect to encounter at the evidence giving stage;
  (iv)   kept informed of progress on a regular basis, which could be as part of a general briefing for all stakeholders in the inquiry;
  (v)   informed in advance on a confidential basis of findings and recommendations so that they are not embarrassed by public disclosure;

(d)   all commissioning agents should specify in their terms of reference:
  (i)   that the interests of the victim and the victim's family are a high priority, not to be subordinated to the interests of others, and
  (ii)   the relationship they wish to be established between the inquiry and the family of the victim;

(e)   whenever possible, inquiries should be held in public as are coroners' inquests for which they are a substitute, but even if held in private, bereaved family members should be entitled to attend hearings as observers and receive transcripts, subject to undertakings as to confidentiality;

(f)   every attempt should be made to include in inquiry panels a person who has direct experience of bereavement in a similar tragedy (not necessary homicide by mentally ill people, e.g. the Marchioness, Clapham Rail or Manchester Airport disasters);

(g)   the secretariat, counsel and professional adviser to inquiries should be persons whose location and normal professional or business activities are such that they have not had and would not be expected to have past, present or future contact with witnesses;

(h) it should be mandatory that an independent barrister from another region be appointed to assess the information gathered by the secretariat and lead the questioning of witnesses in accordance with the wishes of the inquiry panel;

(i) all members of inquiries should be of equal status, with the chairman only as first among equals, and act on a collegiate basis in reaching collective decisions on all matters relating to inquiry processes as well as findings;

(j) all members should attend all hearings with the sole exception of interviews with the perpetrator of the homicide if medical requirements dictate a restriction on those involved;

(k) inquiries should be required to minimise the formality and legalisation of inquiry hearings, and give those appearing transcripts of their evidence with the right to correct errors;

(l) inquiries should have powers to require the production of papers and the attendance of witnesses;

(m) there should be no disparity between the legal resources available to the agencies involved and the victim's family, who should be offered independent legal support in preparing statements and submissions to the inquiry and in any appearances before it;

(n) inquiries should be required by their terms of reference to search out for and publicly identify individual or agency failures in professional competence, commitment to care; or communication, and the responsibility assigned where it is due. Likewise, excellent performance should be identified and praised as an incentive to good performance and to establish a case law of best practice;

(o) inquiries' terms of reference should require them to assess and comment on the management responses of the agencies involved after the event both for the light they cast on the event and as a guide to the way in which recommendations should be framed if they are to be properly implemented;

(p) inquiry recommendations should be specific and action-oriented, identifying who is required to do what and by when. There should be an automatic follow up review 12 months later leading to a summary public statement setting out what has been done and what remains to be done;

(q) commissioning agencies shall be obliged to distribute copies of the final report to:

    (i) all similar institutions (e.g. local hospitals, police stations) within their jurisdiction requiring them to report within three months on any action required within that institution;

    (ii) all similar authorities (e.g. health authorities, chief constables, departments of social services) who should be encouraged by their central agency (e.g. NHS Executive, Home Office) to have an internal assessment carried out to see if it is appropriate for any action to be taken;

     (iii) all relevant central agencies of government;

     (iv) all national and local media (and respond to questions at a media conference);

     (v) the family of the victim and the family of the perpetrator of offences;

     (vi) witnesses;

     (vii) others as requested;

(r)   There should be a central panel (including a victim of a previous tragedy) to monitor the terms of reference, membership, business plans, secretariat arrangements, procedural guidelines of all Inquiries together with the proposed distribution of the Report by the commissioning agents.

References

Coonan, K., Bluglass, R., Halliday, G., Jenkins, M. and Kelly, O. (1998) *Report into the Care and Treatment of Christopher Edwards and Richard Linford*, Chelmsford: Essex County Council, HM Prison Service and Essex Police.

Edwards, A. (2002) *No Truth No Justice*, Winchester: Waterside Press.

Edwards, P. and Edwards, A. (1998) 'Recognising responsibilities to families', in A. Liebling (ed.) *Deaths of Offenders: The Hidden Side of Justice*, Winchester: Waterside Press.

European Court of Human Rights: Edwards v. the UK (Application 46477/99) Judgement 14 March 2002.

Chapter 3

Staff and patient perspectives on the Fallon Inquiry into the Personality Disorder Service at Ashworth High Secure Hospital

Pete Melia

Pete Melia is an experienced mental health nurse and health service manager with a long history of practice in forensic [high and medium security] services. He was drafted in to the Personality Disorder Unit as the Senior Clinical Nurse prior to February 1997 when the Ashworth Inquiry was announced. During the course of the inquiry he held various posts at Ashworth Hospital including those of Clinical Manager and Acting Clinical Director for the Personality Disorder Unit. Throughout the period of the inquiry, and in its aftermath, Pete worked closely with the staff and patients of the Unit to develop a more robust operational framework to enable proper treatment to take place without compromising the well-being or professional integrity of the staff. His achievements were acknowledged in both volumes of the inquiry's findings (Fallon *et al*. 1999a, 1999b).

Pete has since moved on from Ashworth Hospital and is currently working in the North East of England as a Nurse Consultant in Forensic Mental Health. He continues, however, to have considerable involvement in the development of national policy for personality disorder services through his work with the Strategic Health Authority and Department of Health. He maintains the conviction that the developments achieved by the many dedicated staff within Ashworth Hospital's Personality Disorder Unit following the announcement of the Fallon Inquiry offer a bedrock for future development and that the lessons learned are an invaluable source of wisdom for those wise enough to learn.

What follows is an account of Pete's first-hand experience of working in, and managing, the Personality Disorder Unit throughout the period of a highly critical and very public inquiry.

Introduction

Special hospitals have had a somewhat chaotic and turbulent history even within the traditions of psychiatry in Britain. Their inception dates back to 1863 when Broadmoor was commissioned as the first institution to house the 'criminally insane', effectively taking over this role from Bethlem Hospital.

The decision to create a separate asylum for 'criminal lunatics' followed the apparent success of the central criminal asylum in Dundrum near Dublin (which opened in 1852) in aiding recovery.

Broadmoor was originally commissioned to house 500 patients (400 male and 100 female) but by 1903 was housing 750 patients and, as a result of this overcrowding, a second high secure, or 'special', hospital was considered necessary. This led to the commissioning of Rampton Hospital which opened in 1912, the principal aim being to relieve overcrowding. Predictably, Rampton too soon became overcrowded and this led to the establishment of a third special hospital, Moss Side, in 1933. The problems of overcrowding continued, however, and a fourth special hospital, Park Lane, was built on land adjoining Moss Side Hospital and took its first patients in 1974 (although the official opening of the completed Park Lane Hospital was not until 1984).

From the outset there were considerable differences in the functioning of Moss Side and Park Lane Hospitals despite their proximity. Moss Side maintained the traditions of the prison system with staff wearing prison officers' uniform and discharging only the responsibility to contain patients, but giving little or no attention to the offending history of the patients or their underlying psychopathology. The role of Moss Side Hospital was very much focused on security. Park Lane, conversely, was commissioned with the intention of providing a far more therapeutic environment in which staff could work collaboratively with patients to address mental health and criminogenic needs. The difference of philosophies of the two hospitals existing on one site were stark and had a negative polarising impact, recognised in the local culture by the rather crude references to staff as either 'Moss Side meat-heads' or 'Park Lane puffters'. Such language reflected the judgemental and paternalistic values of that period which were based upon prejudice and separatism.

Some efforts were made to address this situation in the early 1990s when the two hospitals amalgamated under one management team and merged to become Ashworth Hospital. Unfortunately, this initiative collided in time with the announcement that, following media allegations of systematic abuse of patients in both Moss Side and Park Lane Hospitals, considerable concerns existed as to the standards of care and treatment. A public inquiry was subsequently established under the leadership of Sir Louis Blom-Cooper, QC.

Following the publication of this inquiry in the summer of 1992 the traditional model for the organisation and delivery of care at Ashworth was changed. Up to this time, Ashworth was a large psychiatric hospital which was managed in an entirely hierarchical fashion with little devolution of responsibility or attention to the particular needs of different client groups. In the aftermath of the Blom-Cooper inquiry (Blom-Cooper et al. 1992) a high level task force worked with the managers of Ashworth Hospital to reorganise Ashworth into four units with local management responsibility, one of which was to be dedicated to the care and treatment of clients whose health or functional deficit related to personality. Or, as the Mental Health Act (1983), defines it:

> A disorder or disability of mind (whether or not including significant impairment of intelligence) which results in abnormally aggressive or seriously irresponsible conduct on the part of the person concerned.
>
> (part 1, para 2.4)

By the end of 1993, the Personality Disorder Unit had been established within six wards in a discrete corner of the high secure compound, housing about 130 adult men whose primary diagnosis was within the Mental Health Act's definition of psychopathic disorder. This constituted about a quarter of the hospital's patient population (at that time Ashworth was contracted to provide 500 high secure beds) and took up about one-third of the wards available in the North site (the maximum secure enclosure referred to as Ashworth North).

A culture of inquiry

The 'special hospitals' have been dogged by problems of culture and practice throughout their existence. In 1980 Sir John Boynton chaired an inquiry into Rampton Hospital and pointed to serious problems described as:

> The isolation, geographically, professionally and culturally, of the special hospitals; a general lack of medical and nursing professional leadership, a vacuum which, in the case of nursing staff, was filled by the prison officers association; recruitment difficulties, notably of clinical psychologists; a focus on containment rather than therapy; a poor complaints procedure; and poor facilities for visitors, particularly relatives.
>
> (Boynton 1980: iv)

In 1988 the Health Advisory Service (HAS) visited Broadmoor and raised similar criticisms. In 1992 Blom-Cooper and his team concluded the first of two inquiries into Ashworth Hospital during that decade and recommended a 'thorough-going change in the culture of the hospital' (Blom-Cooper *et al.* 1992: para 1.19.3). Sir Louis and his colleagues went so far as to question the need for the special hospitals and at this time Professor Robert Bluglass, an eminent forensic psychiatrist, called for the closure of the special hospitals (Bluglass 1992).

Following the publication of the Blom-Cooper Report (1992) there was a wave of liberalisation within Ashworth and the other special hospitals in an attempt to bring them more into line with the practices of mainstream psychiatric facilities. Whilst to some extent this greatly increased the degree of freedom and the range of psychiatric treatments available to patients, at Ashworth, security was seriously compromised to the degree that staff felt incapable of exercising any degree of control for fear of being considered dinosaurs and bastions of the past. Whilst the physical security maintained by the perimeter wall continued unchanged, the sense of emotional security found in the presence of clear boundaries and professional relationships was lost. Patients were not confident that staff were in control of the hospital and many reported a sense of extreme vulnerability, to the degree that they feared for their own health and well-being. Indeed many staff felt the regime denied them the opportunity to ensure basic standards of environmental and personal security.

It was against this backdrop of confusion and fear that in September 1996 a patient, on what was supposed to be an escorted shopping trip (that is, accompanied by a single nurse who should have remained within three metres of the patient at all times) from Ashworth Hospital's Personality Disorder Unit, absconded. We now know that this patient, a man with multiple convictions for paedophilic offences, had separated from his escort by 'mutual agreement' and fled the country to Holland, using passport, driving licence and work permit documentation he had been able to gather as a result of the poor security standards existing at that time. This led to widespread publicity and, as a result of the potential risks to the general public brought about by this patient's unauthorised liberty, his photograph, personal details and forensic history were provided to the media by Ashworth Hospital and appeared in many national newspapers.

As a consequence of this, the patient returned and surrendered himself into the custody of the hospital managers. In the months that followed, however, this patient raised objection to the disclosure of personal information by Ashworth Hospital and claimed his actions were a direct result of his lack of faith in the clinicians and care staff to provide even basic standards of care and safety, much less any meaningful therapy. At the same time, this individual outlined serious concerns about the safety of himself and others (both patients and visitors) and made allegations of various staff improprieties, including the marketing of illicit drink, drugs and pornography. He further detailed concerns about contact between various patients, known to have paedophilic interests, and children visiting the unit. He made a number of specific allegations of organised contact between patients with known paedophilic interests and children visiting the unit who, he claimed, had been abused in the course of these visits.

The accuracy of these allegations was perhaps given added credibility by the fact that at around the same time a number of videos were found on the Personality Disorder Unit containing hardcore pornography, including paedophilia and bestiality. In addition, there were also photographs of children visiting the unit with apparently free contact with patients known to have paedophilic predilections. There were also serious concerns about the possibility of staff collusion and, although a widespread search of one particular ward was undertaken in January 1997, the police involved communicated their belief that patients had received advance warning of the search. One senior officer commented that 'there must have been a power drain' during the night before the search due to the number of videotapes that were 'wiped clean'. One particular patient had reformatted the hard disk on his computer in the early hours of the morning immediately before the search took place.

In addition, further allegations came to light including staff involvement in the unauthorised dispensing of prescribed and proscribed drugs, trading in pornography (at least some of it involving children), poor standards of security, poor standards of clinical care, various financial irregularities, the trading and dealing in nefariously obtained mail order catalogue goods and even possible paedophile activity. On 7 February 1997, Stephen Dorrell, the then Home Secretary, announced he was calling for a high level 'judicial review' of the Personality Disorders Services at Ashworth Hospital and so began the Fallon Inquiry.

The process

The announcement of the panel came shortly after the announcement of the inquiry itself and was broadly acknowledged as being composed of individuals with good professional standing. The inclusion of Dr Bluglass, however, signified an almost inevitable conclusion that the high secure hospitals were unworkable and should be closed. As noted earlier, he had previously made public such strong opinions (Bluglass 1992) and it was unlikely his involvement in this inquiry would alter that view. Critics were not disappointed, as indeed this was a recommendation and in fact the only recommendation not publicly accepted by the Secretary of State for Health who considered the final report (Fallon et al. 1999a).

Additionally it was notable here that the terms of reference guiding the panel in this judicial inquiry covered not only the investigation into allegations of professional improprieties, but also questioned the appropriateness of the clinical care and security provided for this group of patients. Furthermore, it was openly acknowledged that these terms of reference constituted a mere baseline and their actual brief was to be much wider. In his final report Peter Fallon and his team commented that both Stephen Dorrell and his successor, Frank Dobson, 'encouraged us to look more widely than our relatively narrow brief'. They noted:

> First, Lawrence Ward was not the only ward within the PDU to have suffered very major problems . . . (we are thinking here in particular of the Owen Ward hostage-taking in June 1994 . . .). Second, we could not

discuss the various security weaknesses of Lawrence Ward without examining the overall security failures of the hospital. Third, this inquiry follows the earlier Blom-Cooper Inquiry of 1991/2, which quite rightly launched a radical change in the nature of the Hospital. But the implementation of its recommendations was fatally flawed . . .

(Fallon *et al.* 1999a: 2)

In effect the inquiry team had a free role to investigate what and how it saw fit, over a period which was equally nebulous in its definition. This whole brief considerably extended the period over which the inquiry took evidence and the time needed to formulate and interpret the team's findings. Most especially, this process was to expose the lack of consensus as to the nature of personality disorders, their cause or causes and the effectiveness or appropriateness of various psychiatric or psychological treatments.

The inquiry gathered evidence during three sittings; the first in London (November/December 1997) when it heard evidence of the background and management arrangements for the unit; the second at Ashworth itself (February/March 1998) when it heard the evidence of patients; and third in Knutsford Crown Court (April/May 1998) when it heard the evidence of staff from the unit. The process of giving evidence was overpowering for most witnesses, with 13 parties being represented by different barristers, all of whom had junior counsel and instructing solicitors.

Even the seemingly simple process of informing individuals they would be called to give evidence took on a sinister appearance when it was decided (by Peter Fallon) that this would be by the so-called 'Salmon letter'. The origins of this lay in the recommendations of the Royal Commission on Tribunals of Inquiry (Salmon 1966) which state:

As soon as possible after he [a witness from whom a statement has been taken] has given his statement, and certainly well in advance, usually not less than seven days before he gives evidence, he shall be supplied with a document setting out the allegations against him and the substance of the evidence in support of those allegations.

(Salmon, 1966, as quoted in Fallon *et al.* 1999a: 7)

Whilst individuals were assured this was in the interests of fairness, the process as a whole was entirely daunting. Indeed some Association (union) representatives advised their members to avoid accepting these 'Salmon letters' (sent by registered delivery) as, if a person could not demonstrate that he had had the prior knowledge of allegations and supporting evidence, as recommended by Lord Salmon, he could not be expected to have his evidence cross-examined. The Clinical Director, who reported he was unable to give evidence due to mental ill health, was subpoenaed and shortly after was awarded early retirement on health grounds.

In January 1999 the final report was published, almost two years from its announcement (Fallon *et al.* 1999a). During this time the attention given to Ashworth Hospital by the press, the professional associations and the politicians waxed and waned. In addition to the formal taking of evidence there was considerable police investigation of various allegations but most especially into the allegations that at least one child had been sexually abused by a patient or patients with previous convictions for paedophilia. Additionally, Peter Fallon instructed a review of policy and practice within the unit by a team of independent clinicians with acknowledged expertise in the management and treatment of people with personality disorders. A team composed of a professor of psychiatry and two leading nurses spent a week in the unit with unrestricted access to all areas and all personnel (staff and patients). This team seemed ever present during that period (day and night), conducted many staff and patient interviews, read case files, attended ward rounds, reviewed decisions, observed the operation of the wards and clinical areas and finally reported directly back to the inquiry team.

Like many other senior staff in and around the unit at that time, I would argue that this intense and exact process of probing, questioning and challenging achieved more in one week than the inquiry achieved in two years. We had previously addressed a number of problems prior to the inquiry being announced but, guided by the expert team's critical eyes we were able to tease out some particularly complex and challenging issues to great effect. The findings and recommendations of this team are referred to extensively in the second volume of the Fallon Inquiry (Fallon *et al.* 1999b).

The patient experience

It was my intention to give an account of the patient experience through direct quote here; unfortunately, the current policy of Ashworth Hospital is to deny any further research involving direct contact with patients and it was not possible to gain consent to take narrative from individual patients which would directly convey the patients' experience of living through the Ashworth Inquiry. The patients' perspective has consequently been extrapolated from the evidence made available to the Fallon Inquiry Panel, including the evidence given by the team of independent clinicians referred to above.

At the time when the Fallon Inquiry was announced, the Personality Disorder Unit provided 130 beds for adult men considered to have a primary diagnosis of psychopathy as defined by the 1983 Mental Health Act. Of these it was noted that a significant number had committed serious sexual offences and primarily had interpersonal deficits involving profound psychosexual dysfunction. Many patients had previously received care and treatment in other hospitals, including other special hospitals, and were described by the review team of independent clinicians as a 'very heterogeneous group of individuals'. The team also noted that these patients required complex and wide-ranging intervention programmes to address disorders involving multiple aspects of personality and to reduce the risk of re-offending. Notwithstanding this, it should be understood that the likelihood was that many if not most would remain in some level of contained security for much of their lives.

This team of acknowledged experts did argue that, despite the many faults of the special hospitals, they still offered an environment within which individual psychological work could be carried out, where research could be undertaken and where people with seriously disturbed personalities could cope. The special hospitals were contrasted with prison environments which were seen as ill-equipped to cope with such individuals and often to greatly increase the environmental stressors, exacerbating aberrant aspects of their interpersonal functioning.

Only a limited number of patients themselves gave evidence to the Fallon Inquiry and the views of those patients differed considerably. One particular patient boasted that he had no belief that he would ever be able to change, irrespective of treatment offered, that he had come to terms with the fact that he would remain in Ashworth Hospital for the remaining part of his life and that he was quite happy to do so. This individual commented on the significant reduction in security that had occurred over previous years and noted that the staff no longer had any significant degree of control over the activities taking place within Lawrence Ward or the Personality Disorder Unit in general. He added that as a result of this the patients themselves had taken steps to ensure their own safety and that a number of 'camps' had arisen.

This patient described the complete collapse of procedures regulating and monitoring patients' possessions. He commented that in his own room he had a number of videos he frequently used for 'pirating' videotapes; he kept a bicycle in his room and frequently rode around the grounds of the hospital, unchecked and unmonitored on this bicycle. This patient's evidence was that there was an unspoken policy among patients on the Personality Disorder Unit that staff within the unit were invited to engage with patients in various activities involving some degree of collusion and that staff who resisted would be subject to verbal complaints and allegations in order to have them moved elsewhere. He told the inquiry that patients were confident that staff on the wards would either 'play the game' or be moved off the ward and out of the Personality Disorder Unit.

Another patient described to the inquiry team the process by which senior staff coming on to the ward would be approached by as many patients as were available at the time of the visit and be bombarded with a barrage of questions, complaints, allegations and general hostility in order to inculcate a sense of foreboding regarding visits to that particular ward. This strategy was designed to dissuade senior staff from coming on to the ward. The principal motive for this was the fear that if senior staff spent any time on the ward the poor security standards and level of collusion between staff and patients would become apparent and might be addressed. The effectiveness of this policy was illustrated when the then Clinical Director commented during his evidence to the inquiry team that he had not been near the wards for some time as he feared he might 'get my head kicked in'.

Similarly, a number of patients reported to the inquiry that they felt the environment was generally unsafe and that staff were not in control. One patient in particular reported that he had had a long-term sexual relationship with a fellow patient which was largely unwanted. This individual described the other patient as a man prone to violence and claimed that staff were clearly frightened of him. He feared that had he refused the advances of this other patient he would have been subjected to victimisation and probably serious physical assault. He did not have confidence in the staff's ability to ensure his safety and well-being had he refused these sexual advances.

All patients felt the potential for therapy being able to make any major impact on their psychological functioning or, in particular, in changing the characteristics of their personality disorder was unlikely if not impossible in that environment. Generally the consensus from patient information was that the benefits in terms of opportunity for subversive activities in the unit were too great to be missed, even though they acknowledged that this was to the detriment of the potential for treatment. A number of patients reported that, since 1992 when the Blom-Cooper Inquiry concluded, patients had continually pushed at the boundaries of what was permissible and many reported that they had been staggered at how far they were able to erode security, subvert relationships and deconstruct professional boundaries.

Some patients described an 'unspoken agreement' amongst the patients on Lawrence Ward that they would not raise formal complaints or otherwise attract the attention of senior managers, Mental Health Act Commissioners, independent advocates or other individuals outside the service. The acknowledged reasoning behind this adopted policy was the fear that any such attention would highlight poor practice and ultimately disrupt the way the ward was managed. Again it needs to be acknowledged that a number of patients had serious concerns about the way Lawrence Ward was run but took no action, partly because they were too afraid of the possible consequences from other patients had they voiced their concerns. They also lacked confidence in the staff's willingness or ability to intervene.

Patients on the unit were well aware that one patient had continually raised similar concerns about serious malpractice on a particular ward (Owen) in the Personality Disorder Service. The health care professionals involved in this individual's care had continually ignored the claims of this man and had even questioned whether he might benefit from psychotropic medication (the suggestion being his claims were a result of some form of paranoid, delusional psychosis). Eventually in the summer of 1994 this patient succumbed to enduring frustrations and opportunistically took the head of psychology and a fellow patient hostage for a period of about three hours.

Whilst this situation ended without physical harm to anybody, both the hostages suffered considerable psychological trauma. The patient was returned to prison without treatment despite the fact that at his trial he was found 'not guilty' for various reasons including provocation. In the aftermath, many staff were disciplined (including one staff member being sacked and struck off the professional register), but the same problems continued unabated. Managers continued to stay away from the clinical areas, senior clinicians continued to blame failures on the ward staff and ward staff continued to be totally confused as to whether they were custodians or saviours.

Patients who sought treatment had little reason to trust the integrity of the system or its administrators. Patients who did not revelled in the chaos. For these patients, who abandoned the possibility of treatment and exploited the opportunity for gain, the process of inviting staff to collude in activities which facilitated the availability of various contrabands was, according to many patients, based on a tried and tested method. The usual routine was to invite staff to engage in 'community' activities, such as having a social evening on the ward, and to encourage staff to participate by buying foodstuffs from money supplied by the patients or attending the social evening as invited guests and even bringing their spouses or partners. Using such techniques, patients were able to gauge the extent to which individual staff could be coerced to surrender their professional roles and responsibilities or conversely, were able to resist environmental persuasions and maintain a detached professional demeanour. It was the reported experience of patients that staff who were willing to be involved in such activities were equally likely to be prepared to engage in the trading of contraband. The task of the patients was then either to target those staff and invite collusion or to have staff who resisted moved off the ward. Broadly, the patient view was that anything could be obtained in Ashworth Hospital that could be (legally or illegally) obtained on the outside. This included pornography in both still and video imagery, alcohol and drugs (prescribed and illicit) and much technological equipment, including computers, videos, televisions and even mobile phones.

Patients were particularly aware that circumventing of the hospital's complaints procedure by going directly to solicitors was a highly effective mechanism for ensuring staff who they did not want on the wards would be moved and it had become fairly routine to threaten staff with solicitors' letters if they attempted to enforce basic security procedures. Generally, patients in their evidence to the inquiry acknowledged that the unit was not in anyway replicant of a treatment facility and that a gang culture largely prevailed.

However, during the course of the inquiry, many patients indicated that the level of press reporting (and the nature of those reports) caused great distress for themselves and, most especially, for members of their families. Family members were reading reports of a unit completely out of control and who feared for the safety of those who were resident in the Personality Disorders Unit. This press attention also brought with it the revisiting of many cases that had hitherto ceased to be of interest to the general public and the media, and revived a curiosity in the criminal and sexual offence histories of many of the patients within the unit. A number of patients in particular were targeted by the popular press and their offences republicised in often graphic detail.

Also during the course of the inquiry, patients reported a sense that security had been reinvented with forceful aggression and many patients who had been in the high security hospital system for long periods (in some cases in excess of 30 years) feared that the authorities were returning to the dark days of the pre-Blom-Cooper Special Hospitals. The principal reported features were that staff were again becoming paternalistic, brutal and over-controlling. Although most patients acknowledged that the unit had been out of control and required a far greater degree of security and therapy to enable the Personality Disorder Unit to serve the purpose for which it was intended, many more patients felt that the imposition of security was simply too great and that the pendulum had swung back to where it had been more than a decade earlier. Another factor heightening the tension and anxieties of patients was the removal of a number of patients from the hospital, either to other high secure psychiatric facilities or back to prison, often without notice or negotiation. As a consequence, many patients feared that their time at Ashworth was limited and that they too would be 'lifted' and removed to prison or some other high secure institution without warning. This again provided one more reason to doubt the integrity of what was already seen as a brutal system.

Staff experience

In many ways the staff perspective is actually a more complex element of the inquiry process on which to comment as staff's experiences were so diverse and largely dependent upon any one individual's level of involvement, and to some degree the extent of criticism or blame received by that individual. Indeed one view from staff working within Ashworth Hospital (but not directly within the Personality Disorder Unit) was typified when the author visited a ward in the Mental Health Unit and, when making reference to the inquiry, was asked by one experienced nurse, 'which inquiry?' It seemed that whilst the inquiry was a major event of considerable significance for anyone working in, or associated with, the Personality Disorder Unit, many staff not concerned with that unit were uninterested and often unaware of the cause, nature and impact of the Fallon Inquiry.

Many more staff outside the Personality Disorders Unit proclaimed some degree of awareness of the inquiry and the allegations leading to its establishment, but took the view that it had little or nothing to do with them and that they were steadfastly determined to keep it that way. An experienced manager and clinician illustrated this perspective, asserting that the circumstances leading to the inquiry were foreseeable and predictable from the time the unit was created and all personality disordered men were grouped together in one unit. He summarised this view with the pithy aphorism that: 'we should not be surprised when psychopaths behave like psychopaths!' For many staff, then, the inquiry simply did not happen. Other staff acknowledged its existence but took the view that it happened to someone else and that it did not affect them or impact on their own practice.

However, for staff working within the Personality Disorder Unit, the inquiry was cataclysmic in its impact. In the build-up to the announcement of the inquiry there were clear (but not always obvious) signs that things were going badly wrong. Tensions amongst staff on the unit were high and splitting amongst care delivery staff and managers was apparent. On one occasion, the then Clinical Director was reported to have addressed a community meeting on one ward and commented to the patients that staff on the unit were 'shite' and that he did not trust them. Although the accuracy of this report was questioned, it was entered in the annals of Ashworth history as an irrefutable truth. Furthermore, there was little or no contact between care staff on the unit and the authority's Directors or board members and generally there was a sense that staff and patients on the unit had been abandoned. Many ward-based staff voiced the opinion that it was a case of 'virtual management' or, more glibly, a case of 'virtually non-existent management'.

During the period immediately preceding the inquiry there were, despite the normally litigious nature of this client group, no formal complaints, incident reports or security alerts. Rather it was the norm for patients to make verbal complaints from numerous sources about specific staff but refuse to 'make it formal' or co-operate with any attempt at investigation. Additionally, it was evident that the amount of time dedicated to this client group by solicitors and independent advocates was far greater than with other (mentally ill) patients at Ashworth Hospital, despite the obvious fact that personality disordered clients were quite able and prepared to advocate for themselves. Ward staff felt they lived under an almost daily threat of litigation and believed themselves completely unsupported by managers, whom they considered to be weak, ineffective and too busy fighting amongst themselves to offer any tangible leadership.

This perhaps more than any other factor exemplifies the extent to which those of us working in the unit had lost our sense of proportion. Staff on the unit would describe at great length how they lived with an almost daily fear of suspension, disciplinary action or litigation. It was often stated that managers had failed to protect ward staff from the unreliable and litigious disposition of personality disordered patients. When we reviewed documented evidence, however, it was evident that for more than three years there had been no complaints, no disciplinary action taken against any staff (prior to the announcement of the inquiry) and no staff had ever received any communication from a solicitor instigating, or even threatening to instigate, legal proceedings. It was apparent that there was a huge disparity between staff's perceptions of what was happening on the unit and what actually was happening. The notion that 'people create their own realities by story telling' (Said 1993: 121) was again demonstrating itself and it was evident that patients had taken control by asserting 'an impression of power' rather than by exerting any real power over staff on the unit.

That said, when any senior staff visited the unit, the amount of verbal complaint, criticism and protest implied by the patients on Lawrence Ward was considerable. No patients, however, were willing to make their allegations formal or to co-operate with any attempted investigation, and it was from this continual iterative of implication that staff had derived the strong impression of being under continual suspicion and imminent suspension. The failure to conduct formal investigation denied staff the opportunity to put their case to any arbiter or investigator and allowed this state of mind to continue to develop. This critical commentary from patients was frequently aimed at those staff attempting to carry out their duties to a high standard and in a professional manner. It was also evident that earlier managers had, in an effort to 'keep the peace' and avoid further damaging allegations, moved these staff from the unit, feeding the perception that the victims were being punished and the perpetrators let off.

Frequently, staff learned they had been accused of various professional improprieties from rumour and gossip, but as these allegations were not made 'formal', these staff had no opportunity to state their case or defend their own clinical credibility. Ultimately, there was a strong sense that those managing the unit could not be trusted. It seemed obvious that there was a gulf between those responsible for the management of the unit and those responsible for the delivery of care. Managers and clinicians were split to the point of disarray. This split was mirrored in the relationship between the Personality Disorder Unit's (PDU) managers and the authority board and even spilt over into the inquiry itself with Peter Fallon later commenting:

> We are satisfied Mr Green (an Executive Director of the Authority Board) and his team fulfilled their duties diligently and honestly. Unfortunately some members of the PDU appear to have been less than cooperative, for whatever reason.
>
> (Fallon *et al.* 1999a: 4)

Despite these remarkable circumstances the announcement of the inquiry by the then Home Secretary, Stephen Dorrell, on 7 February 1997 was regarded by staff on the unit with a mixture of disbelief, amazement and sheer incredulity. The reports which dominated local and national news coverage outlining, *inter alia*, allegations of paedophilia, pornography and trafficking in illicit goods (including alcohol and 'dangerous' drugs) were regarded with simple disbelief. The very suggestion that staff could be involved in such serious, grossly unprofessional and probably illegal activities, was unthinkable for the majority of staff. The initial view internally was that this incredible situation had resulted from a combination of weak management and malicious untruths, perpetrated by patients and seized upon by those seeking to make a name for themselves out of the complex difficulties posed by the very existence of high secure psychiatric facilities.

It became apparent that there was some truth in these allegations (although there were also many untruths), and there began a suspicious and critical sense of questioning the actions and motives of colleagues and one's self. Many practices which had been encouraged (such as the social evenings and community activities) were now being paraded as evidence of collusion and bad practice. As more staff became implicated in practices of questionable standards, so the rumours and fantasies abounded. The news that the escort of the patient first raising these allegations really had knowingly separated from his charge was startling and his dismissal, after disciplinary investigation, was viewed with a mixed sense of 'quite right too' and a fear that it would now be open season for the most spurious of allegations as, if such events had really occurred, anything was believable.

The majority of staff reported feeling a mixture of blame and despair at this time as the realisation dawned that, whilst they thought they were doing a good job, they were in fact unknowingly sustaining a corrupt system. There was additionally a sense of anger that those staff who had voiced concern about practice on the unit had been marginalised and moved by managers who had set the standards for practice but were now 'trying to blame ward staff' for what should have been foreseeable. There was also considerable hostility and derision towards those staff who had transgressed professional and cultural codes of conduct. A smaller number of staff took the view that the inquiry was a misguided response from an ignorant public who didn't understand that what they had been doing was to simply 'gain the trust of the patients' in an effort to work therapeutically.

One particularly well experienced and senior psychologist wrote to the then Executive Nurse intimating that the inquiry was a gross overreaction by people who failed to understand the complexities of the situation. He illustrated this by explaining that he personally had encouraged contact between a patient with multiple convictions for paedophilia and the child of a visitor as he (the psychologist) considered the patient had 'difficulties relating to adults and found contact with children less threatening'. This perspective, which completely excludes any consideration of the interests of the child, highlighted the extent to which collusion was taking place and how seriously minimised and corrupted the understanding of the situation by some staff had become.

Concurrent with the announcement of the inquiry was the news that Ashworth Hospital's Chief Executive Officer was suspended pending the outcome of the inquiry. This was to be the first of many staff who would be suspended, undergo disciplinary investigation and face disciplinary action as a result of those original allegations, allegations which many only heard for the first time when they appeared in the press. The prevailing mood at this time, however, was one of fear and uncertainty. It is quite usual and common for personality disordered people to create havoc by complex processes of complaint, allegation and protest, but in this case no one close to the unit was quite sure why these allegations had been taken so seriously. Added to this, there was confusion as to how the press had got access to so much sensitive material and how or why the Secretary of State had felt the need to call a judicial review, particularly as it was only three months before a general election, a period when traditionally the message to public services is that there must be no embarrassing revelations.

This sense of insecurity and lack of trust was perhaps perpetuated by the fact that the then Clinical Director refused to visit the wards. He later explained, in his evidence to the inquiry, that this was because he feared physical assault by patients on the unit and lacked trust in the ward staff's willingness to protect him. Unfortunately this contributed significantly to the sense of abandonment and desertion felt by staff and patients.

The impact on the culture of the wards was fairly profound as it was perceived that there were serious splits amongst senior managers and that the net result was to leave staff and patients on the wards extremely vulnerable. There was additionally complete inertia in relation to therapeutic and clinical work (supposedly the core business of the unit) as a result of the perception that leadership was lacking and that the only direction would come from the inquiry. One senior member of the care teams operating within the Personality Disorders Service regarded the current situation as being 'management by inquiry' as there was little other evidence of tangible leadership apparent. The general view of care staff was that the 'knives were out' and that this was an 'opportunity to settle old scores'. The impact of this was entirely disabling for staff and particularly disadvantaging for patients as the general feeling was that you did as little as possible, took no risks and made no recommendations. As the staff said, 'if you do nothing, that's all they can blame you for'.

The effect of such divisions on the culture of the wards was an intense polarisation of attitude amongst nursing staff who were expected, by a tacit rather than overt process, to proclaim allegiance to a code of either 'gaoler or saviour' (often colloquially referred to as 'boot boy or messiah'). Generally, those adopting the role of 'gaoler' generated stories to explain how the current situation was entirely foreseeable, given the total liberalisation of the regime imposed by 'weak managers who allow psychopaths to run out of control'. Conversely, those adopting the role of 'saviour' argued that the patients were the innocent victims of the fundamentally flawed system of compulsory psychiatry and the press who were acting as moral voyeurs, imposing a corrupted gaze on an ignorant public to satiate a desire for the macabre. The system, however, very definitely took the view that the first and ultimate priority was to be security not therapy.

Discussion

During the almost two years of the inquiry's life (from its announcement to the publication of its findings), media interest varied and with it the exposure afforded to Ashworth Hospital in newspapers and on the television and radio. Each wave of media interest, however, reopened old wounds and reiterated the growing perception that the hospital was a paradigm of bad practice, bad staff and bad patients. There was no recognition for staff who continued to ply their trade in these difficult conditions and no regard from the media for the mental health needs of the patients.

The ignominy of this situation culminated in the publication of photographs and personal details of directors and senior managers in the tabloid press in what was declared a 'name and shame' initiative, but was more akin to a trial by rumour. One director in particular was highlighted and shortly after had his contract of employment terminated, despite the fact that he received no criticism from the inquiry team and indeed Peter Fallon himself praised his co-operation and contribution, stating:

> We are grateful to Mr Green and his team who at all times have responded to our requests to the very best of their ability . . . he and his team did not enjoy the same level of cooperation from within the hospital and in particular the PDU (Personality Disorder Unit) . . . but just before his final appearance, for some reason he had been relieved of his duties at Ashworth Hospital. We lost a valuable assistant at a critical time.
>
> (Fallon *et al.* 1999a: 4)

Internally, the process and publication of the inquiry led to many more staff being 'relieved of their duties', others underwent disciplinary action and were sacked (some justifiably so) and still more suffered mental health problems related to the stress of the inquiry and have not worked since.

In the aftermath, many skilled, experienced clinical staff and managers lost their employment through disciplinary action, retirement due to ill health or heavy-handed management. In many cases, these individuals were not in any way found lacking nor were they deemed guilty of any professional improprieties. The cost to these individuals and their families has been immense. The cost to the taxpayer has similarly been considerable. The cost to Ashworth Hospital, its patients and staff is incalculable and is still being paid as many 'professionals' not from Ashworth (but often from within the forensic psychiatric system) still cite Ashworth as a paradigm of bad practice, despite its considerable achievements and the fact that many of the original allegations (especially including the allegation that child abuse occurred within Ashworth Hospital) were found to have no validity.

Conversely, the tangible benefits are difficult to discern as, despite the fact that all recommendations were accepted by the government (excepting the recommendation that Ashworth should close), the outcomes of the inquiry have already been forgotten, no criminal charges were ever brought against hospital staff or patients and no staff have ever been called to account to their professional bodies.

Whilst the impetus of the inquiry brought together the leading authoritative figures in the personality disorder debate from Britain and other parts of Europe (especially Holland) it failed to provide any meaningful answers to the question as to how we may best provide care and treatment for such individuals. The inquiry team did publish its findings after hearing these 'expert opinions', drawing conclusions and making recommendations (Fallon 1999b), but already these have been ignored or discarded. One major recommendation was that no personality disorder facility should house more than 50 clients; a number of units in the special hospital and prison systems are currently being built housing up to 100 such individuals.

A perhaps even more catastrophic outcome of the inquiry was that it failed to offer any tangible evidence or indicators of which, if any, treatment approaches were likely to be effective in the care and management of those with personality disorders. The effect of this has magnified the impression that no one really knows what to do with this client group and that in fact they are largely untreatable. In the most extreme manifestation of the debate, some mental health care practitioners have taken the view that personality disorder is a social rather than medical problem. Whilst there may yet be some validity in this argument, the impact has been that many doctors will neither admit nor attempt to treat individuals whose health deficit relates to personality. As a result there is little real progress in our developing understanding as to the cause, progress and maintenance of personality disorders and individuals suffering such disabling conditions are at best left to 'get by', often living wretched unhappy lives and at worst end up committing serious criminal offences for which they are sent to prison.

In conclusion, it seems that the impact of the Ashworth Inquiry has severely disadvantaged the very people it sought to help – people with personality disorders. In seeking answers to an enduringly complex problem the inquiry has only succeeded in highlighting the current state of ignorance and prejudice and further reinforcing the perception that working in the field of personality disorders is a nervous condition which may seriously damage your professional career. Its recommendation that 'more research is needed' is somewhat obvious but the inquiry failed to offer a framework for the nature and impetus of such research. Ironically, in July 1999, only six months after the publication of the Fallon Inquiry Report, Frank Dobson, the then Secretary of State for Health, launched the 'Managing Dangerous People with Severe Personality Disorder' document (Home Office and Department of Health 1999). At this launch, he addressed a professional audience stating his view that the traditional model of psychiatry has both failed to provide effective care and treatment for these clients and to protect the public. He called for radical changes in legislation to dramatically alter the framework of care and intervention for such individuals. Five years later, the human cost and consequences of the inquiry endure but we remain bereft of a policy, professional, medical or social framework for the care and treatment of those with personality disorders.

References

Blom-Cooper, L., Brown, M., Dolan, R. and Murphy, E. (1992) *Report of the Committee of Inquiry into Complaints about Ashworth Hospital*, Volumes I and II, Cm 2028, London: HMSO.

Bluglass, R. (1992) 'The special hospitals should be closed', *British Medical Journal*, 305: 323/4.

Boynton, J. (1980) *Report of the Review of Rampton Hospital*, London: HMSO. Cmnd. 8073.

Fallon, P., Bluglass, R., Edwards, B. and Daniels, G. (1999a) *Report of the Committee of Inquiry into the Personality Disorder Unit, Ashworth Special Hospital. Volume I*, London: HMSO. (www.archive.official-documents.co.uk/document/cm41/4194/ash-01.htm#1.2.0)

Fallon, P., Bluglass, R., Edwards, B. and Daniels, G. (1999b) *Report of the Committee of Inquiry into the Personality Disorder Unit, Ashworth Special Hospital. Volume II*, London: HMSO.

Home Office and Department of Health (1999) *Managing Dangerous People with Severe Personality Disorder, Proposals for Policy Development*, London: HMSO.

Mental Health Act 1983, London: HMSO.

NHS Health Advisory Service/DHSS Social Services Inspectorate (1998) *Report on the Services Provided by Broadmoor Hospital*, London: DHSS, HAS/SSI (88) SH1.

Said, E. (1993) *Culture and Imperialism*, London: Chatto & Windas.

Salmon, Lord Justice (1966) *Royal Commission on Tribunals of Inquiry: Report of the Commission*, Cmnd. 3121. London: HMSO.

Part II

Inquiries into child abuse and deaths

Chapter 4

The impact of child abuse inquiries since 1990

Eileen Munro

Introduction

Public inquiries into child abuse are held when society is seriously worried about the way professionals handled particular cases. Their purpose is to analyse what went wrong (if anything) and to identify lessons to prevent a recurrence. Unfortunately, public concern is biased. Child welfare services have a broad remit, ranging from supporting families who are struggling to care adequately for their children, to protecting children from highly dangerous parents. Public interest is aroused only by certain types of adverse outcomes, predominantly deaths and, occasionally, the removal of children from their parents on what seems insubstantial grounds. Gaps in other areas of service, such as failure to provide adequate preventive and supportive services, get less public scrutiny. They lead to less extreme adverse results and these outcomes have a less clear-cut causal connection to professional actions or omissions. They are a concern to professionals and, intermittently, to politicians but less so to contemporary British society in general where parenting is seen as primarily a private rather than a social responsibility. As a result of this biased interest, the impact of inquiries has been to prioritise the child protective functions against a backdrop of professionals struggling, with varying degrees of success, to continue to meet the broader remit of child welfare.

One might have expected the impact of inquiries to have lessened since 1991 when the stream of inquiries became a trickle as a result of the new *Working Together* guidance which introduced private Part 8 inquiries to be conducted by local agencies, only a few of which have been deemed by the Department of Health to require further, public, scrutiny (Department of Health 1991: 57). This, I shall argue, is not the case. Although there was only one inquiry a year between 1993 and 1997, followed by a silence for five years, the threat of a public inquiry has remained a major influence on professional action, encouraging a defensive style of work and hampering attempts by policy makers to broaden the focus of the services.

Professionals' fears have been realised by three recent reports that have received considerable media attention (Lauren Wright, Norfolk Health

Authority 2002; Ainlee Labonte, Newham ACPC 2002; Victoria Climbié, Laming 2003). To the public, the priority is still to provide a child protection service; broader child welfare concerns take second place. These latest reports, however, also reveal an appalling level of practice. Public pressure, political policy making, and professional endeavour have all focused on improving child protection work. The opposite appears to be happening: morale has fallen, the quality of practice has deteriorated, and there are major problems in recruiting and retaining staff. This chapter explores how this reversal of fortunes has happened.

Developments in the 1970s and 1980s

Dividing history into decades is a neat literary device but, of course, reality is not so tidy. It is, however, possible to see important continuities in the way policy and practice developed during the 1970s and 1980s which have to be understood before we can understand subsequent changes.

In the 1960s, when the pioneering work of Kempe and his colleagues (1962) put child abuse on the political agenda, the problem was presented as a socio-medical issue. It required accurate diagnosis and treatment, albeit with an important role for social work as well as medicine in helping the abusive family. The very first inquiry – into the death of Graham Bagnall, age two (Salop County Council 1973) – stressed the need for better medical diagnosis and improved co-operation and communication between medical and social services personnel. It identified a need for a designated child protection agency that could 'assist both the child and the battering adult', the parent being seen as someone with a 'character disorder'.

The emergence of child abuse as a major public issue in the UK was significantly accelerated by the next public inquiry – into the tragic death of Maria Colwell in 1973. Maria had been taken into care soon after birth because of neglect. She was fostered happily by her aunt from age four months to six years when her birth mother, who had since re-married and had three more children, persuaded the social services that it was in Maria's best interests for her to be returned to her. This was very much against Maria's wishes and she fought against moving from the home where she felt secure. The birth mother's rights to care for her were, however, given greater weight and Maria eventually went to live with her mother, stepfather, and three step-siblings, aged one, two and three. Over the next fifteen months, despite being monitored by social workers and despite many expressions of concern by neighbours and a range of professionals, Maria was systematically maltreated, starved, and physically abused before dying at the age of seven. The case received widespread media coverage with a photo of a happy and healthy, younger Maria being contrasted with the sad and painful life she had then led with her birth mother.

As a result of the inquiry (Department of Health and Social Security 1974), changes were introduced with three main aims:

1 to increase awareness of child abuse and professionals' ability to diagnose it;
2 to improve communication and co-operation between professionals so that a more comprehensive assessment of the child's well-being could be made;
3 to set up at risk registers to improve monitoring so that any professional could check if anyone else had concerns about a particular child.

Approximately 40 more inquiries were published up to 1990, providing a constant reminder to the public of the existence of child abuse and the apparent failure of professionals to protect the victims. A review of inquiry reports found that 25 per cent of the reports were not critical of any professional group and social workers escaped censure in 42 per cent (Munro 1999). Media coverage, however, varied, with more attention being paid to inquiries that castigated professionals and less to the ones that exonerated them, fostering an image of all deaths being, in principle, preventable if only all professionals acted competently. In this coverage, social workers were repeatedly singled out for blame even when other professional groups had played a major role.

The report on the death of Jasmine Beckford in 1985 was particularly emotive and influential (London Borough of Brent 1985). In spite of the growing pressure to identify abuse victims accurately, Dingwall et al.'s (1983) research found that professionals were still reluctant to take a more intrusive approach and operated a 'rule of optimism', looking for the most benign explanation of any signs of abuse and being slow to take action against parents. Jasmine's case demonstrated that public opinion wanted the welfare of children to be given more weight than the rights of parents. Jasmine's case had many echoes of Maria Colwell's story. She too had been taken into care because of abuse and later rehabilitated with her birth mother and stepfather. Like Maria, she steadily lost weight at home and suffered a series of injuries but her social worker failed to notice or see their significance. The inquiry report firmly concluded that the prime task of child protection workers was to protect children; the needs and rights of parents must take second place:

It is the children and not the parents who are their [social workers'] primary concern . . . to treat the parents as the clients is fatally to misdirect the efforts of what is in essence a child protection service.

(London Borough of Brent 1985: 294)

This was a significant shift from the view expressed in the first inquiry (Graham Bagnall 1973) which saw abusers and children equally in need of assessment and help.

The sustained impact of these public criticisms led professionals to place more and more priority on responding to allegations of child abuse. The increased public and professional awareness of abuse led to a rise in referrals to Social Services Departments. No national statistics were kept on referral rates but some indication of the increase can be gauged from numbers placed on the child protection register which rose from 11,844 in 1978 to 45,300 in 1991 (Parton *et al.* 1997: 5). The bulk of the extra work of responding to these referrals fell on social services teams, reducing their ability to meet their other responsibilities in relation to supporting families and looking after children in public care.

It quickly became apparent that the inquiries were reporting similar faults in the management of cases and producing much the same recommendations. Constant themes were the need for good inter-professional collaboration and thorough investigation and assessment of allegations. The procedures for working together and for conducting an investigation were spelt out in more and more detail. This was a major change in social work practice where practitioners had been accustomed to exercising a high degree of autonomy and professional judgement. Increasingly, practice was shaped by central government frameworks, checklists and procedures. The growing rigour of these investigations also had an impact, making the experience more distressing and intrusive for the families with a subsequent effect on their working relationships with professionals.

With the pressure on professionals not to miss a case of abuse, the effort put into investigations increased and the threshold for taking action dropped. More and more families found themselves subject to investigations; a growing number complained that their children were being removed from them without justification. The public became concerned that the child protection system was becoming too powerful and intervening unnecessarily in the privacy of the family. This led to a backlash with child protection workers being accused of 'trampling the rights of innocent victims' and engaging in 'hysterical witchhunts' (Myers 1994). Newspapers have described social workers variously as: 'abusers of authority, hysterical and malignant' (*Daily Mail*, 7 July 1988), 'like the SAS in cardigans and Hush Puppies' (*Sunday People*, 10 March 1991), or 'child stealers' (*Today*, 29 March 1991).

These feelings came to a head in 1987 when two newly appointed paediatricians in Cleveland started diagnosing a high rate of sexual abuse among children taken to hospital, some with no pre-existing suspicion of abuse. Placing strong reliance on a controversial 'anal dilatation' test, the doctors, in a five-month period, diagnosed sexual abuse in 121 children from 57 families. Even with hindsight, it is impossible to say with confidence how many of these were accurate – though evidence suggests a substantial number were. However, the public and media reactions showed that they could not believe sexual abuse was happening on such a scale and the dominant impression was that the child protection system was out of control and breaking up innocent families. The public inquiry was more moderate in its conclusions, acknowledging that child sexual abuse was a real and important problem (Butler-Sloss 1988). It criticised the paediatricians for having too much confidence in an unproven test and for the way the cases were subsequently managed, with the children being hurriedly separated from their parents although resources could not cope with the sudden rise in number.

The Cleveland Report captured the change in the political mood that was exemplified in the 1989 Children Act. The power of professionals was seen to have become too great and the rights of parents needed to be strengthened. This belief was based on little firm evidence but more on media coverage of sensationalist stories that fed into people's paranoia about an all-powerful state eroding liberal freedoms. The overriding philosophy of the legislation is that children are best brought up by their birth family. It encourages professionals to try to work with families through negotiation rather than coercion, involving children and parents in agreed plans. Although the word *partnership* does not appear in the statute, it has a pervasive influence. In view of the value assigned to the birth family, removing children should be an option of last resort with more effort put into making their families safe places to be. David Mellor, the minister who introduced the Bill to the House of Commons, said:

> We hope and believe that it [the new legislation] will bring order, integration, relevance and a better balance to the law – a better balance not just between the rights and responsibilities of individuals and agencies, but most vitally, between the need to protect children and the need to enable parents to challenge intervention in the upbringing of their children.
>
> (Hansard 1989)

Developments in the 1990s

By the late 1980s, it was becoming apparent that the child protection system was becoming unbalanced and needed fundamental reform. While the Cleveland Report was undoubtedly instrumental in epitomising public concern about the level of professional power, empirical research was influential in providing a wider picture of how the system was functioning. This showed that the problem of imbalance lay not only between state and parental power but also between helping families and policing them.

In 1994 the Audit Commission produced a report on health and social services provision of child welfare that noted that the Children Act gave them wider responsibilities to support families that were not yet being met on a significant scale, with priority still being given to child protection work:

> Social services departments must develop a more proactive rather than reactive approach, paying particular attention to Part III section 17 of the Children Act which covers authorities' responsibilities to children in need.
>
> (Audit Commission 1994: 3)

The Department of Health published a summary of research into child protection in 1995 that identified a similar need for re-focusing work:

> The spirit of the *Children Act 1989* is that there should be a balance between child protection and family support services. A significant finding of the researchers was that enquiries were too often characterised as investigations and that better outcomes might be achieved if children's needs were prioritised and matched to appropriate services. The research indicates that real benefits may arise if there is a focus on the needs of children and families rather than a narrow concentration on the alleged incident of abuse.
>
> (Department of Health 1995: Foreword)

The priority and effort put into responding to child protection issues made heavy demands on the social services budget, as the Audit Commission had found, and led to a focus on the incident reported rather than a broader assessment of the child's development and the family functioning. Cleaver and Freeman's (1995) research also found that the experience could be very traumatic for the families investigated who rarely received any service as a result of the professional attention, leading them to question whether it was too high a price to pay for finding the rare cases of serious abuse.

The Department of Health's policy advice was that many referrals should be re-classified and the initial response should not be a child abuse investigation (under Section 47 of the 1989 Children Act) but take the form of an enquiry into whether the child is in need and might benefit from services (under Section 17 of the Act).

> Such an approach to children in need would help rebut the criticism that many investigations are undertaken, many families are visited and case conferences called but, in the end, little support is offered to the family . . . a more balanced service for vulnerable children would encourage professionals to take a wider view. There would be efforts to work along

side families rather than disempower them, to raise their self-esteem rather than reproach families, to promote family relationships where children have their needs met, rather than leave untreated families with an unsatisfactory style.

(Department of Health 1995: 54)

One important strategy for developing a more preventive and comprehensive service was the introduction of additional training for social workers – a Post-Qualifying Child Care Award provided by universities. Basic training, it was considered, provided an inadequate level of specialised knowledge and skill in relation to working with children and families. A review of inquiries in the 1970s and 1980s found that the earlier reports tended to criticise social workers for not collecting the relevant information, while later ones complained that they had failed to interpret it correctly (Munro 1998). The hope is that, when sufficient numbers have this award, it can become a requirement for some child protection posts. The new course aims to improve social workers' ability to assess children's needs, to work with children and their parents, and to devise packages of care to meet identified needs.

Another major strategy in broadening the remit of child welfare services has been the introduction of a new framework for assessing need and a set of related forms (Department of Health 1999). Based on forms developed for assessing the development of children in public care, these materials encourage workers to take a comprehensive look at a child's development and assess whether their needs are being met.

Difficulties in re-focusing services

How is this new policy being implemented? The evidence from research seems persuasive and the case for developing support services is strong. The Department of Health has taken steps to ensure staff have the relevant knowledge and skills to assess and help families in need. The new policy is welcome to most professionals who entered caring professions wanting to help rather than police families. The negative impact of public inquiries into child deaths has also been muted since the introduction of confidential Part 8 inquiries. All signs look favourable yet, a decade later, implementation is still proving severely problematic.

The Social Services Inspectorate, having examined eight local authorities, found that 'departments continue to respond to child protection and looked after children cases to the exclusion of support to other families of children in need' (1997: 1). The Department of Health's review of studies of the implementation of the 1989 Children Act came to a similar conclusion: 'Access to services often related solely to concerns about child abuse or neglect and should be widened to other children in need' (2001: 118).

Colton *et al.*'s (1995) study of eight local authorities found that social workers and managers were not opposed to the policy of developing more support services but believed it could not be done *instead of* child protection work but *as well as*, and so required additional funding which was not yet forthcoming.

One factor that creates a reluctance to shift the focus is the way that public inquiries allocate blame. Although their overt goal is not so punitive, in reality inquiries do reach judgements that name and shame individuals and agencies. The Colwell Report was an exception in making a clear judgement that:

> We think it quite impossible, and indeed unfair, to lay the direct blame for such inadequacies in the care and supervision of Maria upon any individual.
>
> (Department of Health and Social Security 1974: 86)

The system, rather than individuals, was at fault:

> The overall impression created by Maria's sad history is that while individuals made mistakes it was 'the system', using the word in the widest sense, which failed her. Because that system is the product of society it is upon society as a whole that the ultimate blame must rest; indeed the highly emotional and angry reaction of the public in this case may indicate society's troubled conscience.
>
> (Department of Health and Social Security 1974: 86)

In contrast, the Beckford Report (1985) had no hesitation in naming and blaming individuals: 'to the extent that Ms Wahlstrom and Miss Leong were the two workers in the front line of social and health services, they must take some personal responsibility for what happened' (London Borough of Brent 1985: 287). In the Climbié case, the senior social worker's mental health problems, her own difficulties as a parent, and her religious beliefs were mercilessly scrutinised in the press. The front-line social worker was also castigated by the media; her employers added to the punishment by sacking her and placing her name on the Department of Health register of people considered unsuitable to work with children in any capacity, a register usually restricted to individuals suspected of being abusive.

The threat of this kind of personal outcome is understandably going to affect professionals' practice. Another obstacle to re-focusing, however, lies in the complexity of judging whether a referral should be classified as possible abuse or not. In a defensive culture, this leads to an over-estimation of severity. Spratt's (2000, 2001) study provides an interesting and more detailed picture of what is going on and why staff are failing to re-focus practice to the extent wanted by policy makers. He examined how staff try to re-classify more referrals as 'children in need' rather than 'child protection', looking at

whether social workers are managing to shift from a child protection to a child welfare orientation. He found that, while they are willing to do so, they are hindered by professional and organisational concerns to manage risk. He studied 200 consecutive referrals to a Family and Child Care Programme in Northern Ireland. They were each classified by a senior social worker into one of three categories: a 'child protection investigation' (27 per cent), a 'child-care problem' (27 per cent) or 'other', e.g. relationship difficulties, housing, financial (46 per cent). After investigation, 70 per cent of the child protection cases were re-classified, suggesting that a more accurate classification at the beginning would lead to a significant drop in investigations. Examination of these referrals indicated that social workers were classifying any degree of risk, however small, as a child protection case. Only 6 per cent of the cases classified as child-care problem were re-classified later as child protection, i.e. there was a high rate of false positives and a low rate of false negatives in this sample. The researcher checked the consistency of the senior social workers' judgements by creating vignettes of the most ambiguous referrals (those that might indicate harm or need or both) and presenting them to the same workers for classification. Thirty of them had previously been classified child protection and four as child-care problems. Their judgements now differed markedly from the real-life scenario. Only 3 per cent of the cases previously classified as child protection were so classified by all eight senior social workers.

The author suggests as an explanation for this major difference that the vignettes are decontextualised, particularly in relation to the concept of risk. Therefore, the workers are making decisions without any personal vulnerability if they make a mistake. Their preference, in the real-life situation, for opting for investigations makes sense as a defensive measure to protect themselves from possible criticism:

> The safest way, procedurally, of dealing with personal risk is to instigate a personal investigation where such risks are shared both intra- and inter-organizationally. The use of the investigative response as a catch-all for the presenting problems of families may be consequently explained as a rational approach to the management of personal risk.
>
> (2000: 613)

While there appears to be scope for re-classifying referrals, this study found that the senior social workers did not agree on which could be:

> The result was apparent confusion. It was impossible to analyse the data and identify which type of investigations might be re-coded, simply because there was no grouping of responses. The patterns of choice

were more representative of what one might have expected as a result of random allocation rather than professional interpretation.

(2000: 613)

The Social Services Inspectorate has repeatedly recommended clearer criteria for classifying referrals so that families are not drawn unnecessarily into investigations (e.g. 1997: 5). Spratt challenged the feasibility of doing so. He sent his vignettes to eight Social Services Inspectors. Only five responded but the results were interesting: there was 80 per cent disagreement between them in how to classify the vignettes. Although only a small sample, this result, combined with the larger study, does raise serious questions about whether the information contained in a referral is too limited and open to varied interpretation to enable any consistent response. If further research reproduces this finding, then it seriously undermines the claim that front-line workers should be able to classify referrals accurately at the point of initial contact.

Deterioration in child protection services

The history of recent years not only reveals that the system is not re-focusing to the degree policy makers want but also that the quality of child protection services themselves is deteriorating. A major government inspection report on services to safeguard children (Department of Health 2002) expressed continuing concern for how social services were dealing with children in need:

> In most areas there were serious concerns amongst staff of all agencies about the thresholds that social services were applying in their children's services. Professional staff from other agencies considered that social services were not providing an adequate response when they judged a situation did not involve a high risk of serious harm to children and young people.
>
> (2002: 4)

The report identified worries about the services for children at risk. They stress the importance of the quality of the initial social service response, affecting as it does the quality of the assessment and the whole course of work with the family but found that:

> Many staff in agencies in most authorities expressed concern about the accessibility and quality of this initial response by social services . . . duty systems were found to be impersonal and unresponsive.
>
> (2002: 46)

A review of child protection services in Scotland came to worrying conclusions:

> The review findings suggest that many adults and children have little confidence in the child protection system and are considerably reluctant to report concerns about abuse and neglect. . . .
>
> The review findings also suggest that the child protection system does not always work well for those children and adults who become involved in it. Forty children in the audit were not protected or their needs were not met following the intervention of agencies. A further 62 children were only partially protected or their needs partially met. In 77 cases children were protected and their needs met and in 24 of these cases their needs were well met.
>
> (Scottish Executive 2002: 13)

Concerns about the quality of practice have also emerged from the three recent public inquiries. Indeed, the re-emergence of the public inquiry after a lull of five years indicates growing anxiety about what is happening. Of the three reports, the Climbié Report (Laming 2003) is by far the most detailed and therefore the best source of information about what is going on in front-line work.

Reading the Climbié Report is a disturbing experience. As someone who has read all the reports since 1973, I found this report in a class of its own, describing a level of practice that was frighteningly bad. Other reports have revealed incompetence and inadequacies in staff but have conveyed a general impression that people were trying to do a good job. The picture obtained from the Climbié Report is of a set of professionals trying to avoid taking responsibility for Victoria's welfare by minimising their interpretation of their own role as much as possible and relying on someone else doing the necessary work. There were also numerous occasions when the most basic principles of practice were not followed. This criticism applies not only to social workers but also to police officers and to hospital staff. Nurses bathing Victoria in hospital saw how extensive and varied her injuries were (a classic presentation of physical abuse); none recorded this or mentioned it to doctors or social workers. Victoria was an in-patient for two weeks with suspected physical abuse but none of the doctors who saw her did a full physical examination. There were only two occasions when professionals tried to talk to Victoria in any depth but these seem half-hearted because they did not take the elementary step of speaking to her in her native language of French, using English instead, of which Victoria knew only a few words. (In contrast to the professionals' thoughtlessness, the child-minder who became concerned about Victoria had the sense to take her to her son's school and get the French teacher to ask Victoria about her injuries. Her difficulties in explaining them satisfactorily led the childminder to take her to hospital.)

Victoria was not an unusual or complex case but died because of persistent failings in the protection system. The inquiry team were able to identify 12 occasions in the nine months she was in London when professionals *should have* recognised the need to investigate more thoroughly. The most basic inquiries would have quickly led to an assessment of high risk. Lord Laming, the Chair of the inquiry, has forcibly and eloquently expressed how appalled he felt by the story that was unfolded to the inquiry. At the beginning of his report, under a photograph of Victoria, he put a quote from *The Little Prince* by Antoine de Saint-Exupery: 'I have suffered too much grief in setting down these heartrending memories. If I try to describe him, it is to make sure that I shall not forget him'.

It might be hoped that Victoria's care was an extreme and isolated incident, but this seems implausible given the number of agencies involved: four social services departments, three housing departments, two specialist police teams, two hospitals and a voluntary sector specialist family centre.

The probability that the deterioration in services is more widespread is increased by the evidence of a national crisis in recruiting and retaining staff. There has been a sharp drop in the number wanting to become social workers. Applications to training courses fell by 59 per cent between 1996 and 2001 (after an advertising campaign by the government, application rates rose by 8 per cent in 2002, reversing the trend slightly). In 1994, the Audit Commission could write: 'there is a perceived "elitism" in protection work' (1994: 61) but its status has fallen steeply and job satisfaction is declining. In 2002, one in six child-care social work posts were vacant (*Guardian*, 20 February 2002). Three London boroughs had vacancy rates over 50 per cent. Newly qualified staff who, a few years ago, would have been protected from the more serious child abuse, are now dealing with all levels of referral. Reliance on short-term agency staff, even at managerial level, is now also commonplace. Many London boroughs report agency rates of 40–50 per cent at both front-line and senior levels. Moreover, posts are increasingly being filled by workers coming from overseas who, while their training may have been high quality, need additional induction and supervision to operate in a foreign legal and cultural framework. The extra support needs do not seem to be met. In Brent, at the time of Victoria Climbié's referral, all members of the duty team were agency staff who had trained overseas (Laming 2003, para. 5.14). The inquiry was told:

> There were occasions where a person will get off a plane in the morning, arrive in the office just after lunch, be interviewed and start work either in the duty team or the child protection team. It was happening very, very often.

> (Laming 2003, para. 5.60)

To the outsider, relying on such inexperienced people to deal with some of the most challenging aspects of social work seems baffling, but it is a measure of the desperation senior management feel in trying to fill vacancies. The severity of the problem was stressed by Denise Platt, the Chair of the Social Services Inspectorate, in her 11th annual report: 'Recruitment and retention of appropriate staff is the most critical issue that faces social care services in all sectors' (Social Services Inspectorate 2002).

The Audit Commission conducted a study of why staff leave and concluded that most are leaving because of push not pull factors. Their analysis identified six main factors that underpin the decision to leave:

- the sense of being overwhelmed by bureaucracy, paperwork and targets;
- insufficient resources, leading to unmanageable workloads;
- a lack of autonomy;
- feeling undervalued by Government, managers and the public;
- pay that is not 'felt fair'; and
- a change agenda that feels imposed and irrelevant (2002, Section 3).

It is hard to separate out the specific impact public inquiries have had in causing this slump in morale. Their recommendations can, however, be seen as a paradigm example of the types of solutions that have been adopted to try to improve front-line work. Strategies have predominantly taken the form of bureaucratic solutions, increasing formalisation of the tasks and greater managerial oversight and control of all levels of work (Munro, forthcoming). The procedural innovations established as a result of the Colwell report in 1974 were undoubtedly needed because, at that time, there were no formal mechanisms for sharing information among professionals and this is essential for a full assessment of a child's welfare. However, the subsequent stream of re-organisations, at both local and national level, has not been shown to make any significant difference to the quality of front-line work.

The other managerial solution is to develop increasingly detailed procedures, protocols and guidelines to standardise practice and make it visible for monitoring and audit. Again, some formalisation is necessary but the question is how much (Munro 2002). The fundamental problem seems to lie in the nature of the central tasks in child protection. Crucially, the managerial systems that have been developed refer to the more easily described and recorded aspects of practice, with a major bias towards quantity rather than quality. It is easy to record whether a visit was done or a phone call made but more complicated to find a way of measuring the quality of the interaction and the reliability of the information gained. Consequently, it seems to many practitioners that the most challenging and satisfying aspects of their work – the interpersonal skills needed to elicit and interpret information and to engage families – are rendered invisible by an audit system that concentrates on the easily measured. This is noticeable in supervision which, traditionally, paid a lot of attention to the relationship dynamics. Supervisors are tending to shift the focus onto whether practitioners are meeting administrative requirements; there is less time, if any, spent on casework supervision in which front-line staff are helped to stand back and review critically their assessments and plans (Rushton and Nathan 1996). Victoria Climbié's social worker, who had never before conducted a child abuse investigation, was offered little supervision and none of it related to the professional skills and knowledge needed to carry out the work. Peter Reder and Sylvia Duncan's contribution in this book (Chapter 5) stresses the importance of understanding the psychological dimension of practice and shows how it is necessary for accurate assessment of a family and for working with them constructively.

Increasing formalisation also helps agencies defend themselves from public criticism. Hood *et al.* (2000) show how public sector services engage in 'blame prevention engineering'. Formal procedures set out a formal 'correct' way of dealing with a case. Then, if a tragedy occurs, the agency can claim 'due diligence' and show that their employees followed the 'correct' procedures (although they did not lead to the correct outcome in terms of averting the tragedy).

The Climbié Report fitted into the bureaucratic tradition in many respects, recommending the establishment of a new national body for inter-agency working and greater managerial accountability for ensuring the quality of front-line practice. However, it was original in saying that management should be held accountable for the *quality* of front-line work and this is potentially a major change. The report, unfortunately, said little about how quality can be measured – and this is a key point (Munro, forthcoming). Will managers continue to use the performance indicators of the current audit system, indicators that are only a clumsy measure of quality? Alternatively, will they try to develop more sophisticated and accurate ways of monitoring practice? If they choose the latter option, then, although the task is far more challenging, it could make a significant contribution to the development of knowledge and skills in child protection.

Conclusion

Public inquiries into cases of child abuse with tragic outcomes have strongly influenced the development of child welfare services. Three landmark cases have been Maria Colwell (DHSS 1974), Cleveland (Department of Health 1988), and Victoria Climbié (Laming 2003). The report into the care provided to Maria Colwell captured the growing public concern for children who were being abused by their carers and identified the need to increase professional awareness. It also created formal mechanisms for inter-professional collaboration so that a comprehensive, and thus more accurate, picture could be gained of a child's welfare. The public pressure to prevent child deaths led professionals to lower their threshold for action and to intervene more readily, challenging parental authority and disrupting the family unit. This provoked public unease about the increased professional power threatening the privacy of the family, leading to a backlash, exemplified by the Cleveland Report where professionals were seen as having become too quick to identify abuse and to break up families. The Children Act 1989 reflected the desire to change the balance of power, diminishing professional and increasing parental authority. Under pressure to avoid mistakes of both kinds – missing abuse cases or mistakenly classifying safe families as dangerous – professionals, quite rationally, put their efforts into more and more rigorous investigations to increase the accuracy of their assessments. This caused a shift in the allocation of resources, starving other sections of child welfare.

There are persuasive arguments for re-focusing to make a broader assessment of children's needs beyond the need for protection but, despite persistent political directives, change is slow to materialise. This, it is argued, is because there is insufficient additional funding to finance support services *in addition to* protection services. Since the majority of referrals of abuse are not substantiated or not considered serious enough for professional intervention, one option for saving money is to classify cases more accurately at the time of initial referral, thus reducing the time and resources spent on rigorous investigations. One obstacle to this lies in the intellectual difficulties in classifying referrals accurately on the limited knowledge available in the initial referral. Another obstacle comes from the defensive culture now prevalent in child protection agencies. The increasingly punitive attitude of society to mistakes, illustrated by public inquiries, encourages practitioners to err on the side of caution.

The blame culture is also implicated in the shift towards creating more and more formal procedures. Unfortunately, only some dimensions of practice are getting attention in this process. Many of the most difficult aspects of working with families are being excluded and so undervalued. The report into the death of Victoria Climbié described a child protection service that was failing at the most basic level to safeguard children. Like its predecessors, it recommended re-organisation but it also stressed the need for management to measure the *quality* of front-line practice. Developing ways of doing this is intellectually challenging.

Nevertheless the most pressing problem for management at present is recruiting and retaining staff. The public scrutiny and criticism of the child protection service, exemplified by public inquiries, seems to have had the unintended effect of creating a demoralised workforce. Society seems to have recognised the importance of protecting children but underestimates the difficulties of doing so.

References

Audit Commission (1994) *Seen but not Heard: Co-ordinating Community Child Health and Social Services for Children in Need*, London: HMSO.

Audit Commission (2002) *Recruitment and Retention: A Public Service Workforce for the Twenty-First Century*, London: Audit Commission.

Butler-Sloss, E. (1988) *Report of the Inquiry in Child Abuse in Cleveland, 1987*, Cmnd. 412, London: HMSO.

Cleaver, H. and Freeman, P. (1995) *Parental Perspectives in Cases of Suspected Child Abuse*, London: HMSO.

Colton, M., Drury, C. and Williams, M. (1995) *Children in Need: Family Support under the Children Act 1989*, Aldershot: Avebury.

Department of Health (1991) *Working Together under the Children Act 1989*, London: HMSO.

Department of Health (1995) *Child Protection: Messages from Research*, London: HMSO.

Department of Health (1999) *Framework for the Assessment of Children in Need and their Families*, London: Department of Health.

Department of Health (2001) *The Children Act Now. Messages from Research*, London: The Stationery Office.

Department of Health (2002) *Safeguarding Children*, London: Department of Health.

Department of Health and Social Security (1974) *Report of the Committee of Inquiry into the Care and Supervision Provided in Relation to Maria Colwell*. London: HMSO.

Dingwall, R., Eckelar, J. and Murray, T. (1983) *The Protection of Children: State Intervention and Family Life*, Oxford: Blackwell.

Hansard (1989) House of Commons, 27 April, 2nd Reading, col. 1107–1108.

Hood, C., Rothstein, H. and Baldwin, R. (2000) *The Government of Risk: Understanding Risk Regulation Regimes*, Oxford: Oxford University Press.

Kempe, C., Silverman, F., Steele, B., Droegemueller, W. and Silver, H. (1962) 'The battered child syndrome', *Journal of the American Medical Association*, 181: 17–24.

Laming, H. (2003) *The Victoria Climbié Inquiry: Report of an Inquiry by Lord Laming*, London: The Stationery Office.

London Borough of Brent (1985) *A Child in Trust: The Report of the Panel of Inquiry into the Circumstances Surrounding the Death of Jasmine Beckford*, London: London Borough of Brent.

Munro, E. (1998) 'Improving social workers' knowledge base in child protection work', *British Journal of Social Work*, 28: 89–105.

Munro, E. (1999) 'Common errors of reasoning in child protection work', *Child Abuse and Neglect*, 23: 745–58.

Munro, E. (2002) *Effective Child Protection*, London: Sage Publications.

Munro, E. (forthcoming) 'The impact of audit on social work practice', *British Journal of Social Work*.

Myers, J. (ed.) (1994) *The Backlash: Child Protection under Fire*, London: Sage.

Newham Area Child Protection Committee (2002) *Ainlee. Part 8 Review*, Newham: ACPC.

Norfolk Health Authority (2002) *Summary Report of the Independent Health Review*, Norwich: Norfolk Health Authority.

Parton, N., Thorpe, D. and Wattam, C. (1997) *Child Protection: Risk and the Moral Order*, London: Macmillan.

Rushton, A. and Nathan, J. (1996) 'The supervision of child protection work', *British Journal of Social Work*, 26: 357–74.

Salop County Council (1973) *Report of the Inquiry into the Circumstances Surrounding the Death of Graham Bagnall (d.o.b. 20.5.70) and the Role of the County Council's Social Services*, Shrewsbury: Salop County Council.

Scottish Executive (2002) *It's Everyone's Job to Make Sure I'm Alright*, Edinburgh: Scottish Office.

Social Services Inspectorate (1997) *Responding to Families in Need: Inspection of Assessment, Planning and Decision-Making in Family Support Services*, London: Department of Health.

Social Services Inspectorate (2002) *Annual Report*, London: Department of Health.

Spratt, T. (2000) 'Decision making by senior social workers at point of first referral', *British Journal of Social Work*, 30: 597–618.

Spratt, T. (2001) 'The influence of child protection orientation on child welfare practice', *British Journal of Social Work*, 31: 933–54.

Chapter 5

From Colwell to Climbié: Inquiring into fatal child abuse

Peter Reder and Sylvia Duncan

Introduction

It is unusual for society to address concerns about children before it has considered equivalent issues for adults. However, systems to examine cases of fatal child abuse in the United Kingdom preceded inquiries into homicides by adult psychiatric patients by two decades. This may be because care in the community for adult patients has been a relatively recent development, while a culture of criticism has only latterly become directed at health, as opposed to social work, staff. Nonetheless, this longer history provides those involved in child protection with a unique perspective from which to consider the impact and value of the inquiry process.

In this chapter, we shall briefly trace the history of fatal child abuse inquiries and reflect on their benefits and limitations. Their principal findings will be summarised in order to highlight how very similar problems have recurred, implying that key lessons have not been learned. We shall suggest reasons for this that lie within fundamental premises about the inquiry process and conflicting agendas of the procedure. In that light, we shall debate the merits of persisting with current systems.

History

Procedures for scrutinising cases in which a child has died or been severely injured from abuse have changed significantly over the last 30 years. As Eileen Munro notes in her chapter, the inquiry into the death of Graham Bagnall (Salop County Council 1973) was the first of a series of at least 35 public inquiries conducted up to the end of the 1980s (Reder *et al.* 1993; Corby *et al.* 1998; Munro 1999), although it was the Maria Colwell Inquiry Report (Department of Health and Social Security 1974) which was considered a landmark event that fundamentally changed child protection practice. Corby *et al.* (1998) described three main types of public inquiry during that period: statutory inquiries ordered by a Secretary of State, which were conducted in public, in a quasi-judicial way and produced a published report; those sponsored by a health or local authority but carried out by an independent panel, often in the same adversarial manner as the statutory inquiries, and ending with a published report; and those carried out internally but resulting in a report available to the public. It is difficult to ascertain how the style of inquiry was determined for any particular case, or, indeed, how the decision was made to conduct one at all, but many had clearly been prompted by media, public, political or judicial concern about professional practice. Some of the reports were huge, with copious recommendations; others were only a few pages, with circumscribed conclusions.

In anticipation of the forthcoming Children Act 1989, the first *Working Together* document (Department of Health and Social Security and Welsh Office 1988) introduced a more uniform set of procedures, in which internal case reviews would be conducted locally by each involved agency, under the co-ordination of an inter-agency forum – the Area Child Protection Committee (ACPC). The purpose of these reviews was 'to assess whether decisions and actions taken in the case were reasonable and responsible' and 'to check whether established procedures were followed' (p. 46). Successive revisions to *Working Together* (Home Office *et al.* 1991; Department of Health *et al.* 1999) provided fuller guidance in Part 8 of the documents and such reviews became known as 'Part 8 Reviews'. Each involved agency was required to instigate its own internal review, to be integrated into a composite analysis by the ACPC. In practice, this was delegated to an ACPC sub-committee or a specially commissioned impartial outsider. All composite reports had to be submitted to the Department of Health but were otherwise confidential to ACPC member agencies, with an anonymised executive summary made publicly available. The intention was to establish at a local level 'whether there are lessons to be learned from the case . . .' in order 'to improve inter-agency working and better safeguard children' (Department of Health *et al.* 1999: 87). For a short while, reviews were known as 'Chapter 8 Reviews' but are now being referred to as 'Serious Case Reviews' (Sinclair and Bullock 2002). Approximately 50 child abuse related Reviews were submitted to the Department of Health each year during the early 1990s (Reder and Duncan 1999), although the impression is that this number is now closer to ninety (Sinclair and Bullock 2002).

Working Together guidance always allowed for exceptional cases in which the circumstances of a child's death generated so much concern that a more detailed, centrally commissioned inquiry was required. The death of Victoria Climbié in February 2000 from hypothermia, malnutrition and physical abuse suffered at the hands of her carers, a great-aunt and her co-habitee, was such a case and it resulted in the most lengthy public inquiry to date and a massive report, published three years later (Laming 2003).

Relative merits of the inquiry/review systems

Public inquiries

The one clear value of the public inquiries has been to raise society's awareness about the problem of child abuse. Media attention to the most extreme cases of physical abuse and neglect has reminded the public and policy makers alike of the horrors that some children suffer and to the dilemmas that front-line professionals face. Political attention has led to new legislation designed to promote children's welfare, such as the 1975 and 1989 Children Acts (Hill 1990). For practitioners, the reports have identified some important lessons that helped to refine policies and everyday practice (Hallett 1989). However, it was the Maria Colwell Inquiry in 1974 that had a transitional effect, with consolidation of Child Protection Registers (then called At Risk Registers), inter-agency committees (now the ACPC) and case conferences (now called Child Protection Conferences) and prompting the 1975 Children Act. Following this, the impact of public inquiries appears to have declined significantly. As there are no reliable statistics for the number of children killed through abuse each year (Reder and Duncan 2002), it remains an open question as to whether 30 years of inquiries have enabled professionals to reduce the number that occurs.

Despite certain benefits, there have been considerable drawbacks. Even though child abuse deaths are rare, the critical atmosphere of public inquiries and accompanying media reporting has generated wholly unrealistic expectations that such deaths 'should never happen again' and beliefs that front-line professionals are incompetent. Over time, the work of social workers has mainly gained media attention when they were being criticised, so that their public standing sank, impacting significantly on morale and recruitment. Their approach to everyday practice inevitably became defensive (Hill 1990). Also, large public inquiries have been extraordinarily expensive in terms of money and time, with costs spiralling to hundreds of thousands of pounds and an excessive lapse of time before the findings could be announced. Once published, reports' availability has been inconsistent, with differing publishers, no central reference list and discouraging prices. Corby et al. (1998) and Reder et al. (1993) have commented on the considerable difficulty they experienced discovering what inquiries had taken place and obtaining copies of the reports. However, although the full Victoria Climbié Inquiry Report cost £42.50, its free availability on-line did much to increase its accessibility and readership.

Part 8/Serious Case Reviews

The Part 8/Serious Case Reviews system has been a considerable improvement on the public inquiry process. Reviews are carried out locally, on many more cases, more speedily and at much less cost. They tend to be conducted in a more constructive atmosphere and in greater privacy, which increases the possibility that the findings will impact on local practice in a thoughtful way. Responsibility for implementing recommendations in a workable manner and for monitoring progress is held within the ACPC, which brings it closer to each involved agency. At another level, central government has had the opportunity to identify common themes across a more representative practice sample. An early benefit was the recognition of an association between fatal child abuse and parental mental health problems (Falkov 1996), which reinforced initiatives to address the needs of children of psychiatric patients (e.g. Falkov 1998; Reder et al. 2000).

However, the system is not ideal and numerous disadvantages remain. For example, local issues seem to determine which child's death or serious injury receives a formal review and the system is therefore unable to give an accurate picture of the incidence of fatalities across the country. Our study of Part 8 Reviews from 1993/4 (Reder and Duncan 1999) revealed that the focus of many reviewers was limited to whether existing child protection procedures had been followed and this significantly restricted the practice lessons that could emerge. Information which might have provided an understanding of the underlying dynamics was often not available in agency reports and was not sought by the reviewers. The membership and level of expertise of review panels varied considerably and relevant agencies sometimes chose not to participate in the review process. In addition, differing presentation styles rendered some reports very difficult to follow. When Sinclair and Bullock (2002) interviewed selected authors of review reports and ACPC chairs, even though all respondents stressed their value, they also commented that the process could be so exhausting that, once the report was completed, there was a tendency to sit back and say 'that's it'.

Repetitive findings

For practitioners, the critical question is whether the two systems of investigation have significantly contributed to our understanding of child maltreatment and professional responses to it. The declared intention of both processes has been to learn lessons and we shall consider whether this has been achieved by comparing the findings of a series of meta-analyses of reports spanning the last 30 years. The Department of Health sponsored two overview syntheses of the findings of public inquiries (Department of Health and Social Security 1982; Department of Health 1991) and three of Part 8 Reviews (James 1994; Arthurs and Ruddick 2001; Sinclair and Bullock 2002). They also invited Falkov (1996) to focus on the frequency with which parental mental health problems featured in Part 8 Reviews. Independently, other researchers have offered further analysis of groups of cases (Greenland 1987; Reder et al. 1993; Corby et al. 1998; Reder and Duncan

1999; Munro 1999; Brandon *et al.* 1999; Sanders *et al.* 1999; Dale *et al.* 2002a, 2002b), while White (1995) and Fitzgerald (2001) reflected on common themes in the reviews which they have chaired.

Table 5.1 brings together the principal issues identified in these meta-analyses. The consistency between the findings is striking, with particular clusters around: deficiencies in the assessment process; problems with inter-professional communication; inadequate resources; and poor skills acquisition or application. Furthermore, the more recent public inquiry into the death of Victoria Climbié (Laming 2003) found the same problems: they may have been enacted in different ways than before, but the issues remain the same.

Significantly, the Confidential Inquiries into Homicides and Suicides by Mentally Ill People (Boyd 1996; Appleby *et al.* 1999; Appleby *et al.* 2001) have highlighted many equivalent themes, summarised by Prins (1998: 213, see also Chapter 1 in this book) as improved assessment techniques, better contact with patients, better communication between professionals and better liaison between psychiatric professionals and those in close contact with the patient's family and carers.

We are not the first to lament that core lessons about child protection practice have not been learned over the years. Dingwall (1986) and Hallett (1989) concluded that successive reports have failed to make a lasting impact on everyday practice, and Corby *et al.* (1998) wrote of a depressing repetition of the same recommendations and a sense of frustration and saturation. One factor must be that the reports, together with their practice implications, have not been easily available. However, most authors believe that it is primarily the nature of the investigations that has restricted their value. Both Dingwall and Hallett pointed to fundamental limitations in a legal approach to inquiries, where stories are reconstructed in terms of individual actions but not understood within their context and in relation to other people. Similarly, Handley (2001) noted that the Part 8 Review system focuses predominantly on system weaknesses and failures, so that little consideration is given to the dynamics of the serious abuse that occurred.

In contrast with the approaches of formal inquiry/review panels, commentators who have set out to understand the cases from other perspectives have been able to offer more useful insights. It is worth noting the observations of Olive Stevenson, who had been a member of the Maria Colwell Inquiry panel in 1974 and contributed a minority section to the final report in order to ensure that the opportunity for a wider understanding of the case was not lost. Stevenson (1989) considered that social workers lacked suitable theoretical frameworks to guide their assessments and decision making and were inadequately trained in observing and talking with children. Furthermore, their judgements were made more difficult by having to manage within themselves the ambivalence often engendered by competing needs of children and parents.

Re-analysis of the cases themselves has been particularly illuminating and these studies will be considered in more detail.

Our review of 35 public inquiries (Reder *et al.* 1993) suggested that: practice effectiveness depended on the quality of resources, work atmosphere and organisational stability; adequacy of assessments was determined by the way information was sought, collated and integrated and by any preconceptions that were held; and the dynamics of inter-agency and inter-professional relationships and of professionals' interactions with the family all impacted on the development of the case, such as through distortions in communication (see also Reder and Duncan 2003). When we repeated our study with 49 Part 8 Reviews (Reder and Duncan 1999), we were able to suggest that assessments depended on a practitioners having an appropriate mindset, where observations are organised into hypotheses, which require validating or modifying as the result of further observations, together with reference to research and professional experience.

Munro (1999) examined 45 inquiry reports and concluded that many of the recurrent mistakes were due to everyday habits of reasoning, which introduced a bias into assessments and reviews of cases. In particular, professionals had been slow to revise their early judgement about a family, even when faced with subsequent contradictory information. For example, if a case had been initially assessed as being of low risk, later allegations were poorly investigated. A picture was also painted of professionals becoming absorbed in current issues and failing to stand back and consider present-day information in the context of past history. Written information was less valued than verbal, so that some social workers failed to read their files. Munro went on to argue that all these styles of thinking accord with psychological research on human reasoning and that reviewing judgements is hard, not only intellectually but emotionally.

Dale *et al.* (2002a, 2002b) reported similar assessment problems in their re-analysis of 17 Part 8 Reviews (amongst a larger group of serious abuse cases). There was evidence of bias in social services' approach to many of the cases, which could be attributed to expectations that they would apply central government guidance. In response to the drive to refocus the balance of their work, following publication of the Department of Health's (1995) 'Messages from Research', social workers artificially and inappropriately categorised concerning cases as a 'child in need' rather than 'child at risk', which meant that no child protection assessment was undertaken. Social workers also appeared so preoccupied with 'working in partnership' with parents that they failed to explore rigorously details of serious injuries to the child and missed evidence that 'some parents were more skilled and effective in negotiating the basis of this than were their social workers' (2002a: 308).

Brandon *et al.* (1999) studied ten case review reports and included a discussion that tried to go 'beyond the familiar themes'. They concluded that

Table 5.1 Meta-analysis of groups of public inquiry and/or 'Part 8' Review cases in the UK

Source	Cases reviewed	Years	Principal issues identified
Department of Health & Social Security 1982	18 public inquiries, UK	1973–1981	Inter-agency collaboration and co-ordination. Deficiencies in recognition and assessments. Identifiable warning signs. Inadequate professional resources or training. Inadequate use of professional authority.
Greenland 1987	35 public inquiries, UK[1]	1972–1982	Inter-agency communication. Identifiable warning signs. Assessment deficiencies. High risk check lists proposed.
Department of Health 1991	19 public inquiries, UK[2]	1980–1989	Inter-professional communication and co-ordination. Inadequate use of professional authority. Inadequate professional resources. Inadequate professional training or supervision. Deficiencies in assessments. Identifiable warning signs.
Reder et al. 1993	35 public inquiries, UK	1973–1989	Inter-professional communication. Influence of parental 'care and/or control conflicts'. Relevance of the meaning of the child for the parent. Inadequate professional resources. Inadequate integration of information as part of assessments. Identifiable warning signs. Need for training improvements.

Study	Sample	Period	Findings
James 1994	30 'Part 8' Reviews, England	1991–1993	Parental histories of abuse. Parental mental health problems. Chaotic families. Questionable assessments. Questionable resources.
White 1995	8 personally conducted independent case reviews	'before and after' introduction of 'Part 8' Reviews in 1991	Families' 'culture of violence'. Assessment deficiencies and mis-understandings. Inter-agency communication. Inadequate professional experience and supervision.
Falkov 1996	100 'Part 8' Reviews, UK	1993–1994	Parental mental health problems. Inter-agency co-ordination. Need for training improvements.
Corby et al. 1998	70 public inquiries[3] & 'Part 8' Reviews, UK	1945–1997	Inter-agency co-ordination. Training/supervision improvements. Procedure improvements.
Munro 1999	45 public inquiries & 'Part 8' Reviews, UK	1973–1994	Unsystematic reasoning in assessments and monitoring. Inter-professional communication.
Reder & Duncan 1999	49 'Part 8' Reviews, UK	1993–1994	Assessment deficiencies. Parental mental health and substance misuse problems. Parental 'care and/or control conflicts'. Identifiable warning signs. Young age of children. Need for training improvements. Need for screening of risk in peri-natal period. Child Death Review Teams proposed.

continued on next page

Table 5.1 continued

Source	Cases reviewed	Years	Principal issues identified
Sanders et al. 1999	21 'Part 8' Reviews, Wales	1991–1996	Parental mental health problems. Domestic violence. Assessment deficiencies. Inter-agency communication. Over-emphasis on 'partnership'.
Brandon et al. 1999	10 'Part 8' Reviews, Wales	1996–1998	Assessment deficiencies. Inter-agency communication and co-ordination. Inadequate supervision. Inadequate record-keeping. Non-compliance with procedures. Need to enhance professional competence and confidence.
Fitzgerald 2001	Over 40 inquiries and 'Part 8' Reviews conducted by the Bridge Child Care Development Service	Not given	Inter-professional communication and co-ordination. Over-emphasis on family support (vs. assessment of risk). Failure to listen to the children.
Arthurs & Ruddick 2001	30 'Part 8' Reviews, South East England	1998–2000	Assessment deficiencies. Domestic violence. Inter-agency collaboration/communication.

| Dale et al. 2002a, 2002b | 17 'Part 8' Reviews, South of England[4] | 1996–2001 | Assessment deficiencies. Parental mental health and substance misuse problems. Inter-agency co-ordination. Over-emphasis on 'partnership'. Young age of children. Structured evidence-based assessment aids proposed. National Standards for Child Protection proposed. |
| Sinclair & Bullock 2002 | 40 randomly selected 'Serious Case Reviews', UK | 1998–2001 | Young age of children. Parental mental health and substance misuse problems. Domestic violence. Assessment deficiencies. Warning signs ignored. Inconsistent recording of information. Unclear decision making. Training deficiencies. Under-involvement of general practitioners. Need for better evidence-based practice. |

1　Plus 33 fatalities notified to the NSPCC in UK and cases reported in Canada and USA.
2　Including inquiries into responses to sexual abuse concerns.
3　Including inquiries into abuse in residential care and responses to sexual abuse concerns.
4　Plus 21 cases of severe abuse known to the authors.

multi-disciplinary work has to be firmly grounded in competence and confidence in the practice of one's own profession. They emphasised the importance of professional training and supervision in generating confidence to use professional discretion both to contribute to or challenge decisions made by others.

All this leads us to believe that there have been two fundamental failings of inquiries/reviews. Firstly, analysis of the problems and the nature of the recommendations are not at the most useful level, since they mainly focus on bureaucratic, instead of human, factors. Secondly, inquiries/reviews must satisfy multiple agendas, all of which may be necessary yet cannot be fulfilled simultaneously through the same process.

Problem analysis and recommendations

Bureaucratic focus

Inquiries and reviews follow a pattern of targeting recommendations at a bureaucratic level. We mean by this advising modifications to existing policies or the creation of new ones, introducing systems to monitor the work of agencies and to check whether they are following procedures and refining technical aids to practice (such as referral forms, assessment forms, computerised information technology). A preoccupation with procedures was noted by Brandon *et al.* (1999) and Munro (1999), even though there has been little evidence that the problems lay with the procedures themselves (James 1994; Sanders *et al.* 1999; Dale *et al.* 2002a, 2002b). Corby *et al.* (1998) found that the main improvements recommended in 70 reports clustered around training/supervision (49 per cent), inter-agency co-ordination (37 per cent) and staff qualifications/experience (19 per cent), which suggests that the problems were only marginally related to bureaucratic failures.

The report into the death of Victoria Climbié (Laming 2003) is a recent example of this bureaucratic inclination. Its Summary referred to 'sloppy and unprofessional performance' and 'a lack of basic good practice', going on to reflect that the 'gross failure of the system' and 'widespread organisational malaise' was 'hard to understand'. Attempts to make sense of the events included that 'the gap is not a matter of law but in its implementation' and 'it is not just "structures" that are the problem, but the skills of the staff that work in them'. Despite this promising beginning, the recommendations revert to an emphasis on creating new organisational structures at governmental and local levels, refining guidance documents and identifying organisational imperatives.

The inquiry also graphically detailed the gross under-funding, understaffing and low priority given to the child protection agencies involved, together with excessive case loads, low morale and minimal support experienced by key staff. However, the final recommendations only address these superficially with, for example, the proposal that local authorities should publish their budget allocation to children's services. A recommendation to multiply that budget allocation would have been even more welcome! Although many deficiencies in staffing were identified, little is said about how to redress them and create a motivated, enthusiastic and skilled work-force, with the necessary time, facilities, training and support to do one of the hardest jobs in the welfare system. This seems to have been a missed opportunity to focus attention on the skills of practitioners who hold child protection responsibilities and to reflect further on why laws and policies may not be implemented properly. It repeats the findings of previous inquiries and inspections which have acknowledged serious resource deficiencies, skills inadequacies and the stressful nature of the work yet failed to translate this into recommendations that would remedy the problem (Hallett and Birchall 1992).

Inquiries and reviews seem to be driven by a number of related presumptions that reinforce the tendency for a 'top-down' bureaucratic rather than human approach. First, since the outcome is known to have been so undesirable, those practitioners who were most directly involved are presumed to have made errors. The mindset underlying the inquiry/review is that they delivered a below-standard service and may have been incompetent. Second, it is presumed that the only way to identify errors and incompetence and learn lessons is for their work to be scrutinised by someone who is more knowledgeable, more senior and more independent. Third, necessary changes can only come about by imposition from above, since those low in the hierarchy are the ones who made the errors and are believed to be the least capable of identifying them. A fourth presumption is that those low in the hierarchy have the least motivation to learn and to take responsibility for improvements.

Some of the presumptions are spurious. Although many reports aimed their criticisms at individual practitioners, there was little evidence of gross negligence by those involved. In our study of 35 public inquiries, we found only one clear case of unprofessional conduct, where a member of staff falsely claimed that he had made a home visit. Overall, the impression was of professionals working hard and with integrity, albeit making tragic errors of judgement. Sinclair and Bullock (2002) similarly commented that their analysis of 40 Serious Case Reviews revealed only three in which there was evidence of gross incompetence by an individual or agency, but even then the criticisms concerned social services' failure to take co-ordinated and decisive action rather than any non-involvement. In our experience, the strongest desire to learn from undesired events is usually found in those most intimately involved in the case. Sometimes it is guilt which drives this wish, for such practitioners are often horrified by the outcome and fear that they did make mistakes. Furthermore, it is these very professionals who hold the greatest amount of knowledge about their work and its context.

Other presumptions are only partially valid and do not take account of the spectrum of ways that people learn. Certainly, didactic lecturing from those with greater expertise can impart a considerable amount of knowledge and wisdom. However, this needs to be complemented by other learning techniques and it is commonly held that a variety of approaches provides the optimum result. These would include participation in small discussion groups or workshops, individual supervision or mentoring, reading or personal reflection and, importantly, learning from experience. It is this last factor that needs to be capitalised on, by inquiries valuing reflective participation of the involved practitioners. It rarely, if ever, is. The senior social worker who had been centrally involved in the Kimberley Carlile case (London Borough of Greenwich 1987) was referred to in the report as 'the prime candidate for blameworthiness' in failing to prevent her death, with the recommendation that he should no longer perform any statutory child protection functions. Bizarrely, the report continued that 'his written statement is an outstanding document of insight into the nature of a social worker's tasks . . . [and his] employing authority should make the document available as an educational tool for the training of social workers generally, and for those involved in child abuse particularly' (p. 22). We understand that this never happened.

Human focus

As already indicated, we believe that the factors which need addressing in inquiries/reviews are primarily human, not procedural. A human focus demands paying attention to psychological processes, such as individual thinking styles, professional interactions with others and group dynamics within and between agencies. It includes giving due weight to the factors that are known to reduce work efficiency, such as inadequate resources and staffing and high levels of stress. In addition, it means acknowledging that the capacity to make sense of what children say, to understand how their family functions, to assess parenting problems and to take measures to protect those children who need it are highly sophisticated professional activities, requiring considerable skill, knowledge and experience.

These human factors are complex but we shall attempt to summarise them under three main headings: the emotional toll of child protection work; the skills required; and the nature of human error.

The emotional toll of child protection work

The lack of importance given to an analysis of emotional factors by inquiries/reviews is, on the face of it, surprising, since the stressful nature of child protection cases is common knowledge. For example, Hoxter (1983), Tranter and Vizard (1988), MacCarthy (1988) and West (1997) have all described how practitioners working with abused or deprived children may experience the same emotions as the child, perhaps feeling guilt, fear, shock, grief, anger, hate, isolation, confusion, helplessness or dread. Krell and Okin (1984), Pollak and Levy (1989) and Killén (1996) used psychoanalytic concepts to discuss how workers need to defend themselves against such powerful feelings, calling upon survival strategies which have a consequence for their practice. Workers may withdraw emotionally and practically, such as by postponing a home visit, not seeing evident signs of abuse or failing to report the abuse to statutory agencies, or might take on board the family's sense of chaos and become helpless and ineffective. Killén pointed out that these are human survival mechanisms and it would be remarkable if practitioners did not resort to them, while Lewis (1979) argued that they are common phenomena throughout the helping professions and may lead to practice errors. In their review of inquiries into homicides by psychiatric patients, Rumgay and Munro (2001) noted a pattern of professionals' apparently heartless rejection of those patients when they were in severely distressed states. They suggested that professionals may abdicate their ethic of care in circumstances when they feel powerless to alleviate suffering because of resource scarcity and/or personal vulnerability.

According to Anderson (2000), all child protection service staff are at risk of 'compassion fatigue', both from what they directly witness and from the cumulative effects of vicarious trauma experiences. Ultimately, there is the possibility of 'burnout', with emotional exhaustion, depersonalisation of clients and impaired capacity for information processing (Stevens and Higgins 2002). Dale *et al.* (1986) caricatured 'dangerous professionals' as working under chronic stress and in isolation, with no guiding theoretical framework, perhaps suffering from unresolved, but unacknowledged, personal conflicts that mirror those of their client families. They find it more comfortable to dwell on practical, rather than emotional, aspects of the family's problems and tend to sustain an over-optimistic outlook about them.

Furthermore, all these natural reactions to emotional exposure can ripple beyond the individual practitioner and reverberate around their organisation (Main 1957), becoming manifest in inflexible structures and procedures that distance staff from the client (Menzies 1970). At a different level, inter-agency communication and collaboration, a key requirement of child protection practice, may become so problematic as to add another layer of stress to the work (Woodhouse and Pengelly 1991; Morrison 1996; Reder and Duncan 2003).

The skills required

Child protection practice is not only extremely demanding emotionally, it requires considerable professional skill and knowledge. The practitioner must be conversant with, amongst other things, the theory and practice of child development, individual functioning of children and adults, family dynamics, parenting behaviour, management of violent or mentally disordered people, and the law and local policies. These skills are amongst the most exacting in all of the helping services, particularly since parenting behaviours are notoriously difficult to describe or measure and thresholds of concern are particularly difficult to define (Reder *et al.* 2003).

A capacity for self-monitoring and a flexibility in reasoning, described by Munro (2002) as necessary for effective child protection, are probably a product of innate characteristics, appropriate training, ongoing supervision and acquired experience. This is underlined by the numerous investigations of child abuse fatalities which suggest that many of these ingredients were missing and, in particular, that the key workers were very inexperienced and unsupported. However, frequently missing from the analysis and recommendations were references to the core training of front-line child protection staff in such skills as talking with children. It takes many years of training and experience before an adult is comfortable at being with a child in a professional capacity and competent at using language and non-verbal techniques to communicate with them. The Victoria Climbié Inquiry Report (Laming 2003) expressed considerable dismay that no professional spent time talking with Victoria, despite the numerous opportunities that were available. It does not go on to ponder why this might have been. On the face of it, the recurrent omissions seem illogical, if not unforgivable. However, it could be that limited expertise in conversing with a traumatised, frightened, maltreated child, together with an unacknowledged anxiety about exposure to their distress, significantly contributed to this picture.

The nature of human error

The notion of 'human error' introduces a different perspective to the argument, since it acknowledges that helping professionals are only human and that nobody is perfect. It is human to make mistakes through omissions or commissions and for people's actions to be sensitive to the contexts within which they work. Therefore, not only do human errors occur throughout the helping services but an analysis of them reveals familiar themes. For example, a review of inquiries within the National Health Service (Walshe and Higgins 2002: 899) concluded that: '[t]he consistency with which inquiries highlight similar causes suggests that their recommendations are either misdirected or not properly implemented . . . However, many of the problems identified by inquiries are cultural and demand changes in attitudes, values, beliefs, and behaviours – which are difficult to prescribe in any set of recommendations'. Berwick's (2001: 247) answer to the question of how errors in the NHS recur is '. . . surprisingly mundane. It is this: we are human, and humans err. Despite outrage, despite grief, despite experience, despite our best efforts, despite our deepest wishes, we are born fallible and will remain so. . . . Being careful helps, but it brings us nowhere near perfection . . . just "trying harder" makes no one superhuman. Exhortation does not help much, . . . nor will outrage in the headlines, nor even will guilt. . . . The remedy is in changing systems of work. The remedy is in design'.

Reason (2000) also emphasised that the 'person' approach to errors – which takes a moral position and focuses on whether individuals might have been forgetful, inattentive, poorly motivated, careless or reckless – has serious shortcomings compared with the 'system' approach – where the basic premise is that errors are expected and the remedy is to change the conditions under which people work in order to minimise their prevalence. According to Reason, even the best safeguards may be bypassed through a combination of 'active failures' and 'latent conditions': that is, unsafe acts committed by front-line staff within a context of design, building, procedural and strategy decision factors that have provided the accident opportunity. Solutions need to be in the form of a comprehensive management programme aimed at the person, the team, the task, the workplace and the institution as a whole.

Howitt (1992) was more concerned with over-reaction in the child protection system rather than inaction, yet his arguments were consistent with this approach. He considered it important to understand child abuse errors as a process rather than an event, in which a number of error-promoting factors in the system compound each other. Error processes, which do not differ all that much from normal processes, require (a) templating, in which the worker has pre-formed beliefs about the family or their circumstances; (b) justificatory theorising, where the worker uses oversimplified principles to confirm the direction of their work; and (c) ratcheting, whereby it is increasingly difficult for the worker to change direction once they have embarked on a particular course of action. There is equivalence here with the pervasive beliefs discussed by Reder *et al.* (1993) and the errors of reasoning identified by Munro (1999).

Even though the human error approach is widely acknowledged to enhance understanding about the functioning of complex systems, it is not used to investigate individual cases of fatal child abuse. Why is this? In our view, it is because inquiries/reviews are not just about learning and, ultimately, the other functions tend to overtake the intention to identify practice lessons.

Multiple purposes of investigations

Public inquiries seem to have at least four purposes: learning; disciplining; catharsis; and reassurance (Reder and Duncan 1996). Learning what went wrong in order to prevent recurrence of the tragedy is invariably presented as the inquiry's primary purpose. However, as we have shown, actual learning is limited. Disciplining is rarely declared as the aim, yet many inquiries have resulted in severe censure for named individuals, with serious consequences for their professional careers. Catharsis is a natural response to news of a child's suffering and inquiries provide an avenue for public catharsis, especially when taken up by the media. Calling for an inquiry is a common recourse by politicians in order to provide reassurance that they take all the issues seriously and are seen to be doing something. While the review process is less public and the reports less overtly critical of individuals, there is every reason to believe that they attempt to serve the same multiple agendas.

All these purposes are legitimate but they may not be compatible if attempted simultaneously. Most especially, no one can learn when they are under threat of disciplinary measures, nor can they contribute to a learning process. When under censure, everyone becomes defensive and guarded; they select the information they disclose and are cautious not to reveal anything that might be misconstrued or used against them. These are the opposite stances from those required by a learning exercise, in which everyone should feel free to reveal personal thoughts or information that only they might hold and to explore different hypotheses without fear of criticism.

Hill (1990) believed that a significant latent function of inquiries was social control, whereby politicians could regulate their expectations of welfare agencies. The restricted focus of inquiries on a few individuals over a circumscribed period of time manages to deviate attention away from wider social factors that may have contributed and enables authority to be exerted over the involved practitioners as representative public servants. However, it may not be as clear-cut as that. In our opinion, inquiries/reviews are probably set up with the best of intentions and in the genuine hope that practice lessons can be learned. What may not be fully appreciated is that other valid, but competing, purposes co-exist and the unfolding process then faces a dilemma – which agenda to prioritise. The formality of a statutory inquiry, particularly if held in public, is almost bound to resolve the dilemma by paying progressively more critical attention to individuals instead of recognising that 'a focus on the individual makes it harder for systems to learn' (Department of Health 2000: 34). Although local reviews have a greater potential to address inter-agency and other processes, the evidence that many participants experience them as a hurdle to be got through and most reviewers end up focusing on procedural refinements suggests that reassurance plays a large part in their conduct. With both approaches, the requirement to produce a formal document with recommendations at the end is liable to sway the reviewer towards proposing solutions that are focal, practical and capable of being audited.

Furthermore, the cathartic nature of inquiries/reviews tends to be underestimated. Many criticisms of professionals in reports have prompted vitriolic press coverage, alongside pictures of the child taken during happier times. The Victoria Climbié Inquiry Report opens with emotive references to Victoria, such as her 'beautiful smile that lit up the room', and then catalogues the dreadful abuse and neglect that she suffered. The report is dedicated to her memory, her parents were invited to participate in the inquiry and her mother sang Victoria's favourite song at the report's press launch. It seems to us that an important process takes place through such rituals: marking the life of the child who has died, recording their suffering and giving meaning to their life and death. This would be similar to the need of holocaust survivors to bear witness both to their own experiences and to the suffering of those who died and therefore are unable to bear witness themselves. Their most important wish is that their experiences are recorded somewhere and that their suffering is known and no longer hidden. In that way, each person can become an individual again, as someone who existed, had an identity and feelings and was connected to others in the world. Perhaps many inquiries replicate this need, not just for the family but for society generally.

Are there alternatives?

If genuine learning is to be our primary task, then models based on an understanding of human error are available from other enterprises. Reason (2000: 770) argued that '[p]erhaps the most important distinguishing feature of highly reliable organisations is their collective preoccupation with the possibility of failure. They expect to make errors and train their workforce to recognise and recover them. They continually rehearse familiar scenarios of failure and strive hard to imagine novel ones. Instead of isolating failures, they generalise them. Instead of making local repairs, they look for system reforms.'

Helmreich (2000) recommended adapting continuous error management programmes devised in the aviation industry. This requires: detailed knowledge of the organisation, its norms, and its staff; systematic observations of team performance; and analysis of data gathered from confidential and non-judgemental incident reporting systems and details of adverse events. Then, attention needs to be paid to latent factors, such as organisational and professional cultures, to providing clear performance standards and to adopting a non-punitive approach to error (but not to violations of safety procedures). Training is needed in teamwork, the nature of error and human limitations, together with feedback on interpersonal and technical performance.

The helping professions seem to be at something of a cross-roads in adopting this approach. On the one hand, the Department of Health (2000) has published a forward-looking document which argues persuasively for the NHS to become 'an organisation with a memory' which can learn from failure by analysing the systemic context of adverse events. It contains the acknowledgement that '. . . there is a level of risk for which no system can fully compensate. Focussing on correction, recovery or rescue from these complications and failures – on error management as well as on error prevention – is an important and under-recognised way to improve safety' (p. 28) and that one barrier to learning is a 'tendency towards scapegoating and finding individuals to blame' (p. 34). On the other hand, the proliferation of top-down inspections, requiring workers endlessly to justify themselves, creates the sense that they are presumed to be unreliable and irresponsible. Added to that, increased encouragement for service users and employees to invoke complaints procedures, which may lead to immediate staff suspension, has generated a mood of suspicion and self-protection, while clinicians are wary of politicians' readiness to disparage them when it seems expedient to do so and of adverse media coverage (NHS Confederation and National Patient Safety Agency 2003; Goldacre *et al.* 2003). Similarly, social services are subject to stringent government targets that many experience as unrelated to the needs of individual families, with a policy of 'naming and shaming' those local authorities which breach them. Prins (1998) believed that a blame culture has extended across almost every field of human enterprise and that the rapid spread of litigious-mindedness has particularly forced practitioners of medicine and social work into defensive practices. The contrast with an atmosphere of openness necessary for learning organisations could not be more stark and, in the current climate, it seems naive to expect that welfare services (and therefore child protection networks) could operate an error-management system.

A compromise can be found in the growing call in the United Kingdom (e.g. Reder and Duncan 1996, 1998; Creighton 2001; Dale *et al.* 2002a) for the establishment of Child Death Review Teams similar to those functioning in all 50 states of the United States, in New South Wales in Australia and in nine Canadian provinces/territories (Durfee *et al.* 1992; Durfee and Tilton-Durfee 1995; NSW Child Death Review Team 2000; Wilczynski 2001; Durfee *et al.* 2002). Since their inception in those countries, the teams have brought together interested and experienced professionals with a primary mission to prevent child death or injury. Teams have evolved with differing terms of reference, structure, funding arrangements and statutory status and they may variously focus on individual case management, reviews of groups of cases and/or analysis of risk factors. Nonetheless, their value has been wide ranging, including modifying procedures for data collection, highlighting demographic patterns in abuse deaths, recognising misdiagnosed deaths, detecting serial murders, raising coroners' sensitivity to abuse and identifying preventive measures. If created in the UK, such teams could receive confidential details of all child deaths, from whatever cause, identifying those which required further review. The primary intention would be to collate information across cases that could enhance knowledge and practice. Secondary aims might be to identify abuse related deaths that would otherwise have been missed. The Victoria Climbié Inquiry Report also seemed to be making similar recommendations, but at the time of writing the government's response is unknown.

In our view, an ideal system would allow the various agendas of the inquiry process to be fulfilled, but not simultaneously because that is impossible, and would capitalise on the different modalities of learning. We suggest that the first requirement would be for each local agency to consider whether disciplinary measures were necessary. Only then would it be possible to progress to a learning mode with those cases selected for more thorough review and this could be facilitated through the chairmanship of an independent expert supplied by the regional Child Death Review Team. The approach used could, in part, follow the current Serious Case Review system, in which a senior representative of each agency prepares a chronology of its involvement in the case. A composite chronology of events would then be compiled by the independent chair, together with a preliminary analysis of the problems and areas requiring further exploration. These could then be pursued through interviews with individuals or groups of workers.

Parallel to this, there would be local confidential workshops for those closely involved, to allow them to reflect on their own work and their working context and to identify lessons that they have learned or solutions they might propose. All this would be collated by the review's chair. The information would both be made available for local dissemination and (anonymously) submitted to the Child Death Review Team, so that it could identify patterns across cases which are likely to have wider policy and practice implications. These themes would be made public, as would the lessons from each local review.

In order to maximise the potential benefits of such a system, it would be important for reviewers to address the human factors that impact on child protection work, especially the skills and personal qualities of staff, the resources available to them and the organisational culture of their workplace. Then, it would need a commitment from central government and service commissioners to implement the necessary remedies in order to avoid further repetition of the same problems.

References

Anderson, D.G. (2000) 'Coping strategies and burnout among veteran child protection workers', *Child Abuse and Neglect*, 24: 839–48.

Appleby, L., Shaw, J., Amos, T. and McDonnell, R. (1999) *Safer Services: National Confidential Inquiry into Suicide and Homicide by People with Mental Illness*, London: Department of Health.

Appleby, L., Shaw, J., Sherratt, J., Amos, T., Robinson, J. and McDonnell, R. (2001) *Safety First: Five Year Report of the National Confidential Inquiry into Suicide and Homicide by People with Mental Illness*, London: Department of Health.

Arthurs, Y. and Ruddick, J. (2001) *An Analysis of Child Protection 'Part 8' Reviews Carried out over a Two-Year Period in the South-East Region of the N.H.S.* London: South East Regional Office, Department of Health.

Berwick, D.M. (2001) 'Not again! Preventing errors lies in redesign – not exhortation' (editorial), *British Medical Journal*, 322: 247–8.

Boyd, W. (Chair) (1996) *Report of the Confidential Inquiry into Homicides and Suicides by Mentally Ill People*, London: Royal College of Psychiatrists.

Brandon, M., Owers, M. and Black, J. (1999) *Learning How to Make Children Safer: An Analysis for the Welsh Office of Serious Child Abuse Cases in Wales*, Norwich: University of East Anglia/Welsh Office.

Corby, B., Doig, A. and Roberts, V. (1998) 'Inquiries into child abuse', *Journal of Social Welfare and Family Law*, 20: 377–95.

Creighton, S.J. (2001) 'Childhood deaths reported to coroners: an investigation of the contribution of abuse and neglect', in C. Cloke (ed.) *Out of Sight: NSPCC Report on Child Deaths from Abuse 1973 to 2000*, 2nd edn, London: NSPCC.

Dale, P., Davies, M., Morrison, T. and Waters, J. (1986) *Dangerous Families: Assessment and Treatment of Child Abuse*, London: Tavistock.

Dale, P., Green, R. and Fellows, R. (2002a) *What Really Happened? Child Protection Case Management of Infants with Serious Injuries and Discrepant Parental Explanations*, London: NSPCC.

Dale, P., Green, R. and Fellows, R. (2002b) 'Serious and fatal injuries to infants with discrepant parental explanations: some assessment and case management issues', *Child Abuse Review*, 11: 296–312.

Department of Health (1991) *Child Abuse: A Study of Inquiry Reports 1980–1989*, London: HMSO.

Department of Health (1995) *Child Protection: Messages from Research*, London: HMSO.

Department of Health (2000) *An Organisation with a Memory: Report of an Expert Group on Learning from Adverse Events in the NHS*, London: The Stationery Office.

Department of Health, Home Office and Department for Education and Employment (1999) *Working Together to Safeguard Children: A Guide to Inter-agency Working to Safeguard and Promote the Welfare of Children*, London: The Stationery Office.

Department of Health and Social Security (1974) *Report of the Committee of Inquiry into the Care and Supervision Provided in Relation to Maria Colwell*, London: HMSO.

Department of Health and Social Security (1982) *Child Abuse: A Study of Inquiry Reports 1973–1981*, London: HMSO.

Department of Health and Social Security and Welsh Office (1988) *Working Together: A Guide to Arrangements for Inter-Agency Co-operation for the Protection of Children from Abuse*, London: HMSO.

Dingwall, R. (1986) 'The Jasmine Beckford affair', *Modern Law Review*, 49: 489–507.

Durfee, M.J., Gellert, G.A. and Tilton-Durfee, D. (1992) 'Origins and clinical relevance of child death review teams', *Journal of the American Medical Association*, 267: 3172–5.

Durfee, M. and Tilton-Durfee, D. (1995) 'Multi-agency child death review teams: experiences in the United States', *Child Abuse Review*, 4: 377–81.

Durfee, M., Tilton Dufee, D. and West, M.P. (2002) 'Child fatality review: an international movement', *Child Abuse and Neglect*, 26: 619–36.

Falkov, A. (1996) *Study of Working Together 'Part 8' Reports. Fatal Child Abuse and Parental Psychiatric Disorder: An Analysis of 100 Area Child Protection Committee Case Reviews Conducted under the Terms of Part 8 of Working Together under the Children Act 1989*, London: Department of Health.

Falkov, A. (ed.) (1998) *Crossing Bridges: Training Resources for Working with Mentally Ill Parents and their Children*, London: Department of Health.

Fitzgerald, J. (2001) 'Lessons from the past – experience of inquiries and reviews', in C. Cloke (ed.) *Out of Sight: NSPCC Report on Child Deaths from Abuse 1973–2000*, 2nd edn, London: NSPCC.

Goldacre, M.J., Evans, J. and Lambert, T.W. (2003) 'Media criticism of doctors: review of UK junior doctors' concerns raised in surveys', *British Medical Journal*, 326: 629–30.

Greenland, C. (1987) *Preventing CAN Deaths: An International Study of Deaths Due to Child Abuse and Neglect*, London: Tavistock.

Hallett, C. (1989) 'Child-abuse inquiries and public policy', in O. Stevenson (ed.) *Child Abuse: Professional Practice and Public Policy*, Hemel Hempstead: Harvester Wheatsheaf.

Hallett, C. and Birchall, E. (1992) *Coordination and Child Protection: A Review of the Literature*, Edinburgh: HMSO.

Handley, M. (2001) 'Serious incidence case reviews – "Part 8s"', in C. Cloke (ed.) *Out of Sight: NSPCC Report on Child Deaths from Abuse 1973 to 2000*, 2nd edn, London: NSPCC.

Helmreich, R.L. (2000) 'On error management: lessons from aviation', *British Medical Journal*, 320: 781–5.

Hill, M. (1990) 'The manifest and latent lessons of child abuse inquiries', *British Journal of Social Work*, 20: 197–213.

Home Office, Department of Health, Department of Education and Science and Welsh Office (1991) *Working Together Under the Children Act 1989: A Guide to Arrangements for Inter-Agency Co-operation for the Protection of Children from Abuse*, London: HMSO.

Howitt, D. (1992) *Child Abuse Errors: When Good Intentions Go Wrong*, Hemel Hempstead: Harvester Wheatsheaf.

Hoxter, S. (1983) 'Some feelings aroused in working with severely deprived children', in M. Boston and R. Szur (eds), *Psychotherapy with Severely Deprived Children*, London: Routledge & Kegan Paul.

James, G. (1994) *Study of Working Together 'Part 8' Reports: Discussion Report for ACPC Conference 1994*, London: Department of Health.

Killén, K. (1996) 'How far have we come in dealing with the emotional challenge of abuse and neglect?' *Child Abuse and Neglect*, 20: 791–5.

Krell, H.L. and Okin, R.L. (1984) 'Counter transference issues in child abuse and neglect cases', *American Journal of Forensic Psychiatry*, 5: 5–16.

Laming, H. (2003) *The Victoria Climbié Inquiry: Report of an Inquiry by Lord Laming*, London: The Stationery Office.

Lewis, E. (1979) 'Counter-transference problems in hospital practice', *British Journal of Medical Psychology*, 52: 37–42.

London Borough of Greenwich (1987) *A Child in Mind: Protection of Children in a Responsible Society, The Report of the Commission of Inquiry into the Circumstances Surrounding the Death of Kimberley Carlile*, London: London Borough of Greenwich and Greenwich Health Authority.

MacCarthy, B. (1988) 'Are incest victims hated?', *Psychoanalytic Psychotherapy*, 3: 113–20.

Main, T. (1957) 'The ailment', *British Journal of Medical Psychology*, 30: 129–45.

Menzies, I.E.P. (1970) *The Functioning of Social Systems as a Defence against Anxiety*, London: Tavistock Institute of Human Relations.

Morrison, T. (1996) 'Partnership and collaboration: rhetoric and reality', *Child Abuse and Neglect*, 20: 127–40.

Munro, E. (1999) 'Common errors of reasoning in child protection work', *Child Abuse and Neglect*, 23: 745–58.

Munro, E. (2002) *Effective Child Protection*, London: Sage.

NHS Confederation and National Patient Safety Agency (2003) *Creating the Virtuous Circle: Patient Safety, Accountability and an Open and Fair Culture*, London: NHS Confederation.

NSW Child Death Review Team (2000) *1998–99 Report*. Surrey Hills, New South Wales: NSW Child Death Review Team.

Pollak, J. and Levy, S. (1989) 'Countertransference and failure to report child abuse and neglect', *Child Abuse and Neglect*, 13: 515–22.

Prins, H. (1998) 'Inquiries after homicide in England and Wales', *Medicine, Science and the Law*, 38: 211–20.

Reason, J. (2000) 'Human error: models and management', *British Medical Journal*, 320: 768–70.

Reder, P. and Duncan, S. (1996) 'Reflections on child abuse inquiries', in J. Peay (ed.) *Inquiries after Homicide*, London: Duckworth.

Reder, P. and Duncan, S. (1998) 'A proposed system for reviewing child abuse deaths', *Child Abuse Review*, 7: 280–6.

Reder, P. and Duncan, S. (1999) *Lost Innocents: A Follow-up Study of Fatal Child Abuse*, London: Routledge.

Reder, P. and Duncan, S. (2002) 'Predicting fatal child abuse and neglect', in K.D. Browne, H. Hanks, P. Stratton and C. Hamilton (eds) *Early Prediction and Prevention of Child Abuse: A Handbook*, Chichester: Wiley.

Reder, P. and Duncan, S. (2003) 'Understanding communication in child protection networks', *Child Abuse Review*, 12: 82–100.

Reder, P., Duncan, S. and Gray, M. (1993) *Beyond Blame: Child Abuse Tragedies Revisited*, London: Routledge.

Reder, P., McClure, M. and Jolley, A. (eds) (2000) *Family Matters: Interfaces Between Child and Adult Mental Health*, London: Routledge.

Reder, P., Duncan, S. and Lucey, C. (eds) (2003) *Studies in the Assessment of Parenting*, London: Brunner/Routledge.

Rumgay, J. and Munro, E. (2001) 'The lion's den: professional defence in the treatment of dangerous patients', *Journal of Forensic Psychiatry*, 12: 357–78.

Salop County Council (1973) *Report of Inquiry into the Circumstances Surrounding the Death of Graham Bagnall (D.O.B. 20/5/1970) and the Role of the County Council's Social Services*, Shrewsbury: Salop County Council.

Sanders, R., Colton, M. and Roberts, S. (1999) 'Child abuse fatalities and cases of extreme concern: lessons from reviews', *Child Abuse and Neglect*, 23: 257–68.

Sinclair, R. and Bullock, R (2002) *Learning from Past Experience – A Review of Serious Case Reviews*, London: Department of Health.

Stevens, M. and Higgins (2002) 'The influence of risk and protective factors on burnout experienced by those who work with maltreated children', *Child Abuse Review*, 11: 313–31.

Stevenson, O. (1989) 'Reflections on social work practice', in O. Stevenson (ed.) *Child Abuse: Professional Practice and Public Policy*, Hemel Hempstead: Harvester Wheatsheaf.

Tranter, M. and Vizard, E. (1988) 'The professional network and management of disclosure', in A. Bentovim, A. Elton, J. Hildebrand, M. Tranter and E. Vizard (eds) *Child Sexual Abuse within the Family: Assessment and Treatment*, London: Wright.

Walshe, K. and Higgins, J. (2002) 'The use and impact of inquiries in the NHS', *British Medical Journal*, 325: 895–900.

West, J. (1997) 'Caring for ourselves: the impact of working with abused children', *Child Abuse Review*, 6: 291–7.

White, R. (1995) 'A perspective from child death reviews', *Child Abuse Review*, 4: 371–6.

Wilczynski, A. (2001) 'Child deaths: working together', in C. Cloke (ed.) *Out of Sight: NSPCC Report on Child Deaths from Abuse 1973 to 2000*, 2nd edn, London: NSPCC.

Woodhouse, D. and Pengelly, P. (1991) *Anxiety and the Dynamics of Collaboration*, Aberdeen: Aberdeen University Press.

Chapter 6

The costs and benefits of the North Wales Tribunal of Inquiry

Brian Corby

Introduction

The North Wales Tribunal of Inquiry Report (Waterhouse 2000) was published at the end of a long list of public inquiries held into institutional abuse throughout the 1990s. Corby *et al.* (2001) found that there were 15 such inquiries between 1991 and 2000, the concerns of which were widespread, ranging from excessive use of physical punishment, as in the Pindown Inquiry (Staffordshire 1991), to gross sexual abuse as in the Frank Beck Inquiry (Leicestershire 1993) and neglect by failing to provide proper protection as in the case of Aliyah Ismael (Harrow ACPC 1999). Apart from the inquiries themselves there were extensive joint police and social work investigations into allegations of residential abuse across the United Kingdom (see Gallagher 1999) and a series of government-sponsored reports into the extent and causes of abuse of children living away from home (Utting 1991, 1997; Warner 1992). There was in addition widespread media coverage of trials of residential care workers who had abused children.

The concerns about this type of abuse reached levels never before attained. Prior to the 1990s there had been very few concerns raised about the abuse of children in residential care. Only four public inquiries into institutional abuse had been held between 1945 and 1989 (Corby *et al.* 2001). For a comparatively recent short book on the subject Webster (1998) used the title *The Great Children's Homes Panic*. His thesis was that the extent of abuse in children's homes had been exaggerated and that in the process innocent people may well have been unfairly accused of abuse. This viewpoint has been given further support following the recent award of damages to the two care workers in the Shieldfield nursery in Newcastle-upon-Tyne (see Dyer 2002). The purpose of this chapter, however, is not to try to judge the rights and wrongs of the concerns raised about residential abuse, but rather to evaluate how effective a tool public inquiries have been in investigating such abuse, to examine the costs and benefits of such inquiries, and to consider what purposes they have served and whether they have had any dysfunctional influences. The aim is to achieve these goals by examination specifically of the events and circumstances surrounding the North Wales Tribunal of Inquiry.

Before proceeding to do this, however, reference will be made to previous studies examining the usefulness of child abuse inquiries in general. Some of these have concentrated on the impact of individual inquiries (see Greenland 1986; Parton 1986; Aldridge 1994). Others have been concerned with the overall impact of such inquiries (see Shearer 1979; Hallett 1989; Hill 1990; Corby *et al.* 1998). Most of these studies have been critical and several have argued that inquiries have had considerable dysfunctional effects on child protection practice. The main criticisms have been, first, that inquiries are cumbersome tools which take a long time to organise and get under way, resulting in a considerable time-gap between the actual abuse incidents and publication of the recommendations. In many cases this delay is so great that by the time reports are published changes have already been implemented. Second, it has been contested that inquiries have been largely concerned with the actions of individual practitioners rather than with the contexts within which they operate. A third criticism is that inquiries operate on the basis of hindsight without sufficiently taking into account the here-and-now pressures under which practitioners operate, thus adding to the likelihood of their actions being seen as faulty. A fourth criticism relates to the process of carrying out inquiries. It has been argued that because they are mostly conducted according to legalistic rules and adversarial methods of procedure, which often alienate and intimidate those giving evidence, they can as a result have an inhibiting effect on the production of useful information. Fifth, it has been argued that inquiries are a very expensive means of investigating child abuse deaths. Sixth, it has been argued that inquiries have had bad effects on the morale of child protection workers, particularly on social workers (see Ayre 2001) and that, partly as a consequence of this, they have led to the adoption of defensive and bureaucratically constrained practices (see Harris 1987 and Howe 1992a). Finally, it has been argued that the impact of inquiries has been to deflect from focus on research on a wider sample of child abuse interventions which provide evidence of good practice (Thoburn 2001).

There has been very little positive writing about child abuse inquiries, particularly from the perspective of the social work profession. Indeed it could be argued that the lack of value placed on inquiries was the main reason why the Department of Health introduced a new mechanism for reviewing child death cases in Part 8 of the 1991 *Working Together* guidelines (Department of Health 1991). This review system has taken a less public and more routinised approach to investigating events surrounding child deaths by abuse and is aimed at securing a speedy response which can be taken on board by the agencies in question with as little delay as possible.

It is important to note, however, that none of the debates and issues discussed above have been about inquiries into the abuse of children in residential settings. This is not surprising because, as has already been pointed out, it was not until the early 1990s that this type of abuse became a public concern. A key aim of this chapter, therefore, is to consider whether the criticisms levelled at child abuse in the community inquiries are equally applicable to institutional abuse of children.

As already noted, the inquiry being used to test out these questions and concerns is that of the North Wales Tribunal of Inquiry, which, it must be admitted, is probably not a typical example of a child abuse inquiry for the following reasons. First, this is the only time that a Tribunal of Inquiry under the 1921 Tribunals of Inquiry Act has been invoked to examine child abuse matters. A tribunal is the most powerful form of inquiry available to Parliament and is particularly controlled by legal procedures which are deemed to be the surest available mechanisms for establishing the truth about events. Second, the North Wales Tribunal was not concerned with a particular case but with a whole set of concerns about abuse of children in two counties over a period of 22 years from 1974 to 1996.

Getting under way

It has been noted that a major criticism of inquiries has been that they are often rendered useless by virtue of the fact of taking so long to get under way. Thus, it is argued, by the time they reach their conclusions, remedies for the problems which they were set up to tackle have frequently already been put in place. The build-up to the North Wales Tribunal was certainly a long drawn-out one. It followed on from seven years of bitter disputes and wrangling about the seriousness of the problem of abuse in this area of the country and about suspected cover-ups involving people in high places. It also took place at the height of general public concern about institutional abuse and to some extent was viewed as an inquiry whose findings would have broader implications beyond the confines of North Wales itself.

Concerns about child abuse in homes in North Wales stemmed from allegations made in 1989 by Alison Taylor who was a residential care worker in Gwynedd. She was particularly concerned about what she saw as the aggressive and abusive behaviour of a care manager named Nefyn Dodd who was in charge of the home where she worked and who later took over responsibility for residential child care services for the whole of Gwynedd. Her concerns, though referred to the police for investigation, were not substantiated and she was dismissed from her post. Nevertheless, Alison Taylor persisted with these and other claims of abuse involving residents in children's homes in Clwyd as well. Concerns centred around a community home in Wrexham, Bryn Estyn, which had closed in 1984. Nefyn Dodd had also worked there, as had Stephen Norris, who in 1991 was convicted of the sexual abuse of boys while working in another Clwyd residential establishment. Alison Taylor, two influential local politicians and the newly appointed Director of Social Services for Clwyd joined forces at around this time. Looking back through the late 1970s and 1980s they found that there had been several allegations of abuse in residential homes in Clwyd, none of which had been properly investigated or, if they had, then the resulting internal inquiries and reports had been ignored. They took the case to the North Wales police who as a result started a major inquiry involving all residential establishments in both Clwyd and Gwynedd. This investigation was completed in 1993. For those expecting the discovery of a widespread paedophile ring or something of that kind, the results were disappointing. Despite interviewing over 300 people and following a whole host of leads, only six residential workers were prosecuted for abuse offences, three of whom were employed at Bryn Estyn at the time of the offences being committed. To make matters even more complicated there were allegations of police involvement in the abuse activities. Dissatisfaction with these outcomes led Clwyd County Council to set up its own inquiry into events, headed by John Jillings, an ex-Director of Social Services in Derbyshire. However, his report was considered libellous and Clwyd's insurers advised against its publication, raising yet more concerns and suspicions about a cover-up. It was at this point, in 1996, that the Secretary of State for Wales, William Hague, announced the setting-up of a Tribunal of Inquiry.

It was in this context, therefore, that the Tribunal started its investigations. It was asked to look into events in over 80 children's homes over 22 years and much of its focus rested on a home that had closed 12 years prior to the Tribunal's commencement. The criticism that inquiries get overtaken by events is, therefore, particularly true of the North Wales Tribunal of Inquiry. The late 1980s and early 1990s had seen the development of several initiatives to tackle what had come to be accepted as the serious problem of residential abuse, starting with the implementation under the 1989 Children Act of complaints procedures which had not previously existed, and with the 1991 Community Homes Regulations which placed greater restrictions on physical restraint and punishment of children. These developments were followed by the recommendations of the Warner (1992) Report on recruitment and selection and training of residential care staff in 1992, and by recommendations in the Howe Report to improve the pay of residential workers (Howe 1992b). Sir William Utting, who had previously written a report about abuse of children in residential care (Utting 1991) had been asked to carry out a broader survey of the risks to children living away from their own homes which was published in 1997 (Utting 1997). Research sponsored by the Department of Health (Department of Health 1998a) pointed to what was needed to improve regimes in children's homes and the Quality Protects initiative set out new goals and objectives for children in care (Department of Health 1998b). Greater importance was attached to listening to children and championing their rights than ever before. Perhaps more importantly, the use of residential care for children had greatly reduced between 1974 and 1996, falling from 45,000 to 10,500 places.

Many of these developments took place either before the North Wales Tribunal started or while it was sitting. Indeed, the transcripts of the Tribunal have a historical feel about them which is understandable since a large part of the material is concerned with events taking place in Bryn Estyn which closed in 1984. Many of the children placed in care then would most probably have remained at home in the late 1990s. Staff:resident ratios have changed considerably since then and most children's homes have been greatly influenced by a children's rights philosophy. Perhaps the most telling evidence about the outdatedness of the Tribunal's findings is the government's response to its recommendations which largely spells out how much the issues raised have already been addressed (see House of Commons 2000).

Putting individuals under the spotlight

Critics of inquiries into abuse of children in the community have been of the view that individual practitioners (and particularly social workers) have been subjected to unfair exposure and have had to shoulder undue blame for the events in which they were involved. This has been seen to be the case from the Maria Colwell report onwards (Department of Health and Social Services 1974). In the early days of inquiries it was argued that insufficient account was taken of the fact that social work's remit to support families and to work with parents often placed them in a difficult position to police families. The clash of perspectives between these conflicting roles was particularly highlighted in the Darryn Clarke (Department of Health and Social Security 1979) and Jasmine Beckford (London Borough of Brent 1985) reports. It has been further argued that this focus on individuals has detracted from the context in which events are happening, particularly in relation to resources, training, supervision and management. According to this line of argument, inquiries have focused too much on the interplay between front-line professionals and service users, disregarding matters such as staff shortages, the fact that inexperienced workers have been assigned to complex cases and the lack of monitoring of practice by social work managers.

This type of criticism is far less applicable to abuse of children in children's homes by virtue of the fact that social workers are the alleged abusers rather than those deemed to have failed in their responsibilities of protecting children from their parents and carers. There is no question in this type of case of not placing such workers in the frame and the fact that they are professional people adds to the urgency of so doing. The public would expect nothing less. Indeed in the 1990s such was the revulsion against abuse of children in residential care that one could almost argue that inquiries were required to expose individuals.

The North Wales Tribunal clearly set about its task with this in mind. The opening statement made by the Treasury counsel asserted that widespread abuse had taken place in Clwyd and Gwynedd and that the Tribunal was determined to find out the truth about events. It did not take the view that the extent of abuse was an unanswered question and that its aim, therefore, was to keep an open mind about this. As a consequence, residential workers who were asked to provide evidence immediately went on the defensive and the Tribunal took on the appearance of a trial as much as an inquiry (see below). As noted in the previous section, there was a view that previous social services and police inquiries had failed to uncover the true extent of abuse of children in North Wales homes. The Tribunal was determined to remedy this by being proactive in pursuing all abuse allegations – or at least to be seen to do so. This inevitably entailed making judgements about the behaviour of individual workers and it was agreed that if they were considered on the grounds of probability to have carried out the acts of which they were accused they would be named in the report and subject therefore to police investigation. In the serious abuse cases this course of action seemed to be perfectly justified. However, some of the incidents considered by the Tribunal were of a relatively trivial nature including alleged assaults that took place while trying to control angry and aggressive young residents and even allegations that teachers threw board dusters at children in the classroom! In these cases the naming of individuals with the subsequent harm to their professional standing and reputation seemed to be more questionable.

Despite its concerns with the actions of individuals, the North Wales Tribunal was also minded to look beyond those directly involved in alleged abuses. It was concerned to find out whether there were staff within the homes who had turned a blind eye to abusive behaviour. It also aimed to examine the roles of those in authority over residential workers (from homes' advisers right up to directors of social services) to find out whether they were complicit by virtue of trying to keep a lid on events as far as possible and, therefore, to prevent the truth from emerging. In addition it examined the roles of insurers and of the Welsh Office which was responsible for inspection and monitoring of residential care practices.

Thus the criticisms levelled at inquiries into child abuse in the community that contexts, management and resources are frequently overlooked do not hold true in the case of the North Wales Tribunal. Other inquiries into residential abuse, such as Pindown (Staffordshire 1991) and Leicestershire (1993), have similarly concerned themselves with broader issues about management and resources in a way that inquiries into abuse within the community have not. There is a greater awareness in all of these reports that the actions of front-line workers are the responsibility of managers and councillors and that failure to provide a safe environment for children in care is to be shared more broadly than is the case with children abused in their own homes.

The wisdom of hindsight

The criticism of over-reliance on hindsight wisdom does apply to the North Wales Tribunal of inquiry. The inquiry report was particularly critical of the fact that staff who were not involved in the abuse of children did not suspect that some of their colleagues were abusers. The most glaring example of this (as far as the Tribunal was concerned) was in the case of Peter Howarth, Deputy Headmaster of Bryn Estyn in the late 1970s and early 1980s. He instigated a procedure known as the flat list. Boys were invited to his flat in the evening, ostensibly as a treat, to experience a taste of home life by watching television and having snacks and soft drinks. The inquiry, with the knowledge that Howarth had been convicted of sexually abusing several boys in his flat, was incredulous of the fact that other staff were not suspicious about his activities at the time. There were, with hindsight, other factors that should have alerted concerns. For instance, the boys who went to his flat were specifically required to wear pyjamas without underwear (for hygienic reasons, according to Howarth). There was said to have been much talk between the residents about Howarth's 'bumboys'. Yet despite what seemed to be obvious with this hindsight knowledge, none of Howarth's colleagues gave any hint of having suspected him of child abuse. Indeed some could still not bring them-selves to believe this despite his conviction for a series of offences. That none of his colleagues suspected him at the time is not incredible when one bears in mind that child sexual abuse was only beginning to be accepted as a more than rare event in the early 1980s. In addition, Howarth was protected by the fact of his high ranking position at Bryn Estyn. Also his flat-list activities were seen as beneficial to the boys and to some extent took the pressure off other staff. Finally, the rumours about his activities could be interpreted as malicious gossip deriving from a highly untrustworthy source.

The inquiry process

Tribunals and other statutory inquiries do have some leeway with regard to the way in which they carry out their business in that their procedures are not specifically defined. Nevertheless, they can exercise considerable legal powers. For instance, they can subpoena witnesses, enforce the production of written evidence and impose contempt charges where they think fit. They are also peopled by lawyers who are used to seeking the truth by adversarial methods and cross-examination. They do, therefore, seem to the lay person to operate like a court even though those giving testimony are theoretically not on trial, but are providing information to the inquiry about matters of which they have been forewarned in so-called Salmon letters. These letters were introduced following a Royal Commission into the conduct of Tribunals of Inquiry (Salmon, Lord Justice 1966). They set out the main areas about which those giving testimony to an inquiry should be prepared to answer questions so that the notion of being on trial should be reduced.

The North Wales Tribunal of Inquiry operated very much like a court. It concerned itself with a series of abuse incidents and concerns about possible cover-ups. Those giving testimony were subject to cross-examination by various parties. Those making complaints about abuse were taken through their statements by the Treasury counsel acting on behalf of the Chair of the Tribunal and then questioned by lawyers acting on behalf of anyone complained against. Similarly those who were answering complaints went through the same process. Questioning of those giving testimony was deliberately challenging in order to test the reliability of the testimony being provided. The Chair of the Tribunal asked supplementary questions as he felt appropriate and was required to make judgement on each of the incidents and issues that was played out before him. The North Wales inquiry report indeed provides a series of judgements on the basis of the balance of probabilities based around the evidence given and the reliability of the witnesses.

The adversarial nature of the Tribunal seems to have been justified given the nature of the concerns. It could be argued that in the case of abuse in the community, social workers and other child protection professionals should not have to feel that they are on trial for the way in which they carry out their tasks. Such an argument does not carry the same weight where the concerns are about children in care being abused by professional carers.

Financial costs

The argument that inquiries are expensive was certainly true of the North Wales Tribunal. Despite attempts by the Chair, Sir Ronald Waterhouse, to keep a lid on costs, the Tribunal exceeded its allocated budget of £10 million by over £3 million. This sum of money did not include that spent on the legal costs of participating public agencies such as the police, social services departments and health authorities which also came out of the public purse. The main costs incurred were for legal expenses. As noted in the previous section, the adversarial nature of the Tribunal process demands that lawyers dominate proceedings. They are seen to be needed both to ensure smooth running of the process and in order to protect those giving testimony. The Tribunal sat for 209 days regularly attended by 29 barristers and solicitor advocates and on some days by as many as 37. In addition there were normally several instructing solicitors present.

Impact on the morale of residential social workers

Residential social work has always been something of a Cinderella service. Its status as a last resort option when all else has failed has greatly influenced this state of affairs. Despite the development of a professional literature over the last 20 years (see Walton and Elliott 1980; Davis 1981; Wagner 1988; Clough 2000) residential social work has in practice been seen as a task that requires little more than common-sense skills and this has been reflected in the poor pay and training of residential workers (see Howe 1992b). Although children's homes have probably attracted more professionally committed staff than homes for older people and adults with disabilities, nevertheless standards have been very variable. The casual way in which new staff with no experience of child care work were recruited to Bryn Estyn in the late 1970s to work with young boys from very deprived backgrounds and with a whole host of emotional and behavioural problems speaks volumes about how the job was viewed then. While this state of affairs has to some extent been remedied by the recommendations of the Warner Report (1992), levels of qualification among residential child care workers still remain low (see Crimmens 2000) and residential work has more and more come to be seen as a very poor third best alternative for out-of-home child placement (after adoption and fostering).

The morale of residential child care workers has never been high, therefore, and the 'discovery' of institutional abuse in the 1990s has been a major additional blow to the self-esteem of this declining sector. The findings of the North Wales Tribunal of Inquiry have no doubt further added to the negative images of residential workers despite trying to be fair to individuals and to view events within their historical context. The key conclusion reached was that not only had many of the establishments which came under its scrutiny failed to safeguard children but that they had also 'failed to provide an acceptable minimum standard of care for children in dire need of good quality parenting' (p. 825, para 55.09). Furthermore, the reaction of the media to the inquiry has been unequivocal in its condemnation of events in Clwyd and Gwynedd, describing them as shameful and unacceptable (the *Guardian* 2000 and the *Independent* 2000). The morale of residential workers has probably been further dented by debates in Parliament in 2000 about the new Adoption Bill which resound with comments about the need to find alternatives to the potentially damaging effects of living in children's homes.

As a result of the negative impact of the North Wales Tribunal's findings and that of subsequent events, there is likely to be a continuing decline in the range (certainly in the state sector) of residential care for children. Yet Utting (1991) has argued that for many young people residential care may be their first choice and that such provision needs to be maintained. A further negative outcome is the fact that children as a result of this decline may well be at more risk in their own homes because of the lack of available residential places. In addition, it should be noted that although great faith is being pinned on fostering and adoption as preferred alternatives to residential care of children, the potential for abuse in foster homes is higher than previously thought (see Utting 1997). Indeed in some areas it is reported that referrals of abuse of children in foster homes are more common than for abuse in residential care (Hobbs *et al*. 1999). Finally, within children's homes, there is a danger that residential workers will react defensively to the findings of the North Wales Tribunal, avoiding physical contact with children and maintaining a professional distance which could have negative consequences in terms of children's emotional and social development.

Negating research

Linked to the last section is the view that inquiries with their emphasis on cases where abuse has not been prevented tend to overshadow research findings looking at a broader range of practice. Throughout the 1990s there has been a series of research studies into children's homes sponsored by the Department of Health whose findings were summarised in the publication *Caring for Children Away from Home: Messages from Research* (Department of Health 1998a). These studies paint a more balanced and contemporary picture of what happens in children's homes than that provided by the North Wales Tribunal of Inquiry. They point to the existence of a wide range of standards with much depending on the quality of leadership and the development of purposeful cultures within homes settings. They demonstrate that children's homes are much smaller in the 1990s than they were before with good staff:resident ratios. However, they also observe that the children and young people who live in them have very damaged backgrounds and as a result present particularly challenging behaviours to residential staff. As regards abuse, they show that children are much more fearful of being bullied by fellow residents than by the staff of the homes. Overall, however, there is little doubt that as an indicator of what is currently taking place in children's homes these studies provide a much more informative account than does the North Wales Tribunal of Inquiry.

Concluding comments

It should be clear by now that many of the criticisms made of inquiries into the abuse of children in the community are equally applicable to the North Wales Tribunal of Inquiry. This is not to say that the Tribunal did not serve some important purposes. For instance, it dealt in a thorough and fair way with events which had created suspicion and hostility over a long period of time. This airing of controversial issues, particularly if it helps draw a line, is an important function of inquiries. As a result of the North Wales Tribunal some individuals (for instance, Alison Taylor) will feel that their actions have been justified, and some victims of abuse may well feel that their suffering has been done justice to (see, however, Appendix 5 of the Inquiry Report, pp. 883–8, which shows that in the short term being a witness at the Tribunal was a very painful experience for most). Some individuals will feel that they have been criticised for their actions (or, in some cases, lack of action) and others may well have been referred to the police for consideration for prosecution. Of course there may be some victims who still feel that the full picture was not provided by the Tribunal. Nevertheless, there can be little doubt that the Tribunal thoroughly sifted all the evidence that was available to it and made considered judgements on all alleged incidents of abuse that were brought to its notice.

Whether one feels the costs outweighed the benefits of the North Wales Tribunal or vice versa depends to some degree on what the function of inquiries is seen to be. Judged from the point of view of the need to publicly examine events that were a source of continuing local concern, undermining the credibility of a range of public agencies, it is reasonable to argue that the North Wales inquiry did its job and to that extent was worthwhile. It could be argued in connection with this that another function the Tribunal served was to act as an indicator of society's concern more generally about the abuse of children in care homes. If, however, one sees the function of inquiries as to learn the lessons of the past to improve practice in the future, it is more arguable whether the benefits outweighed the costs. As has already been seen, by the time that the North Wales Tribunal inquiry reported, many of the changes that its findings pointed to had already been achieved. Because many of the concerns and allegations examined by the inquiry had taken place several years before it reported, there was an historical feel about many of the issues. In addition, the counties of Clwyd and Gwynedd had been disbanded by the time the inquiry started and replaced by five new unitary authorities. Thus, many of the criticisms rightly raised by the Tribunal about organisational deficiencies had no obvious target. Finally, many of the personnel involved in the earlier allegations of abuse had retired or in some cases were dead.

While none of this is of course the fault of the Tribunal, perhaps it could have broadened its focus in an attempt to provide a more up-to-date analysis of abuse in children's homes and to include that knowledge into its recommendations for the future. There was a two-day seminar held towards the end of the Tribunal hearing involving a group of experts whose aim was to achieve this goal, but only passing reference was made to this in the Inquiry Report (see p. 6 para 1.12 and p. 843 para 56.03). Indeed it is stressed in para 56.03 that the report was determined to confine itself to the facts presented to it by witnesses: 'In the end, however, our recommendations have to be directed to our specific terms of reference and based upon the evidence that we have received'. The extent to which inquiries should use research and expert information to influence their recommendations is an open one. It is notable that the recent Victoria Climbié inquiry (Laming 2003) collected a good deal of written evidence and held several seminars involving experts in order to gather ideas about child protection procedures and practice which it could use to inform its recommendations. By contrast the North Wales inquiry took a very conservative approach in this respect.

The main tangible effect of the North Wales inquiry has been the implementation of its recommendation to appoint an Independent Children's Commissioner for Wales (see Waterhouse 2000: 844) in the Children's Commissioner for Wales Act 2001, though as yet it is still too soon to know how effective this appointment will be. In addition it has also raised awareness of the potential for abuse and reinforced the need for greater vigilance and methods of prevention by encouraging whistleblowing, and strengthening the role of visitors and councillors in engaging with children's homes. These factors too should be borne in mind in calculating the costs and benefits.

Despite having tried to present a balanced picture about the costs and benefits of the North Wales Tribunal of Inquiry, nevertheless it is to be hoped that such a process will not be repeated. It is clear from a consideration of the dysfunctions of the process that it would be much better to systematically inquire into cases of residential abuse as early as possible after the events have happened with a view to using the findings to improve practice and systems in a more immediate way. At present there is a mechanism for this, that of Part 8 reviews referred to earlier which are now known as serious case reviews following the introduction of new child protection guidelines in 1999 (Department of Health 1999). However, there are many problems associated with this method of review. First, there is the issue of independence – these reviews are largely carried out by the agencies involved in the particular case being inquired into, though there are special arrangements for independent agencies to be involved in reviews into abuse of children in residential care. Second, the findings of these reviews are not normally made public. This is a cause of particular concern in relation to the abuse of children in residential care and, as we have seen, was a major source of contention in the events leading up to the North Wales Tribunal of Inquiry. Third, the opportunity for agencies other than those involved in the particular case to learn from the content of these reviews has not been available until recently when the Department of Health announced a biennial overview of reviewed cases (Department of Health 1999, para 8.33). It seems of crucial importance given the events in North Wales to find a more systematic, independent and public way to review or inquire into all cases of abuse in residential care in a more routinised way. Unfortunately, the report of the Tribunal of Inquiry was not reflexive enough to consider this in its recommendations. Perhaps this is a matter that in the first instance, given its history of origin, might be a job for the Children's Commissioner in Wales.

References

Aldridge, M. (1994) *Making Social Work News*, London: Routledge.
Ayre, P. (2001) 'Child protection and the media: Lessons from the last three decades', *British Journal of Social Work*, 31: 887–901.

Corby, B., Doig, A. and Roberts, V. (1998) 'Inquiries into child abuse', *Journal of Social Welfare and Family Law*, 20: 377–95.

Corby, B., Doig, A. and Roberts, V. (2001) *Public Inquiries into Abuse of Children in Residential Care*, London: Jessica Kingsley.

Clough, R. (2000) *The Practice of Residential Care*. Basingstoke: Macmillan.

Crimmens, D. (2000) '"Things can only get better!" An evaluation of developments in the training and qualification of residential child care staff', in D. Crimmens and J. Pitts (eds) *Positive Residential Practice: Learning the Lessons of the 1990s*, Lyme Regis: Russell House Publishing.

Davis, A. (1981) *The Residential Solution: State Alternatives to Family Care*, London: Tavistock.

Department of Health (1991) *Working Together under the Children Act 1989: A Guide to Arrangements for Inter-Agency Cooperation for the Protection of Children from Abuse*, London: HMSO.

Department of Health (1998a) *Caring for Children Away from Home: Messages from Research*, Chichester: Wiley.

Department of Health (1998b) *The Quality Protects Programme: Transforming Children's Services*, LAC (98) 26. London: Department of Health.

Department of Health (1999) *Working Together to Safeguard Children: A Guide to Inter-Agency Working to Safeguard and Promote the Welfare of Children*, London: Department of Health.

Department of Health and Social Security (1974) *Report of the Committee of Inquiry into the Care and Supervision Provided in Relation to Maria Colwell*, London: HMSO.

Department of Health and Social Security (1979) *The Report of the Committee of Inquiry into the Actions of the Authorities and Agencies Relating to James Darryn Clarke*, London: HMSO. Cmnd. 7739.

Dyer, C. (2002) 'Cleared nursery nurses fear vigilante mobs', The *Guardian* 5.8.2002.

Guardian (2000) 'Refuges that turned into purgatory' (A. Gillan), 16 February.

Gallagher, B. (1999) 'The abuse of children in public care', *Child Abuse Review*, 8: 357–65.

Greenland, C. (1986) 'Inquiries into child abuse and neglect (CAN) deaths in the United Kingdom', *British Journal of Criminology*, 26: 164–73.

Hallett, C. (1989) 'Child abuse inquiries and public policy', in O. Stevenson (ed.) *Child Abuse: Public Policy and Professional Practice*, Hemel Hempstead: Harvester Wheatsheaf.

Harris, N. (1987) 'Defensive social work', *British Journal of Social Work*, 17: 61–9.

Harrow Area Child Protection Committee (1999) *Part 8 Review: Summary Report*, Harrow ACPC.

Hill, M. (1990) 'The manifest and latent lessons of child abuse inquiries', *British Journal of Social Work*, 20: 197–213.

Hobbs, G., Hobbs, J. and Wynne, J. (1999) 'Abuse of children in foster and residential care', *Child Abuse and Neglect*, 23: 1239–52.

House of Commons (2000) *Learning the Lessons. The Government's Response to Lost in Care: The Report of the Tribunal of Inquiry into the abuse of Children in Care in the former County Council Areas of Gwynedd and Clwyd since 1974*. London: TSO. Cm 4776.

Howe, D. (1992a) 'Child abuse and the bureaucratization of social work', *Sociological Review*, 40(3): 491–508.

Howe, Lady (1992b) *The Quality of Care: Report of the Residential Staff's Inquiry*, London: Local Government Management Board.

Independent (2000) 'Welsh children's homes in abuse scandal', 15 February.

Laming, Lord (2003) *The Victoria Climbié Inquiry*, London: The Stationery Office. Cm 5730.

Leicestershire County Council (Kirkwood, A.) (1993) *The Leicestershire Inquiry 1992: The Report of an Inquiry into Aspects of the Management of Children's Homes in Leicestershire Between 1973 and 1986*, Leicester: Leicestershire County Council.

London Borough of Brent (1985) *A Child in Trust. The Report of the Panel of Inquiry into the Circumstances Surrounding the Death of Jasmine Beckford*, London: Borough of Brent.

Parton, N. (1986) 'The Beckford Report: A critical appraisal', *British Journal of Social Work*, 16: 511–30.

Salmon, Lord Justice (1966) *Royal Commission on Tribunals of Inquiry: Report of the Commission*, London: HMSO. Cmnd. 3121.

Shearer, A. (1979) Tragedies revisited. (1)(2)(3). *Social Work Today*, 10: 9/16/23, January 1979.

Staffordshire County Council (Levy, A. and Kahan, B.) (1991) *The Pindown Experience and the Protection of Children: The Report of the Staffordshire Child Care Inquiry 1990*, Stafford: Staffordshire County Council.

Thoburn, J. (2001) 'The good news on children's services', *Community Care*, 11–17: 36–7.

Utting, W. (1991) *Children in the Public Care: A Review of Residential Child Care*, London: HMSO.

Utting, W. (1997) *People Like Us: The Report of the Review of the Safeguards for Children Living Away from Home*, London: HMSO.

Wagner, G. (ed.) (1988) *A Positive Choice. Report of the Independent Review of Residential Care*, London: HMSO.

Walton, R. and Elliott, D. (1980) *Residential Care: A Reader in Current Theory and Practice*, Oxford: Pergamon Press.

Warner, N. (1992) *Choosing with Care: The Report of the Committee of Inquiry into the Selection, Development and Management of Staff in Children's Homes*, London: HMSO.

Waterhouse, R. (2000) *Lost in Care: Report of the Tribunal of Inquiry into the Abuse of Children in Care in the Former County Council Areas of Gwynedd and Clwyd Since 1974*, HC 201. London: The Stationery Office.

Webster, R. (1998) *The Great Children's Home Panic*, Chichester: Wiley.

Part III

Inquiries into mental health homicides

Mental health inquiries, assertive outreach and compliance: Is there a relationship?

Andrew McCulloch and Camilla Parker

Introduction

In December 1998 Frank Dobson, the then Secretary of State for Health, announced the publication of the Labour government's new 'vision' for mental health services. In doing so, he declared:

> Care in the community has failed because, while it improved the treatment of many people who were mentally ill, it left far too many walking the streets, often at risk to themselves and a nuisance to others. A small but significant minority have been a threat to others or to themselves.
>
> We are going to bring the laws on mental health up to date. In particular to ensure that patients who might otherwise be a danger to themselves are no longer allowed to refuse to comply with the treatment they need.
>
> (Department of Health 1998: 6)

The government's determination to ensure that future mental health legislation would require individuals receiving care to comply with their treatment plan was made clear when Paul Boateng, then the responsible junior minister, later addressed the members of the independent committee appointed to review the Mental Health Act 1983 (the MHA 1983):

> But if there is a responsibility on statutory authorities to ensure the delivery of quality services to patients through the application of agreed individual care plans, so there is also, increasingly, a responsibility on individual patients to comply with their programmes of care. Non-compliance can no longer be an option when appropriate care in appropriate settings is in place. I have made it clear to the field that this is not negotiable.
>
> (Department of Health 1999a: 142)

Unsurprisingly, therefore, the draft Mental Health Bill provides for compulsory treatment powers to be imposed on individuals living in the community. Despite the widespread opposition to this Bill (Department of Health 2002) the government has made clear that it still intends to introduce such powers shortly.

Alongside these proposed enhanced legislative powers, the government's mental health policy has moved towards a more intensive provision of care, with the introduction of assertive outreach teams, which seek to remain in regular contact with people with severe mental health problems who are difficult to engage with services. *The NHS Plan: A plan for Investment, A plan for Reform*, published in July 2000, stated that by '*2003 all 20,000 people estimated to need assertive outreach will be receiving these services*' (Department of Health 2000: 120) and explained why such services were necessary:

> There are a small number of people who are difficult to engage. They are very high users of services, and often suffer from a dual diagnosis of substance misuse and serious mental illness. A small proportion also have a history of offending. Services to provide assertive outreach and intensive input seven days a week are required to sustain engagement with services, and to protect patient and public.
>
> (Department of Health 2000: 120)

It might be assumed that the development of concepts such as assertive outreach and compulsory treatment outside hospital sprang out of the numerous mental health inquiries during the 1990s.

We would argue that the reality is much more complex, and that the development of various strands of thinking about assertive treatment, safety and new legislation has occurred in parallel with inquiries. Inquiry panels did not initiate such concepts. However, the fact that the need for such inquiries arose (i.e. that a homicide by a person in contact with mental health services occurred) and the conclusions that the inquiries on many occasions reached (such as that there had been a failure in the provision of care) set the context in which ideas such as assertive outreach became attractive to an administration which was concerned with the level of media coverage about the perceived dangers posed by people with mental illness living in the community.

This chapter will explore the relationship between inquiries and the development of mental health policy. In doing so, we will consider the following issues:

- the background to, and remit and limitations of, inquiries;
- themes arising from homicide inquiries;
- inquiries and non-compliance with medication;
- the development of mental health policy through the 1990s.

Inquiries: their background, remit and limitations

Background

Mental health inquiries have a long history. Some sort of independent review of mental health care goes back to Victorian times but the modern system of statutory and non-statutory inquiries came into play in the 1960s (see Martin 1984).

During the 1960s and 1970s there were a series of major inquiries into the quality of care within a number of mental illness and learning disability hospitals. These inquiries uncovered major defects in the management and delivery of care in the old asylums and created a useful momentum towards 'de-institutionalism': the closure of the asylums and providing care in community settings. Thus inquiries played a significant role in ensuring that 'community care' (the provision of care to individuals in the least restrictive setting possible, although not necessarily in an 'ordinary' home) – became an explicit and detailed policy goal. The vast majority of long stay psychiatric beds have now been closed.

The current spate of inquiries into homicides by people with mental health problems started in 1988 with the *Report of the Committee of Inquiry into the Care and Aftercare of Miss Sharon Campbell* (Spokes *et al.* 1988) following the fatal attack on Isabel Schwarz, a social worker, by Sharon Campbell, a former client. This inquiry largely arose out of the strong advocacy of Victor Schwarz, the victim's father, and eventually resulted in the introduction of the Care Programme Approach, a system intended to ensure systematic care planning for people in touch with secondary mental health services. A number of further incidents occurred in the late 1980s and early 1990s, culminating with the killing of Jonathan Zito in 1992 by Christopher Clunis, which aroused considerable public concern, and was accompanied by a further round of policy changes, discussed below.

Remit of inquiries under HSG(94)27

In May 1994, the Department of Health issued Health Circular HSG(94)27 which made inquiries into instances of homicide by people with mental health problems mandatory:

> In cases of homicide, it will always be necessary for the DHA [District Health Authority] to hold an inquiry which is independent of the providers involved.
>
> (Department of Health 1994a, para 34)

This requirement has resulted in a significant number of independent inquiries being carried out each year which at the time of writing still continues unabated, despite regular rumours that the inquiry system will be re-formed.

The remit of inquiries should encompass, at least, the following:

- the care and treatment the patient was receiving at the time of the incident;
- the suitability of that care in view of the patient's history and assessed health and social care needs;
- the extent to which that care corresponded with statutory obligations, relevant guidance from the Department of Health and local operational policies;
- the exercise of professional judgement;
- the adequacy of the care plan and its monitoring by the key worker.

(Department of Health 1995)

Limitations of inquiries

When considering the findings and recommendations of inquiries, it is important to bear in mind the limitations of inquiry reports in providing evidence about community care and its possible failings. The strengths and weaknesses in the inquiry system have been discussed in detail elsewhere (Peay 1996) but they can be summarised as follows:

Strengths

- inquiries focus on a specific incident in detail;
- they usually gather a considerable range of evidence – little is overlooked;
- they are led by a multi-disciplinary and senior team.

Weaknesses

- they are ideographic – analysing only the unique group of individuals who actually commit homicide;
- some seem coloured by the ideology of the Chair or members;
- many examine the life history of the perpetrator in detail, but few attempt to establish causal links between the care given and the incident: it is therefore not clear to what extent the long-term histories are actually relevant to the incident;
- there are no mechanisms for reviewing inquiries nationally or chasing implementation of recommendations, if indeed all recommendations should or can be implemented;
- they rely on the retrospective reporting of those who may be implicated in the poor care associated with the incident;
- the methodology of inquiries is not uniform.

Thus, while individual inquiry reports can provide a rich source of information about the care of the individual who is the subject of that particular inquiry, inquiry reports cannot be relied upon to form judgements about the overall state of mental health services.

Themes arising from homicide inquiries

In 1999 we were commissioned by the voluntary mental health organisation Mind to review the findings of major mental health inquiry reports and examine the factors that inquiry teams considered to be of significance in precipitating the incident. The report, *Key Issues from Homicide Inquiries* (Parker and McCulloch 1999) took into account the main findings and recommendations of the inquiry reports referred to in existing relevant publications (Shepherd 1996; Reith 1998; Howlett 1998; Ward and Applin 1998), but focused specifically on the findings of 14 major homicide inquiries (listed at the end of this chapter in the Appendix) which we consider raise a wide spectrum of issues of concern.

The following (in roughly descending order of importance or frequency) 12 key issues arising from these homicide inquiries were identified:

I. Poor risk management

The most frequent factor identified in the reports examined was the absence or inadequacy of risk assessment, and the subsequent failure to manage risk effectively. All of the reports studied made reference to the importance of risk assessment, with 13 out of the 14 making recommendations in connection with risk management, such as the need for good record keeping, training to improve staff competencies in this area and the integration of risk assessment with care planning.

2. Communication problems

These were very common and were linked to poor risk management. There was often a failure to pass on key information in the right form, at the right time, to the right person. Confusion about confidentiality and public interest issues was sometimes a factor.

3. Inadequate care planning

This was highlighted in the majority of reports. Discharge from hospital, or even from all care, was often premature or haphazard. The Care Programme Approach was often not used fully or effectively. Various inquiry teams made recommendations for improving discharge planning.

4. Lack of inter-agency working

This was again a frequent concern not just across health and social care, but also more widely, for example with the police, housing agencies and the independent sector.

5. Procedural failures – both administrative and legal

In at least two cases there were significant breakdowns in following legal or administrative procedures which were directly connected with the incident.

6. Lack of suitable accommodation

A number of reports referred to this factor. The range of required accommodation, from 24 hour nursed care through supported housing to ordinary living with limited support, was often absent.

7. Resources

A number of inquiries pointed to an inadequate range of services available (e.g. psychiatric beds), or the poor quality of those which are available. Concerns about the level, qualification and workload of staff were also raised; in some cases staff were clearly under great pressure or had caseloads which were too high.

8. Substance misuse

This was present to a greater or lesser extent in a number of those committing homicide. Inquiry reports are weak on teasing out the difficult interface between mental illness, personality disorder and substance misuse. The latter may have been the key factor in some homicides, but the evidence was not always sufficient to draw firm conclusions.

9. Non-compliance

Although non-compliance with medication was a clear factor, particularly in one or two cases where individuals responded well to medication but broke down quickly when left without support, its relevance seems to have been overstated. This is discussed in more detail below.

10. Involvement of carers

Whilst not likely to be causal in respect of homicides a number of reports pointed to a worrying lack of involvement of carers.

11. Ethnic minority issues

These did not come up in reports as much as might be expected. Some inquiries, however, observed that staff may have been too ready to make incorrect and stereotypical assumptions about black service users.

12. The need for reform

A few reports argued that there is a clear need to reform the framework for community care, especially the Mental Health Act 1983, but there was no consistency on this point.

Inquiries and non-compliance with medication

Ten of the inquiry reports considered in the Mind study were referred to in a report by The Zito Trust, *Medication, Non-compliance & Mentally Disordered Offenders* (Shepherd 1996), which stated that on an analysis of 35 inquiry reports, non-compliance with medication was 'a significant contributory factor in the breakdown of care before the homicide was committed' in 20 of them.

However, on analysis of these ten inquiry reports, it would appear that the relevance of non-compliance was overstated:

The Clunis Inquiry

The Clunis Inquiry (Ritchie *et al.* 1994) refers to occasions when Christopher Clunis refused to accept medication. In the months preceding the homicide he failed to attend the out-patient appointments arranged for him following his discharge from Guy's Hospital. While the report places great emphasis on the failure of the agencies to prepare an adequate care plan and follow up arrangements, Clunis' non-compliance does not appear to be considered a significant factor. He was never offered the chance to comply with an adequate care plan in the context of sensitive, but assertive, community care.

The Buchanan Inquiry

Michael Buchanan's unwillingness to comply with medication in the community was highlighted by the inquiry team (Heginbotham *et al.* 1994). The team found that Mr Buchanan was a difficult patient to manage. This combined with the rapid improvement of his psychotic symptoms with medication meant that staff wanted to discharge him from the ward at the earliest opportunity, despite the knowledge that he was likely to refuse medication in the community which would lead to a deterioration of his mental health. The inquiry team was critical of the decision to discharge him to a hostel which was not resourced to deal with his behavioural disturbances and considered that he should not have been discharged from hospital until a suitable, supervised accommodation facility had been arranged.

The Newby Inquiry

At the time of the homicide John Rous, who killed an unqualified care worker Jonathan Newby, was on two weekly depot injections. His depot was due on 8 October but was postponed until 11 October. He fatally attacked Jonathan Newby on 9 October. The inquiry team (Davies *et al.* 1995) considered the evidence for and against positive symptoms of schizophrenia (such as delusions, hallucinations and thought disorder) having arisen on 9 October, concluding that the evidence was rather against an exacerbation of his schizophrenic illness. Although various witnesses had stated that immediately preceding his depot injection, John Rous tended to be over-active, restless and excitable, the inquiry team was informed that there had been no deterioration in John Rous' mental state.

The Woodley team

When SL (the perpetrator) was discharged from Kneesworth House Hospital on 6 December 1993 he had been off medication for over a year. Although the ward manager raised concerns that SL would relapse if he remained medication free, the decision to discontinue his medication was not reversed. The inquiry team (Woodley *et al.* 1995) considered that in such circumstances insufficient attention was given to the need for psychiatric follow-up. However, the inquiry team considered that SL did co-operate with the aftercare arrangements and found 'clear evidence' that with encouragement and support SL kept outpatient appointments.

The Grey Inquiry

Although the report refers to prison medical notes which recorded occasions when Kenneth Grey had refused oral medication, the inquiry team (Mishcon *et al.* 1995) do not comment on his compliance with medication during the time he was cared for at Hackney Hospital. The inquiry team's main concern was the lack of follow-up when he went AWOL (absent without leave).

The Walsh Inquiry

The inquiry report into the care and treatment of Doris Walsh (Mishcon *et al.* 1997) found that during the years of her illness there was a pattern of poor sleep, poor appetite and irritability/aggression prior to a relapse which usually followed Mrs Walsh either stopping or reducing her medication. However, the inquiry team were unable to ascertain whether Mrs Walsh was taking her medication at the time of the incident.

The failure to check that Mrs Walsh was complying with her medication was just one of a series of criticisms the inquiry team raised about Doris Walsh's aftercare. Other inadequacies included the lack of an aftercare plan, the absence of a keyworker and the fact that she had not been allocated to a member of the Community Mental Health Team, despite a referral.

The Witts Inquiry

The inquiry team (Lingham and Candy 1996) found that, in the weeks leading up to the homicide, Damian Witts was not regularly taking his medication. However, the team noted other important factors such as drug abuse and self-neglect and that he was re-exposed to the stresses of his family (his family were described as having a history of 'alcohol misuse, drug abuse and mental illness'). The inquiry team considered that a full clinical review, including a home visit and social circumstances assessment and risk assessment had been seriously overdue:

> We must conclude that if the team had during 1995 provided a more truly multi-disciplinary, focused and reviewed package of care then the growing danger he presented might have been recognised earlier and their actions might have prevented the tragedy. Notably, he might have been assessed and given support in his home and help to cope with his renewed exposure to the emotional stresses of his family and pressures from drug users.
>
> (Lingham *et al.* 1996a: 29)

The Ledgester Inquiry

Although Mr Ledgester's unwillingness to accept medication was referred to, the problem identified by the report (Double *et al.* 1997) is the service's failure to engage him either in the community or in hospital:

> Where a patient discharges himself or is absent without leave as occurred in this case, it is not easy to comply with the usual discharge and Care Programme Approach requirements. However, the only positive measure taken to engage DL was the suggestion of an out-patient appointment (which in the event was not instituted) and a letter sent to his GP.
>
> (Double *et al.* 1997: 30)

The Hampshire Inquiry

Frank Hampshire stabbed his wife to death. The inquiry team (Mishcon *et al.* 1996) found that the refusal to take medication was a repeated feature of Mr Hampshire's illness. They noted that Mr Hampshire had been prescribed Prozac and he had stopped taking any anti-psychotic drugs because he did not like the side effects. The team raised concerns about the failure to check Prozac's effectiveness or appropriateness and commented that anti-psychotic medication seemed to have worked in the past. However, the inquiry team found that no one could have predicted the attack and Frank Hampshire was solely responsible for his wife's death.

The Robinson Inquiry

Although Andrew Robinson (Blom-Cooper *et al.* 1995) had refused to comply with his treatment plan in the past, at the time of the incident he was an in-patient (had been for ten weeks) and had been on depot medication for over two months. Accordingly non-compliance with medication was not immediately relevant to the homicide.

Thus, in the research carried out for Mind (Parker and McCulloch 1999), we found that while non-compliance was clearly an issue in homicide inquiries, its significance seems to be over-emphasised in current policy. From the analysis of inquiry reports, it is clear that non-compliance does not exist in a vacuum but occurs because of a combination of a service user's wishes and attitudes, based on past experience, and the level of support and information offered by services.

Development of mental health policy through the 1990s

Community treatment orders

The idea of community treatment orders is not new. With the move from institutional care to 'care in the community' and in the light of the Hallstrom case in 1985 (R v. Hallstrom) which 'effectively outlawed the practice of using prolonged leave as a means of ensuring that patients who did not need to be in hospital could be obliged to go on taking their medication outside it' (Hoggett 1996), the question of the need to introduce community treatment orders has been debated on many occasions (Royal College of Psychiatrists 1993a).

In January 1993, the Royal College of Psychiatrists (RCP) published its report *Community Supervision Orders* which called for the introduction of powers to require individuals who had previously been compulsorily detained in hospital to accept treatment and receive supervision when they were discharged from hospital. The RCP believed that such powers were necessary because of difficulties in the management of patients with chronic mental illness:

> The problem with management and care for more people has been their tendency to stop taking treatment once back in the community, thus getting themselves into difficulties and as a consequence falling through the Community Care net. This debate has recently been highlighted by the tragic case of Ben Silcock.
>
> (Royal College of Psychiatrists 1993b: 1)

Ben Silcock, a young man with a diagnosis of schizophrenia, had climbed into the lions' den at London Zoo in December 1992. This incident happened to have been captured on video and was then widely publicised. In the same month Christopher Clunis fatally stabbed Jonathan Zito on Finsbury Park tube station.

The day after the RCPs' report was published, Virginia Bottomley, the then Secretary of State for Health, announced that the Department of Health would conduct a review of mental health legislation, with the following terms of reference:

> To consider urgently, in the light of the Royal College of Psychiatrists' proposals:
>
> • whether new legal powers are needed to ensure that mentally ill people in the community get the care that they need; and
> • whether the present legal powers in the 1983 Mental Health Act are being used as effectively as they can be, and what action could be taken in advance of any new legislation to ensure that they are.
>
> (Department of Health 1993a: 3)

The resulting report was published in August 1993, alongside Mrs Bottomley's Ten Point Plan (see Box 7.1). This plan included a new power of supervised discharge. Under this power, which was introduced under the Mental Health (Patients in the Community) Act 1995, patients who have been compulsorily detained in hospital under the MHA 1983 can be required to comply with conditions on their discharge from hospital, such as residing in a specified place or keeping appointments for medical treatment. The power falls short of compulsory treatment in the community as there is no power to require individuals to comply with their treatment plan but there is a 'power to take and convey' individuals subject to supervised discharge to the place that they were required to be (for instance, an out-patient clinic where the person has an appointment for medical treatment).

Box 7.1 Mrs Bottomley's Ten Point Plan (1993)

1. Introduction of supervised discharge and extended leave
2. Review of the 1983 Mental Health Act
3. Improved Code of Practice relating to the 1983 Act
4. Guidance on discharge (includes the introduction of compulsory inquiries in the case of homicides)
5. Better training for key workers
6. Development of information systems including supervision registers
7. Clinical Standards Advisory Group review of schizophrenia
8. Implementation programme for the Mental Health Task Force to drive community care
9. Ensuring all commissioning plans adequately cover mental health
10. Specific action plan for London.

(Reproduced in Harrison 1994)

Another item on the plan was the introduction of 'supervision registers' – mental health service providers were required to establish and maintain registers which identified 'people with a severe mental illness who may be a significant risk to themselves or to others' (Department of Health 1994b). Both these measures were subject to widespread criticism (Parker 1997).

It is clear from statements issued by the Department of Health that these measures were driven by two major concerns. The first concern was that some patients fail to comply with their treatment plan:

> [the needs and care of some mentally ill people] is a debate with origins long before events in the closing days of 1992 brought it into prominence. Since then, a number of tragic incidents have added to the pressing questions surrounding the care and treatment of a small and vulnerable group of people with a history of relapse and deterioration of their condition and consequent compulsory re-admission to hospital. This often resulted from a failure or refusal to comply with their care and treatment programme whilst in the community.
>
> (Department of Health 1999c)

The second is the perceived consequence of non-compliance – a concern about public safety, which Virginia Bottomley described when introducing the Ten Point Plan:

> Health and safety must be the paramount considerations. The recent cases underlined the importance of the review which I established in January. I am pleased to be able to bring forward positive proposals which will

bring added protection to the public and to mentally ill people themselves, as well as bolstering confidence in the policy [of providing care in the community] as a whole.

(Department of Health 1993)

Key policy themes

The main policy themes that underpinned the Ten Point Plan were as follows:

- reform of mental health legislation to reflect community care and to give greater powers of compulsion;
- an emphasis on engagement, supervision and compliance – carrying both positive, caring overtones and overtones of control;
- training;
- information systems as a tool for control and engagement;
- whole systems development of community care.

The underlying thinking was to create a greater structure for community care in terms of services, staff behaviour and powers over service users, in the hope that this would address public safety issues. However, there is no strong evidence base to support the hypotheses that:

- safety is endangered by community care – there is no evidence that the number of incidents rose as a result of de-institutionalisation, on the contrary the proportion of homicides committed by mentally ill people seems to be on a historic downward trend (Taylor and Gunn 1999);
- safety can be measurably improved by national policies of this type.

Nonetheless, the new Labour governments have followed broadly the same agenda, albeit fleshed out considerably into the most comprehensive policy package we have ever had in mental health. The new policies map on to the same thinking that underpinned the Ten Point Plan:

- legislative reform – the proposals to reform the mental health legislation (Department of Health 2002) include preventative detention and treatment orders which apply across all settings. The elements of these proposals which address dangerous people are focused largely on public safety;
- engagement, supervision and compliance – the National Service Framework (NSF) for Mental Health (Department of Health 1999c) has a lot to say about this, and assertive outreach (one of the few evidence based service models in mental health) is seen as bringing these functions together, although the moral and practical tensions in this have not been resolved;

- training – the workforce agenda is set out most recently in the Workforce Action Team report (Department of Health 2001a) and covers the development of training in areas such as assertive outreach;
- information – the Mental Health Information Strategy (Department of Health 2001b) was launched in 2001 and, although little progress has been made in implementing it, in London at least this is being extended to the creation of a central London risk register (a project funded by the Treasury as part of its value for money programme) which effectively represents a rebirth of a more comprehensive and accessible supervision register;
- whole systems development – a central theme of the NSF which proposes a complex system of interlocking specialist community care teams – carrying perhaps the risk of breakdowns in seamlessness.

Within this, themes of engagement, compliance and supervision form an important strand. The Sainsbury Centre for Mental Health report *Keys to Engagement* (1998) made the case for assertive outreach at a critical time during policy formulation and it was seen as a way of squaring the circle of engagement, supervision and compliance for the 'hard to engage' group. This drive came more from the international evidence and experiences within Birmingham, central London and elsewhere than from inquiries.

Assertive community treatment

Assertive community treatment or assertive outreach is a much more sophisticated policy response to the compliance/safety issue than what went before, because it apparently offers the possibility of bringing together safety with more positive engagement. The Sainsbury Centre report *Keys to Engagement* (1998) emphasised the latter agenda, whereas early new Labour policy under Frank Dobson's leadership emphasised the former. Current detailed policy offers a more balanced model where assertive outreach is seen as having benefits for both users and society.

It could be argued that the policy push towards assertive outreach is as near a perfect solution to the political problem of anxieties around public safety in mental health as it is possible to achieve in an imperfect world because:

- it is an evidence based intervention which can deliver genuine benefits to a neglected client group;
- at best it could genuinely bring together care with an appropriate form of 'supervision' as required;
- it can form part of a comprehensive and balanced system of intensive community care which approximates to international best practice in the delivery of mental health care.

But there are dangers. Rapid pressure to create assertive outreach teams leads to staff being leached out of other services, and there is also evidence that some teams labelled as 'assertive outreach' are not following the assertive outreach model as described in government's policy and the international literature. The introduction of compulsion in the community could skew teams towards the safety agenda and lead to a breakdown of trust with clients and/or the infringement of their human rights if the care plan is overly intrusive.

Conclusion

The link between policy and inquiries

A few inquiries have demonstrably directly influenced policy – for example the inquiry into the care and treatment of Sharon Campbell (Spokes *et al.* 1998) led to the Care Programme Approach. However, while the report into the care and treatment of Christopher Clunis (Ritchie *et al.* 1994) brought in some policy changes (such as the introduction of section 117 registers), the major policy changes were announced in August 1993 six months before the inquiry panel's report was published (February 1994). Most inquiries have had few direct policy implications. The policy analysis in inquiries is usually weak and naive, and the influence is mediated by media driven anxiety around the incident leading to a policy response generated by the Department of Health rather than borrowed from the inquiry team. Thus, inquiries are therefore only one factor in the political landscape leading to mental health policy.

That there are often a number of factors involved in the development of mental health policy, with media coverage being highly influential, is illustrated by the comments made in the Department of Health's (1993a) internal review report – *Legal Powers of the Care of Mentally Ill People in the Community.* The introduction makes clear that the decision to set up the internal review was a response to a number of factors. The widely publicised case of Ben Silcock and the RCP's proposals for a community supervision order were two important factors. However, they occurred at a time when the newly appointed Secretary of State for Health, Virginia Bottomley, was expressing her own concerns that people with mental health problems were falling through 'the net' of care services.

In the case of assertive outreach, there appears to be no direct link to inquiries; rather assertive outreach forms part of a natural migration of policy towards a more comprehensive and evidence based system of care (albeit with a long way to go on the evidence base), coupled with the political aptness of assertive outreach to be all things to all people.

What of the future?

It seems certain that, whatever the future of mandatory inquiries, some inquiries will continue and the media will continue to report incidents. These in turn will affect mental health policy, particularly mental health legislation. The current proposals from government for new mental health legislation are skewed more strongly towards control than any since the Second World War, so clearly anxiety around mental health 'incidents' continues unabated, despite our more comprehensive mental health policy.

Acknowledgements

This chapter draws significantly on the Mind report 'What are the key issues raised by homicide inquiries?' (Parker and McCulloch 1999). Mind's support in producing that report and its permission for the reproduction of its findings here are gratefully acknowledged.

References

Department of Health (1993a) *Legal Powers on the Care of the Mentally Ill People in the Community, Report of the Internal Review*, London: Department of Health.

Department of Health (1993b) *Legislation Planned for Supervised Discharge of Psychiatric Patients: Virginia Bottomley Announces Ten Point Plan for Developing Successful and Safe Community Care*, Press Release, 12 August 1993.

Department of Health (1994a) HSG(94)27 *Guidance on the Discharge of Mentally Disordered People and their Continuing Care in the Community*, London: Department of Health.

Department of Health (1994b) HSG(94)5 *Guidance on the Introduction of Supervision Registers*, London: Department of Health.

Department of Health (1995) *Building Bridges: A Guide to the Arrangements for Inter-Agency Working for the Care and Protection of Mentally Ill People*, London: Department of Health.

Department of Health (1998) *Modernising Mental Health Services: Safe, Sound, Supportive*, London: Department of Health.

Department of Health (1999a) *Review of the Mental Health Act 1983: Report of the Expert Committee, Appendix C*, London: Department of Health.

Department of Health (1999b) *Community Supervision Orders – Government response to the 5th Report from the Health Committee, 1992–93 session*, Cm 2333. London: The Stationery Office.

Department of Health (1999c) *National Service Framework for Mental Health*, London: Department of Health.

Department of Health (2000) *The NHS Plan: A Plan for Investment, A Plan for Reform*, London: The Stationery Office.

Department of Health (2001a) *Workforce Action Team Report*, London: Department of Health.

Department of Health (2001b) *Mental Health Information Strategy*, London: Department of Health.

Department of Health (2002) *Draft Mental Health Bill*, London: The Stationery Office. Cm 5538–1.

Harrison, A. (ed.) (1994) *Health Care UK: 1993/94*, London: King's Fund Institute.

Hoggett, B. (1996) *Mental Health Law*, 160, 4th edn, London: Sweet & Maxwell.

Howlett, M. (1998) *Medication, Non-compliance and Mentally Disordered Offenders – The Role of Non-Compliance in Homicide by People with Mental Illness and Proposals for Future Policy – A study of Independent Inquiry Reports*, London: The Zito Trust.

Martin, J.P. (1984) *Hospitals in Trouble*, Oxford: Basil Blackwell.

The National Association of Health Authorities and Trusts in association with the Sainsbury Centre for Mental Health (1997) *Mental Health Care: From Problems to Solutions*, Research Paper 23. London: NAHAT.

Parker, C. (1997) Mental Health Act: Aftercare under supervision, *Clinical Risk*, 3: 182.

Parker, C. and McCulloch, A. (1999) *Key Issues from Homicide Inquiries*, London: Mind.

Peay, J. (ed.) (1996) *Inquiries After Homicide*, London: Duckworth.

Reith, M. (1998) *Community Care Tragedies: A Practice Guide to Mental Health Inquiries*, Birmingham: Venture Press.

Royal College of Psychiatrists (1993a) *Community Supervision Orders*, London: Royal College of Psychiatrists.

Royal College of Psychiatrists (1993b) *Community Supervision Orders, Press Release*, London: Royal College of Psychiatrists.

The Sainsbury Centre for Mental Health (1998) *Keys to Engagement: Review of Care for People with Severe Mental Illness who are hard to Engage with Services*, London: The Sainsbury Centre for Mental Health.

Shepherd, D. (1996) *Learning the Lessons – Mental Health Inquiry Reports Published in England and Wales Between 1969 and 1996 and their Recommendations for Improving Practice*, 2nd edn, London: The Zito Trust.

Taylor, P.J. and Gunn, J. (1999) 'Homicides by people with mental illness', *British Journal of Psychiatry*, 174: 9–14.

Ward, M. and Applin, C. (1998) *The Unlearned Lesson: The Role of Alcohol and Drug Misuse in Inquiries*. London: Wynne Howard Publishing.

Appendix: Inquiry reports examined in detail in this chapter

Baroness Scotland of Asthal, Kelly, H. and Devaux, M. (1998) *The Report of the Luke Warm Luke Health Inquiry*, London: Lambeth, Southwark & Lewisham Health Authority.

Blom-Cooper, L., Hally, H. and Murphy, E. (1995) *The Falling Shadow: One Patient's Mental Health Care 1978–1993*, London: Duckworth.

Davies, N., Lingham, R., Prior, C. and Sims, A. (1995) *Report of the Inquiry into the Circumstances Leading to the Death of Jonathan Newby (a volunteer worker) on 9th October in Oxford*. Oxford: Oxfordshire Health Authority.

Double, V.J., McGinnis, P., Nelson, T. and Pritlove, J. (1997) 'Sharing the Burden' – An Independent Inquiry into the Care and Treatment of Desmond Ledgester, A Report

Commissioned by Calderdale & Kirklees Health Authority, Huddersfield: Calderdale & Kirklees Health Authority.

Heginbotham, C., Hale, R., Warren, L., Walsh, T. and Carr, J. (1994) *The Report of the Inquiry of the Independent Panel examining the case of Michael Buchanan*, London: North West London Mental Health Trust.

Lingham, R. and Candy, J. (1996) *Inquiry into the Treatment and Care of Damian Witts – Summary of the Report Commissioned by Gloucester Health Authority*, Gloucester: Gloucester Health Authority.

Mishcon, J., Dick, D., Welch, N., Sheehan, A. and Mackay, J. (1995) *The Grey Report – Report of the Independent Inquiry into the Care and Treatment of Kenneth Grey to East London and The City Health Authority*, London: East London and the City Health Authority.

Mishcon, J., Dick, D., Milne, I., Beard, P. and Mackay, J. (1996) *The Hampshire Report – Report of the Independent Inquiry team into the Care and Treatment of Francis Hampshire to Redbridge and Waltham Forest Health Authority*, London: Redbridge and Waltham Forest Health Authority.

Mishcon, J., Mason, L., Stanmer, S. and Dick, D. (1997) *Report of the Independent Inquiry into the Treatment and Care of Doris Walsh*, Coventry: Coventry Health Authority.

Ritchie, J., Dick, D. and Lingham, R. (1994) *The Report of the Inquiry into the Care and Treatment of Christopher Clunis*, London: HMSO.

Spokes, J., Pare, M. and Royle, G. (1988) *The Report of the Committee of Inquiry into the Care and Aftercare of Miss Sharon Campbell*, London: HMSO.

Woodley, L., Dixon, K., Lindow, V., Oyebode, O., Sandford, T. and Simblet, S. (1995) *The Woodley Team Report – Report of the Independent Review Panel to East London and The City Health Authority and Newham Council following a homicide in July 1994 by a person suffering with a severe mental illness*. London: East London and the City Health Authority.

Court judgements referred to

R v. Hallstrom, ex p. W: R v. Gardner, ex p. L [1986] Q.B. 1090.

Chapter 8

Women and mental health inquiries

Nicky Stanley

Introduction

An analysis of inquiries that addresses the dimension of gender offers an alternative approach to the form. Rather than considering the inquiry as an interrogative tool which seeks to establish a sequence of events and ascribe accountability, the report can be viewed as a social document. From this perspective, inquiries can be used as source material for an analysis of how mental health services interact with their users. Despite an increasing emphasis on psychosocial theories and models in mental health work and literature, services still struggle to recognise and respond to the particular needs of different social groups. This is especially the case for service users who are women, people from minority ethnic groups and those who are learning disabled. This chapter examines what the inquiries communicate about the ways in which services conceptualise and meet the needs of women, as service users, carers and professionals.

The National Service Framework for Mental Health (Department of Health 1999) has provided the impetus for providers of health and social care services in all settings to study the needs of different social groups more closely and to offer services that are sensitive and relevant to those needs. For women, this approach at the level of national policy has comprised mainly a drive towards single sex accommodation. The first National Visit undertaken by The Mental Health Commission in 1996 found that 94 per cent of the mental health wards surveyed still had mixed accommodation. Over half the staff participating in this review reported that women had been sexually harassed on their unit (Sainsbury Centre and Mental Health Commission 1997). This finding fuelled a commitment from central government (Department of Health 2000) to provide single sex accommodation on 95 per cent of all mental health units by 2002. A similar preoccupation with segregated provision is also evident in the consultation document on a national strategy for women's mental health services (Department of Health 2002). While this publication does identify the needs of women as a social group and recognises differences within that group, the proposal for women only day services is likely to dominate the resulting strategy. However, the consultation paper does represent a turning-point in what may prove to be a prolonged process of acknowledging the extent to which mental health services reproduce structural inequalities and reinforce the oppression of one group by another.

Women appear in mental health inquiries in a variety of different roles. Although the violent mentally disordered offender is usually portrayed as male (see, for example, Prior 1999), just under 20 per cent of perpetrators of homicides committed by those who have been mental health service users are female (Appleby et al. 2001). Women are particularly evident in inquiries as victims with 60 per cent of the victims being female in homicides committed by those with symptoms of mental illness at the time (Appleby et al. 2001). While most perpetrators of mental health homicides are men, the majority of victims of homicides committed by those with mental health problems are female spouses, partners or carers (Appleby et al. 2001). However, women also predominate in the professional groups most likely to have high levels of one-to-one contact with mental health service users: nursing and social work. Female professionals from these groups also figure among the those killed and constitute five of the six professionals who died and are identified in the inquiries listed by Sheppard in Chapter 9 of this book.

Women also appear in inquiries as carers or relatives who may be seeking to understand why services failed to protect the victim (see Paul and Audrey Edwards' Chapter 2 in this book). In addition, they may also participate in the process as the carer or the relative of the perpetrator who can also convey a sense of having 'lost' a family member (see, for example, the Robinson family in Blom-Cooper et al. 1995). Women are likely to figure as informants to inquiries since, as noted earlier, they dominate the professions of nursing and social work. However, they are less likely to be represented among the service managers who may be called upon to account for the work of their organisation. Women have also chaired inquiries and, although female chairs of mental health inquiries are in a minority, 46 of the 144 published inquiries included in Sheppard's chapter were chaired by a woman: two barristers, Jane Mishcon and Nicola Davies, have both chaired a number of inquiries.

An inquiry which is headed by a female chair may be more likely than others to demonstrate an awareness of gender issues. There are few inquiries that explicitly explore the issue of women's needs and the service response to them, consequently, those that do so are striking in this respect. This chapter will first consider how the themes of gender and women's needs in relation to mental health services are addressed in the accounts provided by mental health inquiries. In many reports, gender is invisible, but in some the inquiry team specifically addresses women's needs. Elsewhere, the evidence concerning women's experiences of both the process of inquiry and mental health services has to be gleaned by careful reading of the evidence and the inquiry panel's conclusions. This approach to inquiry reports will inform discussions of women as perpetrators of homicides, women's experience of abuse and violence as revealed by the inquiries, and women as carers. Finally, this chapter will focus on inquiries where female professionals have died to consider how the inquiries depict the experiences of women as practitioners engaged in delivering services.

Perspectives on female perpetrators

The inquiry (Double *et al.* 1998) reporting on the homicide committed by Alfina Magdalena Gabriel, who wounded and killed two men when she suspected them of abusing her daughter, is unusual in its emphasis on Alfina Magdalena Gabriel's identity as a black woman. In a section headed 'Gender', the inquiry team suggested that Gabriel's gender was a factor which contributed to professionals under-estimating her potential for violence: serious incidents were never fully investigated and, despite her numerous previous convictions, she continued to avoid custodial sentences. The inquiry, which was chaired by a woman – Valerie Double – also noted that Gabriel was a single parent and concluded that: 'The overall approach to AMG's care would have been different, given the risks and concerns, had AMG been a man' (Double *et al.* 1998: 32).

A similar concern that mental health services focus on the assessment and treatment of men is discernible in the inquiry report on Ms B (Dimond *et al.* 1997) who killed her father. The inquiry team (chaired by a woman) expressed concern that Ms B was the only woman accommodated on an acute ward in a medium secure unit. Although the theme is not particularly relevant to the case examined by the *Woodley Team Report* (Woodley *et al.* 1995), gender was also raised as an issue in the broad approach taken by this inquiry team to issues of commissioning. This report also drew attention to the safety of women in secure units and emphasised the need for single sex accommodation to be available in all psychiatric in-patient settings.

Inquiries into homicides perpetrated by women only rarely explicitly address gender issues. For example, the inquiry reporting on the care and after-care of Sharon Campbell (Spokes *et al.* 1988) who killed Isobel Schwarz, a social worker at Bexley Hospital, emphasised Campbell's ethnicity and her youth but did not comment on her gender. The inquiry team speculated that her age and race may have contributed to a reluctance among professionals to allocate her a diagnosis of schizophrenia (Spokes *et al.* 1988: 16.29), but did not address gender as a factor affecting her diagnosis or treatment. Other inquiries involving women perpetrators are similar in betraying little interest in how gender might shape professionals' perceptions and assessments.

An examination of the evidence from inquiry reports where women were the perpetrators of homicides suggests that gender can function to distort perceptions of risk. Alfina Magdalena Gabriel was not the only female perpetrator of homicide featured in a mental health inquiry report who had a long history of violent behaviour well known to the professionals treating her. Ms B, who killed her father while on leave from a regional secure unit, had committed a number of serious attacks on staff and others (Dimond *et al.*1997). The inquiry team note that the doctors caring for Ms B did not argue for her to be prosecuted for any of these incidents.

Sharon Campbell had a history of violent behaviour towards professionals which included an assault on Isabel Schwarz whilst a passenger in her car and she was known to regularly carry a knife. In their analysis of the public response to this inquiry, Butler and Drakeford (2003) suggest that Campbell's status as a young woman may have been a factor which prevented this inquiry escalating into a public scandal. Gender can thus act to mitigate perceptions of dangerousness both among professionals and in the wider arena of the press and public reactions.

In these three cases, it appears that long histories of violent behaviour were viewed through the veil of gender, and professionals significantly under-estimated risks of violence. A failure to view potential for violence as compatible with female identity is the product of an objectifying, reductive conceptualisation of the mental health service user, a perception which relies heavily on stereotypes. Wilczynski (1997) identified similar processes at work in the criminal justice system's response to women who were charged with filicide: she found that women were more likely than men to receive bail and less likely to be prosecuted or convicted for murder. Coontz *et al.*'s (1994) study of clinicians' assessments of dangerousness in the emergency room of a psychiatric hospital provides evidence of mental health professionals' perception of violence as a male characteristic. Their observations revealed that the issue of violence was raised more frequently with male patients and, even when a violent incident had precipitated a patient's referral to the emergency room, the topic of violence was pursued in more depth with men than with women. Gender appears to be a key, if rarely acknowledged, factor in shaping assessments of dangerousness.

Women's experience of violence and the inquiries

The inquiries involving female perpetrators also provide evidence of professionals failing to acknowledge the significance of the experience of abuse for women. A number of female perpetrators appear to have committed homicide in response to their perceptions or experience of abuse. Ms B had consistently claimed throughout her involvement with mental health services that she had been abused by her father. The inquiry report (Dimond *et al.* 1997) notes the continuing confusion among professionals as to whether her belief was based on fact or was a product of her psychosis. The report also identifies the failure to address Ms B's belief in her experience of abuse as part of a care plan.

Likewise, the inquiry into the care of Justine Cummings (Laming *et al.* 2000) found that the deliberate self-harm services she received from Avalon NHS Trust were inadequate (para 11.5). Justine Cummings had a history of experiencing serious sexual assault and had become involved in a sexual relationship with a nurse involved in her treatment. This latter fact was not communicated by the Bethlem and Maudsley NHS Trust where Ian Kew, the nurse, was later employed and where Justine Cummings was also a patient. The implications of this relationship for Cummings, who later killed her fiancé, Peter Lewis, do not seem to have been acknowledged by services.

Alfina Magdalena Gabriel killed a man and assaulted another whom she believed to have abused her daughter. The inquiry team (Double *et al.* 1998) found that mental health professionals had failed to take account of these allegations and the ensuing investigations on Gabriel. Similarly, the inquiry team (Taylor *et al.* 2000) reporting on Marie Alawode's killing of her three-year-old daughter, Joanne, noted the failure of community mental health services to give sufficient weight to Alawode's belief that Joanne had been sexually abused by her father. The inquiry team also judged that the child protection assessment was incomplete and that liaison between child care social work and mental health services was poor.

The inquiry into the care of Anne Murrie (Williams and Hennessey 1999) who killed her nine-year-old daughter found that services had responded to her as an individual rather than seeing her 'within the context of her family' (Williams and Hennessey 1999: 61). Professionals were judged to have failed to take account of the impact of Anne Murrie's ex-husband's new relationship on her state of mind and to have been unaware of the vulnerability of her daughter in relation to these feelings. In these cases, it appears that professionals saw these women primarily as users of mental health services. This identity excluded consideration of other roles such as survivor of abuse, single mother or rejected wife and mother.

A failure on the part of services to acknowledge an individual's multiple roles can have particularly serious consequences for women who are mothers. A number of these inquiries, including that into the care of Marie Alawode, the inquiry into the care of Anne Murrie, and that into the deaths of Jason and Natalia Henry (Gabbott and Hill 1994) who were killed by their mother, Sharon Dalson, found a lack of communication and co-ordination between adult mental health services and children's services. Falkov's (1996) review of Part 8 Reviews found a similar lack of co-ordination between services characterised child deaths where parents had mental health problems. Stanley *et al.*'s (2003) study identified particular problems in interprofessional work between adult psychiatrists and child care social workers which included failures in co-ordination and difficulties concerning confidentiality. Problems in communication between these two professional groups are likely to limit the capacity of either service to assess risks to women and children.

The inquiries also offer evidence of the failure of mental health services to acknowledge women's experience of domestic violence and abuse. The report investigating the care and treatment of Patient T (Galbraith *et al.* 2000), who killed her former boyfriend, emphasised his history of violence towards her. She had experienced a number of violent relationships which the inquiry panel considered relevant to their investigation of her mental health needs and care. The report commented on the failure of services to engage in any depth with Patient T's family and relationships and concluded that:

> the treatment and care offered to Patient T was constrained by lack of knowledge and understanding about her home circumstances and lack of contact with her family and partner.
>
> (Galbraith *et al.* 2000: 29)

Such comments resonate with those quoted above from the inquiry team investigating the care of Anne Murrie (Williams and Hennessey 1999).

A failure to engage with the issue of domestic violence is also evident in *Bridging the Gaps* (Bhatoa *et al.* 1999), which reports on the care of Naseer Aslam who killed his sister-in-law. The inquiry revealed that Aslam had a long history of domestic violence which involved both his wives and his sister-in-law. The risks he posed to women were never fully assessed by the mental health services who treated him in hospital; there was no communication between the psychiatric ward where Aslam was an in-patient and the medical ward in the same hospital where his wife was treated following his assault on her. No community follow-up was arranged for Aslam and no support was offered his family. On discharge, he was advised to attend a (probably inappropriate) community project which worked with violent men, but the team treating him in hospital made no contact with that project.

A lack of contact with the victim of domestic violence is also highlighted by the inquiry into the deaths of Michael and Hazel Horner (Williams 1997). Horner had a long history of domestic violence towards his wife and daughters, which was known to community mental health staff and ward staff but not communicated to those responsible for his discharge. Mrs Horner was not consulted concerning this discharge, which was badly timed as she was planning to move out in three days time. The inquiry team reporting on the care of Mr K.K. (Gulliver *et al.* 1999), who also killed his wife following a long history of domestic violence towards her, noted the failure of mental health professionals to assess the risk Mr K.K. posed to his wife when drunk, and recommended that social services should allocate 'resources to offer counselling and support in cases of serious domestic violence' (Gulliver *et al.* 1999: paras 139 and 158).

Mental health services are not alone in their failure to recognise the risks that domestic violence may pose to family members. Child care services have been similarly criticised for their tardiness in identifying and responding to this issue (Social Services Inspectorate 1995; Mullender 1996). Those commenting on this issue have tended to focus on the gap between children's and adults' services in the UK, the differing theoretical and research models which have reinforced this gap, and the failure of child care practice and studies to fully acknowledge men's role in and responsibility for the abuse of children (Stanley 1997). Similarly, the structural and theoretical distance between adult mental health services and child care services can be seen to shape the way in which mental health services view domestic violence.

In the case of both services, the construction of the service user's identity can be seen to affect perceptions of the significance of domestic violence. In child care services and studies, the family is conceptualised as consisting primarily of women and children. By contrast, the inquiries depict the mental health service user as decontextualised and stripped of family relations in his or her relationship with services. Furthermore, just as child care services failed to acknowledge the risks posed by domestic violence in the past (see Maynard 1985), so mental health professionals may still regard domestic violence as constituting a less severe risk and as more acceptable than other forms of violence. The inquiries provide some evidence to reinforce this hypothesis and Humphreys and Thiara's (2003) study of women's perceptions of mental health services suggests that awareness of the impact of domestic violence on women remains undeveloped amongst mental health professionals. Such attitudes continue in the face of the evidence provided by inquiries and discussed at the beginning of this chapter that family members are the most likely victims of mental health homicides. The following section moves on to consider the light shed by inquiries on female carers' experiences of mental health services.

Inquiry perspectives on female carers

The inquiries have consistently identified the failure of mental health services to consult and communicate with a range of female carers who have included mothers, wives and sisters. This was a key theme to emerge from the Clunis Report (Ritchie et al. 1994) which noted the lack of communication between agencies and Clunis' sister who maintained regular contact with him as he ricocheted from one mental health agency to another:

> Health and social services workers took few, if any, steps to contact members of his family, and thereby they lost touch with some of the basic realities of his personal history as well as losing the family's potentially valuable support in his treatment and its aftermath. They treated him as single, homeless and itinerant with no family ties, and the more they treated him as such the more he began to fulfil that role.
>
> (Ritchie et al. 1994: 3.1.6)

As in the accounts of the female perpetrators discussed above, the response of mental health services served to strip Clunis of his social relations and family history. For mental health services, the service user's identity appears at times to be restricted to that of patient.

The inquiry into the care of Martin Mursell (Crawford *et al.* 1997) was even more scathing in its criticism of professionals' attitudes to and treatment of carers. Mursell was left without an allocated social worker and without accommodation of his own while he waited for the tenancy of his new flat to become available. He was sleeping in his mother's (Mrs Collins) flat when he killed his step-father and attacked her with a knife. The inquiry team commented on the extent to which services had relied on the support provided by female carers, while failing to value it:

> There was little value placed upon or consideration given to Mrs Collins's contribution as a carer. These professionals who should have worked more closely with Martin when he was well seemed to regard her contribution as a convenient substitute for the after-care plan which they ought to have prepared.
>
> (Crawford *et al.* 1997: 86)

In contrast, the inquiry report into the circumstances surrounding the deaths of Ellen and Alan Boland (Hughes *et al.* 1995) had little to say about the way in which services had liaised with carers, although the report did note the failure to refer Alan Boland to a community psychiatric nurse or social worker who might have focused on his psychosocial needs. However, the glimpses into Boland's case records afforded by the inquiry illuminates the readiness of mental health professionals to pathologise carers. Boland lived with his mother who was 62 years old at the time he was first referred to mental health services. Medical staff recorded in Boland's notes that his mother 'nags him which he finds very depressing. . . .' (p. 2). When she came to outpatients with him, at his request:

> She was noted by the doctor to be domineering and demanding. She alleged he was drinking heavily every day and needed help. She showed surprise when asked to let her son answer the doctors' questions.
>
> (Hughes *et al.* 1995: 9)

Not only were Mrs Boland's needs as a carer not identified or addressed but what was clearly a conflictual relationship was minimised, and her behaviour attributed a stereotypical female label of 'nagging'. Following his discharge from day hospital care, Boland killed his mother, whom he was still living with, as applications to secure him accommodation of his own had been unsuccessful. He later hanged himself while in prison.

The negative constructions placed by professionals on Mrs Boland's relationship to her son and on her role in his care are characteristic of attitudes towards service users' families which were prevalent in mental health services from the 1960s through to the early 1990s. A number of the new theoretical models emerging in psychiatry during this period had the effect of blaming parents for their children's disorders. Laing's (Laing and Esterson 1964) theory of family dysfunction is the most frequently cited culprit in this respect but as Jones (2002) points out, family therapy research and practice together with interpretations of Leff and Vaughan's (1985) early work on expressed emotion had all contributed to a widely held view among mental health professionals that families constituted the root of the problem for many mental health service users. Since women are the family members most likely to undertake the actual tasks involved in caring (Ungerson 1990) and are most likely to have contact with mental health professionals in the course of discharging their caring roles, the potential for female carers to experience hostile attitudes from mental health staff has been considerable. However, the 1990s saw an increasing emphasis on carers' rights, culminating in The Carers (Recognition and Services) Act 1995 which enabled carers to request a community care assessment in their own right. Together with the insistence in the *National Service Framework for Mental Health* (Department of Health 1999) on services consulting and working in partnership with carers, some progress may have been achieved towards dispelling such attitudes.

Older female carers may attract the sympathy of professionals but find it difficult to communicate their situation, perhaps from a sense of duty or because they identify so closely with the cared-for person that it becomes impossible for them to distinguish their own separate and conflicting needs. The experience of Muriel Viner, who was killed by her son Robert who then took his own life, fits Twigg and Atkin's (1994: 122–3) 'engulfment mode' of caring. Carers in this mode are described as remaining 'invisible to service providers, obscured behind the needs of the person they looked after' (Twigg and Atkin 1994: 123). The inquiry report (Harbour *et al.* 1996) notes that, although Muriel Viner, who was 76 at the time of her death, did not formally request help, she did express her distress to professionals who failed to assess her needs or provide adequate support. Robert Viner had a diagnosis of schizophrenia and drank heavily; his mother clearly found his care stressful and had told professionals that she could no longer cope with having him at home.

The *Falling Shadow* inquiry report (Blom-Cooper *et al.* 1995) demonstrated that even carers such as Andrew Robinson's parents, who expressed their needs and concerns forcefully, might fail to elicit a response from services. Jennifer and Peter Robinson were articulate, middle-class professionals who clearly asked for support and services but were frustrated in their attempts to obtain information and resources. Jones' (2002) detailed study of families' experiences of caring for a relative with mental health problems found that it was common for families to receive very limited information from psychiatrists or other professionals. In the absence of expert knowledge or advice, families were left to construct a meaning for their relative's mental health problem for themselves.

Caring professionals and inquiries

The disciplining of staff is one of the key functions of inquiries identified by Reder and Duncan (1996) and some high profile inquiries have resulted in individual professionals being exposed to significant levels of criticism, both in the original inquiry reports and subsequently in the press. Female professionals may be particularly vulnerable to such criticism, both because they are more likely than men to be engaged in delivering community mental health services at the ground level and because their gender renders them more susceptible to press interest in their appearance and their private or family lives. Campbell's (1988) analysis of the events which surrounded the Cleveland Inquiry (Butler-Sloss 1988) into child sexual abuse emphasises the extent to which the gender of the key female protagonists, Dr Higgs and Sue Richardson, acted to attract high levels of opprobrium from the media and their critics.

As front-line workers in health and social care, women are also vulnerable to threats and assault from service users. While men working in social care are more likely to experience all types of violence than women, the incidence of attacks experienced by female members of the social care workforce is still high (Brockman and McLean 2000). In mental health services, high levels of disturbance and distress in service users which occur in the context of situations where they are threatened with detention or coercive powers can increase the likelihood of violence directed towards practitioners (Lindow and McGeorge 2000). A limited number of inquiries have involved the deaths of professionals who provided services to mental health service users; most of these professionals were women working in community settings.

An analysis of the findings of inquiry teams in these cases reveals some differences in approach. The Sharon Campbell Inquiry (Spokes *et al.* 1988) devoted space to examining the training, supervision and experience of Isabel Schwarz, the social worker who died. The report emphasised Isabel Schwarz's inexperience (para 8.20) and recommended specialist training for mental health social workers. The report into the care of Anthony Joseph (Herbert *et al.* 2000) was at pains to stress the extensive experience of Jenny Morrison, the social worker attacked and killed by Joseph. However, the inquiry team did question whether the supervision she was offered was appropriate to her level of experience. The team also suggested that Morrison could have had more direct contact with Joseph than was the case (para 178).

In contrast, the *Dixon Team Inquiry Report* (Dixon *et al.* 1999) did not question the training, management or supervision of PC Nina Mackay who was fatally stabbed by Magdi E. after she entered his flat at the head of a group of police officers. She had removed her protective vest in order to be able to use a ramming device to force open his flat door; she was the only member of the group of nine police officers who had received the training required to operate this device. The inquiry team did suggest that improved inter-agency communication between the police and social services might have resulted in alternative ways of gaining entry to the flat being considered and noted the failure to involve a mediator or negotiator. A lack of attention to police guidelines which warned against conveying an impression of aggression to mentally disordered offenders was also flagged up (Dixon *et al.* 1999: para 510). In this report, the attention was less on the individual practitioner and her manager or supervisor but rather on the extent to which guidelines were followed. The 'masculine' occupation of police officer can be seen to act to protect PC Mackay from the individualised criticism directed at Isabel Schwarz and Jenny Morrison. Indeed, the *Dixon Team Inquiry Report* adopted a particularly respectful tone towards the Metropolitan Police and reported the force's 'firm view' that policy and practice were appropriately implemented in this case (Dixon *et al.* 1999: para 519).

Conclusion

A gender analysis of inquiries demonstrates the value of these reports as commentaries on the way in which mental health services relate to both service users and carers. While a small number of inquiries have an explicit focus on gender, the majority do not acknowledge the issue but may reveal the influence of gender stereotypes in both the practice described and in the judgements reached by the inquiry panel. The view of the inquiry report is usually top-down. Only occasionally, when the inquiry team engage with the viewpoint of family members, does the perspective shift to encompass the user's or carer's view of services. However, even from the somewhat remote perspective of the inquiry team, it is possible to learn much about how mental health services perceive users and carers.

This chapter has emphasised the extent to which mental health services appear to strip users of their family and social identity. This process carries echoes of Goffman's (1961) labelling theory, and this chapter picks up themes from his account of the depersonalisation of the individual who enters the asylum. However, here the focus has been on the ways in which the identity of those who use mental health services both as in-patients and in the community is restricted by the reductive perspective of services. The inquiry reports reveal professional judgement and service delivery to be shaped by stereotyping and a lack of attention to the whole person. Consequently, the capacity of female service users for violent behaviour is not acknowledged, the stresses inherent in their multiple roles are not identified, and the significance of abusive experiences, such as domestic violence, goes unrecognised.

The national strategy for women's mental health services (Department of Health 2002) should have the effect of putting gender issues 'on the map' for mental health services. At the time of writing, the strategy is available in consultation form only, but one of the themes it raises is the question of whether mental health services should be more family oriented. A family friendly mental health service may seem a long way from the world of high risk and danger depicted by mental health inquiries, but one of the aims of this chapter has been to demonstrate how the events recounted by mental health inquiries cannot be dissociated from the real world where people who use mental health services have a social identity. They have families and children whose welfare affects theirs and who are involved in their care. The inquiries suggest that the failure to acknowledge this reality may actually contribute to some of the tragedies described by inquiries. While psychosocial approaches are increasingly advocated within mental health services, they are less frequently used with those service users who attract a 'high risk' label. A focus on women in inquiries allows the social dimension of service users' lives to emerge and reminds us that the protagonists in mental health tragedies have identities as full and as complex as our own.

References

Appleby, L., Shaw, J., Sherrat, J., Amos, T., Robinson, J. and McDonnell, R. (2001) *Safety First: Five Year Report of the National Confidential Inquiry into Suicide and Homicide by People with Mental Illness*, London: Department of Health.

Bhatoa, J.S., Collins, P., McNichol, E. and Whittle, K. (1999) *Bridging the Gaps: Independent Inquiry into the Care and Treatment of Naseer Aslam*, Shipley: Bradford Health Authority.

Blom-Cooper, L., Hally, H. and Murphy, E. (1995) *The Falling Shadow: One Patient's Mental Health Care (1978–1993)*, London: Duckworth.

Brockman, M. and McLean, J. (2000) *Review Paper for the National Task Force: Violence Against Social Care Staff*, London: National Institute for Social Work.

Butler, I. and Drakeford, M. (2003) *Social Policy, Social Welfare and Scandal: How British Public Policy is Made*, London: Palgrave.

Butler-Sloss, Lord Justice E. (1988) *Report on the Inquiry into Child Abuse in Cleveland 1987*, Cmnd. 412. London: HMSO.

Campbell, B. (1988) *Unofficial Secrets*, London: Virago Press.

Coontz, P.D., Lidz, C.W. and Mulvey, E.P. (1994) 'Gender and the assessment of dangerousness in the psychiatric emergency room', *International Journal of Law and Psychiatry*, 17(4): 369–76.

Crawford, L., Devaux, M., Ferris, R. and Hayward, P. (1997) *The Report into the Care and Treatment of Martin Mursell*, London: Camden and Islington Health Authority.

Department of Health (1999) *National Service Framework for Mental Health*, London: Department of Health.

Department of Health (2000) *Safety, Privacy and Dignity in Mental Health Units*, London: Department of Health.

Department of Health (2002) *Women's Mental Health: Into the Mainstream – Strategic Development of Mental Health Care for Women*, London: Department of Health.

Dimond, B., Bowden, P., Sallah, D., Holden, R. and Lingham, R. (1997) *Summary of the Report into the Care and Treatment of Ms. B*, Bristol: Avon Health Authority.

Dixon, K., Herbert, P., Marshall, S., Pinto, R. and Wilkinson, R. (1999) *Dixon Team Inquiry Report: Report of the Independent Inquiry Team to Kensington and Chelsea and Westminster Health Authority, Westminster City Council, Newham Council and East London and the City Health Authority*, London: Kensington and Chelsea and Westminster Health Authority.

Double, V.J., Beilby, C., Rugg, T. and Wilk, R. (1998) *A Difficult Engagement: A Report of the Independent Inquiry into the Care and Treatment of Alfina Magdelena Gabriel*, Huddersfield: Calderdale and Kirklees Health Authority.

Falkov, A. (1996) *Study of Working Together 'Part 8' Reports. Fatal Child Abuse and Parental Psychiatric Disorder: An Analysis of 100 Area Child Protection Committee Case Reviews Conducted under the Terms of Part 8 of Working Together under the Children Act 1989*, London: Department of Health.

Gabbott, J. and Hill, O. (1994) *Inquiry into the Deaths of Jason and Natalia Henry*, London: Haringey Area Child Protection Committee.

Galbraith, A., Humphries, S., Shewan, M. and Southall, C. (2000) *Report of the Independent Inquiry into the Care and Treatment of Patient T*, Durham: County Durham Health Authority.

Goffman, E. (1961) *Asylums: Essays on the Social Situation of Mental Patients and Other Inmates*, New York: Anchor/Doubleday.

Gulliver, A., Buchanan, A., Mason, L. and Makay, J. (1999) *Report of an Independent Inquiry into the Care and Treatment of Mr K.K.*, London: Enfield and Haringey Health Authority.

Harbour, A., Brunning, J., Bolter, L. and Hally, H. (1996) *The Viner Report*, Ferndown, Dorset: Dorset Health Commission.

Herbert, P., Brand, D. and Bird, A. (2000) *Report of the Independent Inquiry into the Care and Treatment of Anthony Joseph*, London: Merton, Sutton and Wandsworth Health Authority and Wandsworth Borough Council.

Hughes, J., Mason, L., Pinto, R. and Williams, P. (1995) *Independent Panel of Inquiry into the Circumstances Surrounding the Deaths of Ellen and Alan Boland*, London: North West London Mental Health NHS Trust.

Humphreys, C. and Thiara, R. (2003) 'Mental health and domestic violence: "I call it symptoms of abuse"', *British Journal of Social Work*, 33(2): 209–26.

Jones, D.W. (2002) *Myths, Madness and the Family: The Impact of Mental Illness on Families*, Basingstoke: Palgrave.

Laing, R.D. and Esterson, A. (1964) *Sanity, Madness and the Family*, London: Tavistock.

Laming, H., Claydon, D. and Davies, C. (2000) *Report of the Independent Inquiry into the Care and Treatment of Ms Justine Cummings: A Report Commissioned by Somerset Health Authority and Somerset Social Services*, Taunton: Somerset Health Authority and Somerset Social Services.

Leff, J. and Vaughan, C. (1985) *Expressed Emotion*, London: Guildford.

Lindow, V. and McGeorge, M. (2000) *Research Review on Violence Against Staff in Mental Health In-patient and Community Settings*, London: Department of Health,

National Task Force Against Social Care Staff. (http://www.doh.gov.uk/violence-taskforce/knowledge.htm)

Maynard, M. (1985) 'The responses of social workers to domestic violence', in J. Pahl (ed.) *Private Violence and Public Policy: The Needs of Battered Women and the Response of the Public Services*, London: Routledge & Kegan Paul.

Mullender, A. (1996) 'Children living with domestic violence', *Adoption and Fostering*, 20, 8–15.

Prior, P.M. (1999) *Gender and Mental Health*, Basingstoke: Macmillan Press.

Reder, P. and Duncan, S. (1996) 'Reflections on child abuse inquiries', in J. Peay (ed.) *Inquiries After Homicide*, London: Duckworth.

Ritchie, J., Q.C., Dick, D. and Lingham, R. (1994) *The Report of the Inquiry into the Care and Treatment of Christopher Clunis*, London: HMSO.

Sainsbury Centre for Mental Health and Mental Health Commission (1997) *The National Visit: A One-day Visit to 309 Acute Psychiatric Wards by the Mental Health Act Commission with the Sainsbury Centre for Mental Health*, London: The Sainsbury Centre for Mental Health.

Social Services Inspectorate (1995) *Domestic Violence and Social Care: A Report on Two Conferences held by the Social Services Inspectorate*, London: Department of Health.

Spokes, J.C., Pare, M. and Royle, G. (1988) *Report to the Committee of Inquiry into the After-Care of Miss Sharon Campbell*, London: HMSO. Cmnd. 440.

Stanley, N. (1997) 'Domestic violence and child abuse: developing social work practice', *Child and Family Social Work*, 2(3): 135–45.

Stanley, N., Penhale, B., Riordan, D., Barbour, R.S. and Holden, S. (2003) *Child Protection and Mental Health Services: Interprofessional Responses to the Needs of Mothers*, Bristol: Policy Press.

Taylor, J., Longhurst, N., Oldridge, P. and Brown, T. (2000) *Report of the Independent Inquiry into the Care and Treatment of Mrs Marie Alawode*, Huntingdon: Cambridgeshire Health Authority.

Twigg, J. and Atkin, K. (1994) *Carers Perceived*, Buckingham: Open University Press.

Ungerson, C. (1990) *Gender and Caring: Work and Welfare in Britain and Scandinavia*, London: Harvester Wheatsheaf.

Wilczynski, A. (1997) *Child Homicide*, London: Greenwich Medical Media Ltd.

Williams, R. and Hennessey, M. (1999) *Strengthening the Net: An Independent Inquiry into the Mental Health and Social Services Care Given to Mrs Anne Murrie*, Reading: Berkshire Health Authority.

Williams, W.J. (1997) *Inquiry into the Circumstances Surrounding the Deaths of Mr Michael Horner and Mrs Hazel Horner*, Nelson: East Lancashire Health Authority.

Chapter 9

Mental health inquiries 1985–2003

Dave Sheppard

Introduction

This chapter attempts to make mental health inquiries more widely known and accessible. While details for obtaining the most recent reports are included here, the disappearance of health authorities has made the task of locating and tracking down inquiries more demanding. However, in many cases, inquiries which were not published by central government can be found in the libraries of the relevant Strategic Health Authorities or hospital trust. Staff there will usually be prepared to provide a copy.

For details of inquiries published since 2003 and of forthcoming inquiries, organizations can subscribe to the IMHL website at http://www.imhl.com

Report to the Secretary of State for Social Services Concerning the Death of Michael Martin at Broadmoor Hospital

Ritchie, S., Higgins, J. and McLoughlin, C.

Michael Martin was born in 1961. He formally came to the attention of the psychiatric services in 1976. In June 1978 he was detained in Bexley Hospital and in November 1979 was transferred to Broadmoor Hospital. He was placed in a seclusion room on 6 July 1984 and given an injection of 500mg of Sodium Amytal and 200mg of Sparine. He was found dead in the seclusion room less than two hours later.

(Published by: DHSS, 1985)

Report of the Committee of Inquiry into the Care and After-care of Sharon Campbell

Spoke, J., Pare, M. and Royle, G.

Isabel Schwarz, a social worker employed by Bexley Social Services Department was killed at her office in Bexley Hospital on 6 July 1984 by Sharon

Campbell (then aged 22), a former client of hers. Pressure from Dr Victor Schwarz finally led to an inquiry into the death of his daughter.

(Published by: HMSO, 1988)

Regional Fact Finding Committee of Inquiry: Care and Treatment of Psychiatric Patients in North Lincolnshire

Unwin, C., Hughes, P., Monahan, A., Morgan, D. and Pattie, A.

Between January 1985 and July 1986, a number of deaths (13 by suicide, two accidental, one case of misadventure and two open verdicts) occurred among patients of St John's Hospital, Lincoln. They were aged between 25 and 79 and were mainly in-patients with the others attending as out-patients or day patients.

(Shortened version published by: Trent Regional Health Authority, 1988)

Report of the Panel of Inquiry Appointed by the North Staffordshire Health Authority to Investigate the Circumstances of the Death of Alma Simpson

Burke, J., Crossfield, E., Gordon, E., Higgins, J. and Taylor, A.

Alma Simpson was born in 1932. She was an in-patient at St Edward's Hospital on a number of occasions between 1982 and 1988. She suffered a number of assaults from other patients and was also the perpetrator of a number of assaults. Her husband complained to the hospital staff and to the local MP of his fears for his wife's safety. During the evening of 31 May 1988, Alma Simpson was brutally assaulted by another patient. She died, aged 53, on 6 June 1988.

(Published by: West Midlands Regional Health Authority, 1990)

Report of the Inquiry into the Circumstances Leading to the Death in Broadmoor Hospital of Joseph Watts

Atha, D., Hunter, C., Newton, K., Williams, T. and Downham, D.

Joseph Watts was born in Jamaica in 1958 and came to England when he was two years old. He was convicted of indecent assault in 1984 and admitted under ss.37/41, Mental Health Act (MHA) 1983 to Broadmoor Hospital. He was placed in a seclusion room on 23 August 1988 and injected with 200mg of Chlorpromazine. Within two minutes of the room being vacated, he was seen to be motionless. Staff re-entered the room but attempts at resuscitation were unsuccessful.

(Published by: Special Hospitals Service Authority (SHSA), 1990)

Inquiry into the NHS Care, Treatment and Management of Stephen Findley

FitzGerald, H., Gatiss, C., Holroyd, A., Johnston, J., Swan, M. and Thompson, T.

Stephen Findley was born in 1968. He was admitted to hospital under s.2, Mental Health Act 1983 in November 1990 after being arrested by police following an incident at a night club where he was found to have in his possession a loaded air pistol and two knives. It was decided that there were no grounds to detain him beyond the expiry of the s.2 order. He left hospital, against medical advice, the following day. Five days later he attacked Oliver Dickens, aged 67, a passer-by in the street, stabbing him 32 times. In June 1991, Stephen Findley was found guilty of manslaughter by reason of diminished responsibility and was made the subject of a Hospital Order with restrictions on discharge.

(Published by: East Cumbria Health Authority, 1991)

Regional Fact Finding Committee of Enquiry into the Admission, Care, Treatment and Discharge of Carol Barratt

Unwin, C., Morgan, D. and Smith, B.

Carol Barratt was admitted under s.2, MHA 1983, to the Psychiatric Unit at Doncaster Royal Infirmary in March 1991 after threatening a young woman with a knife. On 14 April, Carol Barratt was visited by her mother who complained about some bruising on Carol's arms and demanded she be discharged. Dr Silvester, the Responsible Medical Officer, allowed Carol to leave 'against medical advice' after her mother gave an undertaking that she would take full responsibility for her. On 16 April 1991, Carol Barratt visited the Frenchgate Centre Shopping Precinct where she stabbed Emma Brodie, aged 11, in the chest and who subsequently died.

(Summary published by: Trent Regional Health Authority, 1991)

Report of the Panel of Inquiry Appointed by the West Midlands Regional Health Authority, South Birmingham Health Authority and the Special Hospitals Service Authority to Investigate the Case of Kim Kirkman

Dick, D., Shuttleworth, B. and Charlton, J.

Kim Kirkman was born in 1955. He was detained under ss.60/65, MHA 1959 following an assault whilst in hospital and admitted to Broadmoor Hospital in 1973. He was later transferred to Park Lane Hospital in 1983 and to the Reaside Regional Secure Unit in 1989. In February 1990, the Home Secretary agreed to a conditional discharge and Kim Kirkman and his fiancée were offered the tenancy of a flat. On 1 June 1990 he went to the flat for the day and returned to Reaside that evening. Later that day the body of Elizabeth Ford was found in her flat in the same house. Kim Kirkman was arrested and subsequently confessed. He was remanded to Winson Green Prison where he hanged himself in his cell on 5 September 1990.

(Published by: West Midlands RHA, 1991)

Report of the Investigation into Serious Incidents Occurring at the Shrodells Psychiatric Unit: October 1989–November 1990

This investigation followed an earlier inquiry in 1991 which was set up following the death of Margaret Price, aged 67, in December 1990 following an assault by a fellow patient. This second inquiry revealed that in the 15 months prior to December 1990, a further nine serious incidents had taken place. These were: the death of a male patient aged 61 from an aspirin overdose; the treatment of a female patient aged 23 with anorexia who developed neuroleptic malignant syndrome; the arrest by police at the hospital of a male patient aged 28 who objected to being discharged; the absconding and death of a male patient aged 54 who had been assessed as a high suicide risk; the death from untreated hypertension of a female patient aged 42 with manic depression; self-injury by a depressed female patient aged 64 whilst under close observation; death from endocarditis of a male patient aged 46 with a cardiac pacemaker who was suffering from a paranoid illness; death of a male patient aged 39 with epilepsy and encephalitis who died while taking an unsupervised bath; death of a male patient aged 25 who absconded from hospital the day after admission and jumped from a bridge.

(Published by: S.W. Hertfordshire DHA, 1992)

Review of Deaths among Patients of Oxfordshire Health Authority Mental Health Unit: 1990–1991

Rubenstein, V.

This inquiry followed an internal review carried out with the assistance of Professor Morgan, University of Bristol. It examined the circumstances surrounding the death of seven patients of the Mental Health Unit between July 1990 and July 1991.

(Published by: Oxfordshire Health Authority, 1992)

Report of the Committee of Inquiry into Complaints about Ashworth Hospital

Blom-Cooper, L., Brown, M., Dolan, R. and Murphy, E.

The terms of reference of the inquiry, set up in April 1991, were to: investigate allegations of improper care and treatment at Ashworth Hospital contained within the 'Cutting Edge' documentary, *A Special Hospital*, transmitted on 4 May 1991, and any other relevant allegations brought to their attention; and to review the arrangements for handling complaints about the care or treatment provided at Ashworth Hospital, including arrangements for the reference of complaints to the relevant police force.

In September 1991 the Inquiry was put on a statutory footing (s.125, Mental Health Act 1983) and the terms of reference were minimally amended to take into account the fact that some evidence had already been taken. The SHSA subsequently requested the Health Advisory Service (HAS) to look at the hospital two years on from the Inquiry, and to assess current strategy and achievements in the interval. The HAS report, *With Care in Mind Secure*, was published in 1995 by the Health Advisory Service.

(Published by: HMSO, 1992 in two parts)

Report of the Committee of Inquiry into the Death of Freda Latham at Stallington Hospital

Bell, T., Caswell, D., Summerly, M., Thornley, W. and Bishop, P.

Freda Latham, aged 43, a long-standing patient in Stallington Hospital, was taken to the toilet area by a staff nurse at approximately 1pm on 13 May 1992. After she was washed she was taken to a toilet cubicle and seated on the toilet and the tapes of her bib were secured to the inlet pipe of the toilet cistern. She was left unattended and later given her medication while still secured to the toilet. After 45 minutes a member of the domestic staff discovered Freda Latham in the toilet and she was certified dead. The cause of death was inhalation of vomit and suspension.

(Published by: North Staffordshire Health Authority, 1992)

Findings of the Independent Review on the Management of the Case of Erieyune Inweh

Langley, G. and Willis, R.

Erieyune (Erhi) Inweh was born in 1970. She was first admitted to hospital in July 1991 and, after treatment under section, was discharged to a short-term aftercare hostel run by Kingston MIND. In August 1992 she was detained by police under s.136, Mental Health Act 1983 and taken to hospital. She was discharged from section and returned to the MIND hostel in September 1992.

On 30 October 1992, Catherine (Katy) Sullivan, aged 23, a voluntary worker at the MIND hostel, was fatally stabbed 14 times. Erhi Inweh was subsequently detained in Broadmoor Hospital.

(Published: 1992)

Independent Inquiry into the Care and Treatment of Kevin Rooney

Collins, A., Hill, O. and Taylor, M.

Kevin Rooney was born in 1963. He was first admitted in September 1985 under s.4, MHA 1983 to Claybury Hospital after he threatened his family with a pair of scissors and a hatchet. He was compulsorily readmitted to psychiatric hospitals on a number of occasions in the following years. On 4 May 1991 he was admitted informally following threats he made to a woman in a lift but was found to be missing at 4.30pm the following day. On 7 May he was discharged in his absence following a discussion in the course of the routine ward round. On 11 May 1991, Kevin Rooney stabbed Grace Quigley, whom he had known from the previous year when she had also been a patient at Hackney Hospital, 28 times with a lock knife in the presence of her children and a neighbour. He was charged with murder and he pleaded guilty to manslaughter on the grounds of diminished responsibility and sent to Rampton Hospital under ss.37/41, Mental Health Act 1983.

(Published by: North Thames Regional Health Authority, 1992)

Report of the Committee of Inquiry into the Death in Broadmoor Hospital of Orville Blackwood and a Review of the Deaths of Two other Afro-Caribbean Patients. 'Big, Black and Dangerous?'

Prins, H., Backer-Holst, T., Francis, E. and Keitch, I.

Orville Blackwood was born in Jamaica in 1960 and came to the UK at an early age with his mother. He was compulsorily admitted to psychiatric hospitals on eight occasions before being sentenced to prison following conviction for robbery and possession of an imitation firearm in 1986. He was transferred to HMP Grendon Underwood, admitted to a Regional Secure Unit and transferred to Broadmoor in 1987. On the morning of 28 August 1991, Orville Blackwood went voluntarily into a seclusion room in Broadmoor Hospital and, when reviewed that afternoon, was restrained and injected with 150mg Sparine and 150mg Modecate. He died almost immediately. The pathologist gave the cause of death as 'cardiac failure associated with the administration of phenothiazine drugs'.

The terms of reference of the Inquiry, were to: investigate the circumstances leading to the death of Orville Blackwood and to examine the reports of the inquiries into the deaths of Michael Martin and Joseph Watts in the same hospital to identify any significant common factors between all three deaths.

(Published by: SHSA, 1993)

Report of the Inquiry Panel to Investigate the Serious Untoward Incident at the Tudor Rest Home, Nottingham

Tumbull, P., Oyebode, O. and Archer, J.

David Usoro was born in 1965. Between March 1990 and September 1992 he was admitted to Mapperley Hospital, Nottingham, on seven occasions, including under s.3, Mental Health Act 1983. The clinical diagnosis was bipolar affective disorder, complicated by a persistent history of solvent abuse. In 1992 he was discharged to live in his own flat but in April 1993 he moved into the Tudor Rest Home, registered to take seven residents, as he was not coping very well. On 2 August 1993 he was visited by a Senior Registrar in Psychiatry and a Community Psychiatric Nurse. He would not agree to informal admission and was assessed as not meeting the criteria for formal admission. The following evening he attacked two residents with a knife, fatally wounding Samuel Vernon, aged 59. He was subsequently detained in a Special Hospital.

(Published by: Nottingham Health Authority, 1993)

Report of the Inquiry into the Care and Treatment of Christopher Clunis

Ritchie, J., Dick, D. and Lingham, R.

Christopher Clunis was born in 1963. Both his parents came from Jamaica. He began to show odd behaviour in 1986 and went to stay with his father in Jamaica. He was subsequently admitted to Bellevue Hospital, Kingston, Jamaica, where he was diagnosed as having paranoid schizophrenia. He returned to London the following year and was admitted to various psychiatric hospitals on a number of occasions in the following years. In August 1992, Christopher Clunis was detained under s.3, MHA 1983 and was transferred from Kneesworth House to Guy's Hospital. He was discharged in September 1992 to accommodation in Haringey. On 17 December 1992, Christopher Clunis stabbed Jonathan Zito, a complete stranger, to death at Finsbury Park Tube Station. He pleaded guilty to manslaughter on 28 June 1993 and sent to Rampton Hospital under ss.37/41, Mental Health Act 1983.

(Published by: HMSO, 1994)

North West London Mental Health Services Inquiry

Goose, M., McLoughlin, C. and Owens, D.

The inquiry arose from the concerns of the General Manager of the then Parkside Health Authority that there appeared to have been an unduly high number of 'serious incidents' within the Mental Health Unit, Parkside District. Of the 21 incidents examined, ten of these involved deaths which were definite or probable suicides and four were episodes of non-fatal self-harm. There were four deaths of patients from a physical illness, two cases involved alleged sexual assault by one patient on another and the final case involved attacks on staff.

(Published by: North West London Mental Health NHS Trust, 1994)

Report of the Review into the Mental Health Services of South Devon Healthcare Trust

Blom-Cooper, L., Hally, H. and Murphy, E.

A cluster of ten suicides of patients and former patients of the service between June 1988 and June 1989 caused local concern about the style of service and about the management of the Edith Morgan Unit. Various review reports over the preceding seven years had commented on: the fragmentation and lack of co-ordination between the in-patient and community based parts of the service; the lack of professional leadership, especially in the in-patient services; the unsuitability of the unit for acute psychiatric in-patient work in terms of its siting, lay-out, size and integration with community services; the inability of the services to manage seriously disturbed people with difficult behaviours and the lack of appropriate facilities for this group.

(Published by: South Devon Healthcare Trust, 1994)

Report of the Inquiry into Aspects of Learning Disabilities Services Managed by Thameside Community Healthcare NHS Trust

Warner, N., Rendle, H. and Freeman, T.

This followed concerns raised by relatives and the local Community Health Council in respect of six patients with learning difficulties. Complaints included issues surrounding the investigation of complaints and communications with relatives.

(Published by: Thameside Community Healthcare, 1994)

Report of the Independent Panel of Inquiry Examining the Case of Michael Buchanan

Heginbotham, C., Carr, J., Hale, R., Walsh, T. and Warren, L.

Michael Buchanan was born in 1964. He was first admitted to a psychiatric hospital in 1983 and was subsequently admitted on a further 12 occasions. He was last admitted in 1992 to Shenley Hospital under s.37, MHA 1983. Following an aftercare meeting, he was discharged on 21 August 1992 after 22 days on the ward to a Church Army Hostel. On 10 September 1992, Michael Buchanan entered an underground car park on the Stonebridge Park Estate, Harlesden, where Frederick Graver, a 54-year-old former policeman, had just parked his car. Michael Buchanan attacked him with a piece of wood, knocking him to the ground. Frederick Graver died two days later.

(Published by: North West London Mental Health NHS Trust, 1994)

Inquiry into the Deaths of Jason and Natalia Henry

Gabbott, J. and Hill, O.

Sharon Dalson was born in 1969. Her two children, Jason and Natalia Henry, were placed on the Child Protection Register in 1988 after they were left on their own but removed from the Register in June 1991. In 1991, Sharon was taken to hospital by the police and subsequently detained under s.2, MHA 1983. She was discharged a week later but arrested later that month after she held a knife to the children's throats and threatened suicide. In 1992 she was detained in hospital under s.37, MHA 1983. In April 1992 she was given 'trial leave' and returned home and began attending the day hospital. Her children, who were being cared for by their grandmother, were placed on the Child Protection Register again in June 1992. In August 1992, Sharon Dalson strangled Jason, aged six and suffocated Natalia, aged five. She admitted the manslaughter of her children and was sent to Rampton Hospital.

(Published by: Haringey Area Child Protection Committee, 1994)

The Falling Shadow: One Patient's Mental Health Care 1978–1993

Blom-Cooper, L., Hally, H. and Murphy, E.

Andrew Robinson was born in 1957. He was first admitted to a psychiatric unit in 1977. In 1978, following conviction for carrying a firearm with intent to endanger the life of a female university student and assault occasioning actual bodily harm, he was made the subject of a Hospital Order with restrictions and admitted to Broadmoor Hospital. He was transferred to a local hospital in 1981 and conditionally discharged in 1983. Andrew Robinson was admitted on seven occasions to the Edith Morgan Centre between 1986 and his last admission on 9 June 1993 when he was detained for treatment. On 1 September 1993, Georgina Robinson, aged 27, an occupational therapist at the Edith Morgan Centre at Torbay District Hospital, was fatally wounded by Andrew Robinson who was still detained under s.3, Mental Health Act 1983. She subsequently died on 7 October 1993. Andrew Robinson pleaded guilty to manslaughter on the grounds of diminished responsibility and was detained under a Hospital Order with restrictions (ss.37/41, Mental Health Act 1983) and readmitted to Broadmoor Hospital.

(Published by: Duckworth, 1995)

Report of the Independent Panel of Inquiry into the Circumstances Surrounding the Deaths of Ellen and Alan Boland

Hughes, J., Mason, L., Pinto, R. and Williams, P.

Alan Boland suffered from depression and alcoholism. He was, over a period of nine years, seen by over 20 doctors whilst an outpatient at the Paterson Wing, North West London Mental Health NHS Trust. He commenced attending the day hospital in 1993. On the evening of 5 March 1994, it is alleged that he came home to the flat which he shared with his mother, aged 71, strangled her and hit her repeatedly about the head with a hammer. He spent the rest of the night in the flat, though upstairs in his own bedroom, leaving around midday on 6 March by the fire escape, which meant he did not have to pass his mother's body in the hall. On 25 July 1994, whilst on remand, he was found dead in his cell at Wandsworth Prison, having hanged himself.

(Published by: North West London Mental Health NHS Trust, 1995)

Report of the Inquiry into the Circumstances Leading to the Death of Jonathan Newby (a Volunteer Worker)

Davies, N., Lingham, R., Prior, C. and Sims, A.

John Rous was born in 1946. He was first admitted to a psychiatric hospital in 1965 for an amphetamine psychosis, when a diagnosis of personality disorder was made. He had several further formal admissions. He had a street life of some 20 years before he took up residence in Jacqui Porter House, run by Oxford Cyrenians, in 1992. Jonathan Newby began working for the Cyrenians as a volunteer in April 1993 and was the only person on duty when he was attacked by John Rous in the office of the hostel. He was 22 years old when he died. John Rous was sent to Broadmoor Hospital.

(Published by: Oxfordshire Health, 1995)

The Woodley Team Report: Report of the Independent Review Panel to East London and the City Health Authority and Newham Council

Woodley, L., Dixon, K., Lindow, V., Oyebode, O., Sandford, T. and Simblet, S.

Stephen Laudat was born in 1968. His mother suffered from mental illness. In 1991 he was jailed for four years for thefts and robberies, one involving a knife. His mental health deteriorated in prison and he was transferred under ss.47/49, MHA1983, initially to the Interim Secure Unit at Hackney Hospital and, in June 1992, to Kneesworth House Hospital. He was discharged in December 1993. In July 1994, he stabbed to death Bryan Bennett, aged 56, at a Day Centre in Newham where both attended. He was sent to Rampton Hospital.
(Published by: East London and The City Health Authority, 1995)

The Brian Doherty Inquiry: Report of the Inquiry Team to the Western Health and Social Services Board

Fenton, G., Deane, E., Herron, S. and Mullen, B.

Brian Doherty was born in 1974. He had contact with 20 different caring agencies over a ten-year period prior to the killing. These included special schools, children's homes, a training school, various young offender institutions, the Probation Service, and various hospitals. There was no evidence of a formal mental illness but a diagnosis of severe personality disorder of the dissocial type and mild learning disability. This dual diagnosis caused placement problems. He had a number of admissions to various hospitals as both a formal and informal patient. He was admitted to Tyrone and Fermanagh Hospital on 13 January 1994 (his second informal admission that month) following referral from the Accident and Emergency Department of Tyrone County Hospital. He discharged himself, contrary to medical advice on 18 January 1994. Later that day he abducted and killed Kieran Hegarty, aged 11. He was sentenced to life imprisonment for manslaughter and ten years for kidnapping.
(Published by: Western Health and Social Services Board, 1995)

Report of the Enquiry into the Care and Treatment of Philip McFadden

Dyer, J., McCall-Smith, E., Sutherland, J. and Malcolm, J.

Philip McFadden was born in 1975. He began to show signs of mental illness in 1990 and was, for eight months, a patient in the adolescent unit of

Gartnavel Royal Hospital. He continued to have medication and psychiatric contact for the next two years. He was living with his family and his mother contacted the GP practice on several times on 17 June 1994 concerned about his mental state. The police went to the home the same day which resulted in the death of a 28-year-old police constable, Lewis Fulton, and a knife wound to another policeman. Philip McFadden was to have been tried on murder charges but, at the High Court in Edinburgh in September 1994, was found insane in bar of trial and was sent to the State Hospital at Carstairs.

The Secretary of State for Scotland told the Mental Welfare Commission for Scotland that as Philip McFadden had been found insane in bar of trial, the Commission's enquiry was required to avoid any possibility of prejudice to a future trial, and that it should concern itself only with the psychiatric care and treatment received by Philip McFadden and not with the circumstances of the incident involving the police.

(Published by: the Scottish Office, 1995)

The Grey Report: Report of the Independent Inquiry Team into the Care and Treatment of Kenneth Grey

Mishcon, J., Dick, D., Welch, N., Sheehan, A. and Mackay, A.

Kenneth Grey was born in 1970. From the age of about 13, he started to use cannabis and then began to steal in order to buy drugs. The majority of his convictions were for burglary and theft and he had also been convicted for possessing cannabis on a number of occasions. He had three convictions for offences of violence. While in custody in Pentonville Prison he was diagnosed as mentally ill and he was transferred to the Psychiatric Intensive Care Unit (PICU) of Hackney Hospital on 23 November 1994 under s.47 of the MHA 1983 which was replaced two days later by a s.2 MHA Order, which was discharged prior to his transfer to an open ward. Within two hours of arriving on the open ward, he went missing and never returned. On the evening of 1 January 1995, Kenneth Grey murdered his mother, apparently following an argument with her about religion. He was charged with the murder of his mother and on 25 July 1995 he appeared at the Old Bailey where his guilty plea to manslaughter on the grounds of diminished responsibility was accepted. Expert psychiatric evidence was called by both the Prosecution and the Defence, but the sentencing Judge was persuaded by the evidence of the Prosecution expert that Kenneth Grey was suffering from a drug induced psychosis at the time of the murder and that he was no longer showing any signs of mental illness. He was sentenced to seven years imprisonment.

(Published by: East London & The City Health Authority, 1995)

Report of an Independent Joint Agency Review for Southampton Community Health Services NHS Trust and Hampshire County Social Services Department into the Circumstances Surrounding the Deaths of GC, PJ AND TA

Muijen, M.

GC, PJ and TA all died alone at home during the months of June and July 1995. Each of the three men was known to the Waterside and Romsey Community Mental Health Team, to the Department of Psychiatry, and to Hampshire Social Services. An open verdict was delivered on the deaths of TA and GC. A verdict of suicide was made in respect of PJ.

The published part of the review gives no details of the three men but an article headed, 'Starving man died while dog was cared for', appeared in the *Daily Telegraph* on 2 September 1995 describing, 'A man who gave away his dog because he could not afford to feed it'. According to the article, the RSPCA dog warden and the police reported the man's condition to social services but care workers failed to visit Mr Anstey at his home in Southampton. His body was found by police more than two weeks later. TA was under a supervision order after being convicted of assaulting two police officers in June 1994. But probation officers had not visited him since April 1995 – three months before he was found dead.

(Published by: Hampshire County Council Social Services Committee, 1996)

The Case of Jason Mitchell: Report of the Independent Panel of Inquiry

Blom-Cooper, L., Grounds, A., Guinan, P., Parker, A. and Taylor, M.

Jason Mitchell was born in 1970. He was seen by a psychiatrist on a number of occasions whilst he was serving a period of two years' youth custody for robbery and other offences. In 1990 he attacked a cleaner at St Barnabas Church, Epsom, and was charged with attempted murder and other offences. He subsequently pleaded guilty to common assault and possession of offensive weapons and he was made the subject of a hospital order with restrictions. In May 1994 he moved to shared accommodation run by MIND in Felixstowe but, following disruptive behaviour, was readmitted to Easton House as an informal patient. On 9 December 1994 he left the unit and failed to return. On 20 December 1994 he was arrested following the discovery by police of the bodies of his father, aged 54, and neighbours, Arthur and Shirley Wilson, both aged 65.

In July 1995, Jason Mitchell was sentenced to three terms of life imprisonment for manslaughter on the grounds of diminished responsibility. In May

1996 he successfully appealed and was instead made the subject of a hospital order with restrictions (ss.37/41).

(Published by: Duckworth, 1996)

The Viner Report: The Report of the Independent Inquiry into the Circumstances Surrounding the Deaths of Robert and Muriel Viner

Harbour, A., Brunning, J., Bolter, L. and Hally, H.

Robert Viner was born in 1953. He first received treatment for mental illness in 1971 and, in 1976 he moved to Dorset to live with his mother. Apart from two brief in-patient admissions as an informal patient in 1981 and 1982, he lived with and was cared for by his mother with varying levels of contact with mental health services varied over the years. On 19 April 1995, a community psychiatric nurse visited and, because of the deteriorating situation, contacted a psychiatrist and requested that the offer of a hospital bed be made to Robert to give his mother a break. Later that day, while sitting in an armchair in her living room, Muriel Viner, aged 76, died from blows to the head. Robert Viner died some time later from an overdose of drugs. His body was found in the bath upstairs.

(Published by: Dorset Health Commission, 1996)

Report of the Independent Inquiry Team into the Care and Treatment of Nilesh Gadher

Main, J., Wilkins, J., Pope, D. and Manikon, S.

Nilesh Gadher was born in 1958. He qualified as a pharmacist and worked in this capacity for about five years. He was first referred to a psychiatrist in 1984 when a diagnosis of paranoid schizophrenia was made. In May 1985 he was charged with forging prescriptions and placed on probation and the following year he was struck off the Pharmaceutical Register. He was admitted to hospital on three occasions under the provisions of the Mental Health Act 1983.

On 6 September 1994, Nilesh Gadher ran over and killed Sanita Kaura, aged 27, a complete stranger. He was found unfit to plead at the Old Bailey in July 1995 and sent to Ashworth Special Hospital. On 2 October 1997 he admitted manslaughter at the Old Bailey and returned to Ashworth Hospital after the court imposed a hospital order with restrictions on discharge.

(Published by: Ealing, Hammersmith and Hounslow Health Authority, 1996)

The Hampshire Report: Report of the Independent Inquiry into the Care and Treatment of Francis Hampshire

Mishcon, J., Dick, D., Milne, L., Beard, P. and Mackay, J.

Frank Hampshire was born in 1933 and he married Catherine in 1957. They were both teachers. In June 1985 he was referred by his GP to the psychiatric services at Goodmayes Hospital. Over the next nine years he was admitted to hospital on two occasions, once under section. He was also seen as an out-patient and was visited by a Community Psychiatric Nurse. At about midnight on 31 May 1994, Frank Hampshire killed his wife, aged 62, stabbing her over 300 times in the head and neck.

On 5 December 1994, his plea of guilty to manslaughter on the grounds of diminished responsibility was accepted and he was detained in Rampton Hospital. Although Frank Hampshire was an out-patient at the time of his wife's death, there was no internal inquiry. Furthermore, there was confusion as to whether or not there was a requirement to hold an independent inquiry, as a result of which this inquiry was not set up until the end of 1995.

(Published by: Redbridge and Waltham Forest Health Authority, 1996)

The Report of the Inquiry into the Care and Treatment of Shaun Armstrong

Freeman, C., Brown, A., Dunleavy, D. and Graham, F.

Shaun Armstrong was born in 1962. He had received in-patient care on three different wards at Hartlepool General Hospital during his five informal admissions between March 1992 and June 1993. He subsequently attended three out-patient appointments but failed to keep his appointment on 5 May 1994. On the afternoon of 30 June 1994 Rose (Rosie) Palmer, aged three, left her home in Hartlepool to buy an ice cream. On 3 July 1994 her body was found by the Police in a plastic bag at the home of Shaun Armstrong who lived approximately 50 yards away. Rosie had been raped, otherwise sexually abused and her body had been mutilated following her death.

Shaun Armstrong was arrested and pleaded guilty to murder and was sentenced to life imprisonment. In passing sentence, the Judge stated that Shaun Armstrong was a severely disordered personality but had been fully responsible for his actions at the time of the murder. He was detained at Wakefield Prison.

(Published by: Tees Health Authority, 1996)

Report of the Inquiry into the Treatment and Care of Raymond Sinclair

Lingham, R., Candy, J. and Bray, J.

Raymond Sinclair was born in 1961. He was informally admitted to Joyce Green Hospital in April 1994 when an initial diagnosis of a 'hypomanic episode' was made. He was returned to the ward by the police on three occasions (once under s.136, MHA 1983). He was discharged in June 1994 but readmitted for one week in August 1994 after he threatened his brother with a bread knife. He returned to live with his mother in her one-bedroomed flat. He was seen as an out-patient and supported by community psychiatric nurses and a social worker. On 3 November 1994, Raymond Sinclair fatally stabbed his mother, Mary Povey, 15 times with a vegetable knife. On 10 November 1995 he was convicted of manslaughter and detained in Broadmoor Hospital.

(Published by: West Kent Health Authority, 1996)

Report of the Independent Inquiry Team into the Care and Treatment of Kumbi Mabota

Holwill, D., Ndegwa, D., Stanner, S., Welch, N. and Mackay, J.

Kumbi Mabota was born in 1964 and came to the UK in 1993. On 6 April 1994, he went to the flat of his girlfriend, Lidie Diema, age 22, where there was a struggle during which time her nose was broken. By the time the Police had arrived, he had swallowed a large quantity of bleach in an attempt to commit suicide. He was arrested and initially taken to casualty where he was assessed and formally detained at Claybury Hospital. On 14 April 1994 he was transferred to an open ward but absconded from hospital the following day. Two days later Lidie Diema was found murdered, having been kicked and beaten to death. There was a large number of stab wounds on her back. In October 1995 Kumbi Mabota was convicted of murder.

(Published by: Redbridge & Waltham Forest Health Authority, 1996)

Caring for the Carer – Report of the Inquiry into the Care of Keith Taylor

Barlow, R., Crook, J., Kingdon, D. and McGinnis, P.

Keith Taylor was born in 1948. He was first admitted to hospital in April 1994 under section due to a psychotic illness. He was discharged the following month but readmitted informally a couple of weeks later as he was feeling suicidal. In September 1994, he was again admitted informally and discharged a few days later. He returned to live with his father who suffered from Alzheimer's disease but on 16 February 1995 he stabbed his father, aged 74, to death. On 17 July 1995 he pleaded to manslaughter on the grounds of diminished responsibility and was made the subject of a hospital order with restrictions on discharge.

(Published by: Tees Health Authority, Poole House, 1996)

West Cheshire NHS Trust – Report into Seven Unexpected Deaths and One Serious Incident of Self-Harm between January 1994 and January 1996

Horne, J., Brooker, C. and Seager, P.

The inquiry examined issues relating to five deaths which involved in-patients (although two of the deaths took place off the ward), and two deaths which occurred following discharge. Four of the deaths were by hanging (two off the ward), two on the railway line and one by asphyxiation.

(Published by: West Cheshire NHS Trust, 1996)

Report of the Inquiry into the Care of Anthony Smith

Wood, J., Ashman, M., Davies, C., Lloyd, H. and Lockett, K.

Anthony Smith was born in 1971. He was referred by his GP in May 1995 for an urgent out-patient appointment after he disclosed auditory hallucinations and paranoid features. He was admitted informally on 14 June. He was discharged on 6 July 1995 and visited twice by a community support nurse. On 8 August, he killed his mother, Gwendoline Smith, and his half-brother, David, aged 12, and then went to his GP's surgery and reported their deaths.

In March 1996 he was convicted of manslaughter on the grounds of diminished responsibility and was made the subject of a hospital order with restrictions on discharge.

(Published by: Southern Derbyshire Health Authority, 1996)

Report to City of York Council following the Death of Zoe Fairley

Myers, M., Maughan, J., Freeman, T. and Eliatamby, A.

Zoe Fairley, aged 21, who had a learning disability, died in September 1995 whilst being restrained for 50 minutes in a local authority care home where she was receiving respite care. She suffocated whilst being restrained in a 'prone restraint procedure' by four workers with a combined weight of 54 stone.

(Published by: City of York Council, 1996)

Report of the Independent Inquiry into the Treatment and Care of Richard John Burton

Chapman, H., Ashman, M., Oyebode, O. and Rogers, B.

Richard Burton was born in 1964. He first received in-patient care as an informal patient for depression in 1983 whilst he was a university student. He was admitted following an overdose in 1987 and briefly attended a day hospital. In April 1995, he was seen by his GP and prescribed Fluoxetine for depression. On 5 May he attended Leicestershire Royal Infirmary following an overdose of Fluoxetine the previous day. An out-patient appointment with a psychiatrist was arranged. On 11 May, Richard Burton stabbed to death Janice Symons, aged 57, whose home he had moved into a couple of months before. He was made the subject of a hospital order, with restrictions on 31 July 1996 after he pleaded guilty to manslaughter on the grounds of diminished responsibility.

(Published by: Leicestershire Health Authority, 1996)

Report of the Independent Inquiry into the Care and Treatment of Richard Stoker

Brown, A., Harrop, F., Cronin, H. and Harman, J.

Richard Stoker was born in 1936. In 1976 he was convicted of manslaughter on the grounds of diminished responsibility following the death of his mother-in-law and admitted to Rampton Hospital. In July 1985 he was transferred to a Regional Secure Unit and admitted to St Georges Hospital, Morpeth, in November 1986. In June 1987 he obtained a conditional discharge and left hospital in January 1988.

In March 1996 he was convicted of manslaughter on the grounds of diminished responsibility, following the death in her flat of his neighbour, Halina Szymczuk, aged 48, who was repeatedly stabbed. At the time of her death he was still a conditionally discharged restricted patient. He was made the subject of a further hospital order with restrictions (ss.37/41) and sent to Rampton Hospital.

(Published by: Northumberland Health Authority, 1996)

Learning Lessons: Report into the Events Leading to the Incident at St John's Way Medical Centre in December 1995

Nicholson, R., Pevsner, F., Schwabenland, C. and Babulall, M.

Maria Caseiro was born in 1966. In September 1994, she was admitted informally to hospital after expressing suicidal thoughts and auditory hallucinations. She was later detained under s.3. She unsuccessfully appealed to a

Mental Health Review Tribunal in December 1994. At her appeal to a Mental Health Review Tribunal on 24 November 1995, the RMO reported that although her mental illness was not of a nature or degree to warrant continued detention, it was recommended that discharge be deferred until 1 December to enable aftercare arrangements to be made. The tribunal however discharged her immediately to bed and breakfast accommodation.

On 12 December she attended her GP's surgery at St John's Way Medical Centre requesting medication and threatened her GP with a knife. Another GP, Dr Inwald, aged 59, came to the GP's aid and was stabbed twice. In May 1996, Maria Caseiro was made the subject of a hospital order with restrictions on discharge (ss.37/41).

(Published by: Camden and Islington Health Authority, 1996)

Bolton Hospitals NHS Trust – Independent External Review into Mental Health Services

Hetherington, S., Whybourn, L. and Junaid, O.

The report describes a review carried out in December 1996 of patient care and management arrangements.

(Published by: Bolton Hospitals NHS Trust, 1997)

The Report into the Care and Treatment of Martin Mursell

Crawford, L., Devaux, M., Ferris, R. and Hayward, P.

Martin Mursell was born in 1967. His mental illness began at about the age of 17 but was not diagnosed until his first admission to hospital four years later. In May 1988 he seriously assaulted his girlfriend. He was sentenced to two months imprisonment, suspended for one year, for actual bodily harm.

In February 1989 he was admitted to hospital under s.2 and further detained under s.3. He was given leave under s.17 at the end of March which continued until discharged in July 1989. He was subsequently admitted to hospital on four further occasions under s.3.

In October 1994 while waiting for housing of his own to become available, he killed his step-father, Joseph Collins, aged 37, and attempted to kill his mother Mary Collins. In January 1996, he pleaded guilty to murder and attempted murder and was sentenced to life, and ten years imprisonment to run concurrently. He was subsequently transferred to Rampton Hospital.

(Published by: Camden and Islington Health Authority, 1997)

Practice, Planning and Partnership: The Lessons to be Learned from the Case of Susan Patricia Joughin

Leslie, A.

Susan Joughin had an extensive and complex history of mental illness and had been admitted to hospital 14 times between 1980 and 1992. In February 1995, Susan Joughin, then aged 41, went to the police station and told them that she had injured her two daughters, then aged 7 years and 4 years. The younger child was pronounced dead on arrival at hospital but the older child survived. In March 1996 Susan Joughin pleaded guilty to manslaughter on the grounds of diminished responsibility and was made the subject of a hospital order with restrictions on discharge.

(Published by: the Isle of Man Government, 1997)

Report of the Independent Inquiry into the Major Employment and Ethical Issues Arising from the Events Leading to the Trial of Amanda Jenkinson

Bullock, R., Edwards, C. and Farrand, I.

Amanda Jenkinson, aged 37, was employed from 1990 to 1995 on the Intensive Therapy Unit at Bassetlaw Hospital. In November 1996 she received a sentence of five years imprisonment for causing grievous bodily harm to Kathleen Temple, aged 67. She had tampered with the patient's life-support equipment to discredit a colleague on her unit. She had hidden from hospital authorities a history of mental illness.

(Published by: North Nottinghamshire Health Authority, 1997)

Report of the Independent Inquiry Team – Presented to Bromley Health Authority, South East London Probation Service, and Bromley SSD

Dixon, K., Gulliver, A., Reed, J., Rhys, M. and Mackay, J.

Evan B. was born in 1954. Half his early life was spent in custodial/institutional care. On 23 April 1996, Evan B. killed his estranged wife Susan. He pleaded guilty to manslaughter in August 1996. Prior to her death, he had been living in a probation hostel in Bromley and had been admitted and discharged from a psychiatric unit.

(Published by: Bromley Health Authority, 1997)

Report of the Inquiry into the Treatment and Care of Darren Carr

Richardson, G., Chiswick, D. and Nutting, I.

Darren Carr was convicted in April 1996 for manslaughter on the grounds of diminished responsibility, after setting fire to the home of his landlady. Susan Hearmon, aged 25, and her two children, Kylie, aged 6 and Julie, aged 4, died in the fire. He was sentenced to life imprisonment.

(Published by Berkshire Health Authority, 1997)

Report of the Independent Inquiry into the Treatment and Care of Peter Richard Winship

Chapman, H., Higgins, J. and Sandford, T.

Peter Winship was born in 1976. He admitted manslaughter on the grounds of diminished responsibility after stabbing his father and hitting him repeatedly with a hammer in July 1996. He appeared at Nottingham Crown Court in December 1996 and was made the subject of a hospital order with restrictions (ss.37/41).

(Published by: Nottingham Health Authority, 1997)

Report of an Investigation into the Learning Disability Service at Earls House and Recommendations for Action

Brockington, J. and McDonough, J.

The investigation followed serious misconduct allegations against 16 staff. Six staff have been dismissed (two were reported to and are now the subject of investigation by their professional body), three received written warnings. Five are still ongoing and two have resulted in no disciplinary action being taken.

(Published by: Community Health Care: North Durham, 1997)

Scourie Inquiry – Report of the Investigating Team

Scourie Inquiry Team

Donald MacLeod, aged 54, who suffered from schizophrenia, attacked the Rev. John MacPherson at a Remembrance Day service in Scourie, Sutherland.

(Published by: Highland Health Board, 1997)

Report of the Independent Panel of Inquiry into the Treatment and Care of Paul Smith

Mishcon, J., Hayes, L., Lowe, M. and Talbot, M.

Paul Smith was born in 1966. He was found guilty of manslaughter on the grounds of diminished responsibility after killing his mother's boyfriend, John McCluskey, in November 1995. He was made the subject of a hospital order with restrictions (ss.37/41).

(Published by North West Anglia Health Authority, 1997)

Report of the Inquiry into the Events Leading to the Death of David Howell

Chambers, J., Taylor, T., McGowran, T., Roy, D. and Hendley, B.

David Howell, aged 40, was shot dead in November 1996 by Police who feared he was about to kill a store manager during a hold-up at a supermarket.

(Published by: Birmingham Health Authority, 1997)

Report of the Inquiry into the Care and Treatment of Gilbert Kopernik-Steckel

Greenwell, J., Proctor, A. and Jones, A.

Gilbert Kopernik-Steckel stabbed his mother, Suzanne, aged 57, to death in January 1996 and then cut his own throat.

(Published by: Croydon Health Authority, 1997)

Report of the Independent Panel of Inquiry into the Circumstances Surrounding the Absconsion of Trevor Holland from the Care of Horizon NHS Trust on 29 August 1996

Prins, H., Marshall, A. and Day, K.

Trevor Holland was made the subject of a hospital order (s.37) on 4 June 1996. He was detained at the Eric Shepherd Unit, a medium secure unit. He absconded whilst on a supervised visit to Chessington World of Adventures on 29 August 1996 and subsequently apprehended two days later.

(Published by: Horizon NHS Trust, 1997)

Report of the Inquiry into the Treatment and Care of Five Individual Patients by Oldham NHS Trust Mental Health Services Commissioned by West Pennine Health Authority

Sedgman, J., Graham, M., Moran, J. and Wilkins, J.

This inquiry was triggered by the death of Harry Johnstone, aged 79, who was killed by Paul Medley, aged 36, after he walked out of the Royal Oldham Hospital in September 1994. The remit of the inquiry was subsequently extended to include the suicide of two in-patients and one out-patient, as well as the death of a unit resident in the following 20 months.

(Published by: West Pennine Health Authority, 1997)

Report of the Independent Inquiry into the Treatment and Care of Doris Walsh

Mishcon, J., Mason, L., Stanner, S., Dick, D. and Mackay, J.

In July 1995, Doris Walsh, aged 51, started a fire in her flat which led to the deaths of her neighbour Tom Redshaw and his son, Richard, aged 13.

(Published by: Coventry Health Authority, 1997)

Summary of the Report of the Inquiry into the Treatment and Care of Ms B

Dimond, B., Bowden, P., Sallah, D., Holden, R. and Lingham, R.

Ms B pleaded guilty in May 1996 to manslaughter on the grounds of diminished responsibility after the death of her father, aged 56, in August 1995. At the time of the homicide she was subject to s.3 and had been granted s.17 leave from Fromeside Regional Secure Unit. She was subsequently made the subject of a hospital order with restrictions (ss.37/41) and admitted to Broadmoor Hospital.

(Published by: Avon Health Authority, 1997)

Inquiry into the Circumstances Surrounding the Deaths of Michael and Hazel Horner

Williams, W.J., Campbell, A., Hayward, T. and Tallentire, P.

Michael Horner was discharged from an acute psychiatric ward in March 1996. The following evening he telephoned the ward to tell them he had killed his wife Hazel. By the time the police got to the house he had hanged himself.

(Published by: East Lancashire Health Authority, 1997)

The Report of the Independent Inquiry into the Care and Treatment of William Scott

Price, C., Dick, D., Milne, I. and Mackay, J.

William Scott killed his ex-girlfriend, Denise Palmacci, in July 1996. He subsequently pleaded guilty to manslaughter and in April 1997 was made the subject of a hospital order with restrictions (ss.37/41).

(Published by: Bedfordshire Health Authority, 1997)

Inquiry into the Treatment and Care of Damian Witts

Lingham, R. and Candy, J.

Damian Witts killed his brother in September 1995. He subsequently pleaded guilty to manslaughter and in July 1996 was made the subject of a hospital order with restrictions (ss.37/41).

(Published by: Gloucestershire Health Authority, 1997)

Report of the Independent Inquiry into the Treatment and Care of Norman Dunn

Keating, D., Collins, P. and Walmsley, S.

Norman Dunn was convicted in June 1996 of manslaughter on the grounds of diminished responsibility, following the death of his mother, Eileen McLachlan, aged 73, in July 1995. He was made the subject of a hospital order with restrictions (ss.37/41).

(Published by: Newcastle and North Tyneside Health Authority, 1997)

Report of the Independent Inquiry into the Care and Treatment of James Ross Stemp

Adams, J., Douglas, P., McIntegart, J. and Mitchell, S.

James Stemp was convicted in July 1996 of killing John Dawson. He was sentenced to life imprisonment, 12 years for kidnapping and 7 years each for possessing a firearm and attempted robbery, all running concurrently.

(Published by: Leicestershire Health Authority, 1997)

'Sharing the Burden' – An Independent Inquiry into the Care and Treatment of Desmond Ledgester

Double, V.J., McGinnis, P., Nelson, T. and Pritlove, J.

Desmond Ledgester, aged 26, killed a neighbour, Malcolm Hodgson, aged 60, in June 1995, three months after he was discharged, whilst absent without leave, from a psychiatric ward at Halifax General Hospital where he had been an informal patient. In December 1995, Desmond Ledgester pleaded guilty to manslaughter and was made the subject of a hospital order with restrictions on discharge (ss.37/41).

(Published by: Calderdale and Kirklees Health Authority, 1998)

Report of the Independent Inquiry into the Treatment and Care of Sanjay Kumar Patel

Prins, H., Swan, M., Ashman, M. and Steele, G.

Sanjay Patel (then aged 19) killed Patrick Cullen, aged 58, in October 1995. He pleaded guilty to manslaughter on the grounds of diminished responsibility and was sentenced to life imprisonment in December 1996.

(Published by: Leicestershire Health Authority, 1998)

Report of the Inquiry into the Care and Treatment of Christopher Edwards and Richard Linford

Coonan, K., Bluglass, R., Halliday, G., Jenkins, M. and Kelly, O.

Richard Linford was made the subject of a hospital order with restrictions (ss.37/41) in April 1995 after he was convicted of the manslaughter of Christopher Edwards, aged 30, in November 1994, whilst in Chelmsford Prison.

(Published by: North Essex Health Authority, 1998)

Independent Longcare Inquiry

Burgner, T., Russell, P., Whitehead, S., Tinnion, J. and Phipps, L.

The inquiry was set up in September 1997 following the conviction of staff members for abusing residents at Stoke Place Mansion and Stoke Green House, Stoke Poges, Buckinghamshire.

(Published by: Buckinghamshire County Council, 1998)

Report of the Inquiry into the Treatment and Care of Mr D Eske

Johns, G., Ovshinsky, G. and Wood, S.

Daniel Eske was made the subject of a hospital order with restrictions (ss.37/41) in July 1997 after he admitted the manslaughter of his mother, Patricia, aged 48, in November 1996.

(Published by: Southampton and SW Hampshire Health Authority, 1998)

Report of the Independent Inquiry into the Circumstances Leading to the Death of Brenda Horrod

Armstrong, W., Calloway, P., Arnold, M. and Schofield, T.

Peter Horrod was made the subject of a hospital order with restrictions (ss.37/41) in December 1995 after he admitted the manslaughter of his wife Brenda, aged 60, in May 1995.

(Published by: East Norfolk Health Authority, 1998)

Report of the Inquiry into the Treatment and Care of Malcolm Calladine

Gunn, M., Beswick, J. and Hauck, A.

In January 1997 Malcolm Calladine stabbed Ashleigh Baker, aged 12 months, after absconding from Highbury Hospital where he was detained under s.3, Mental Health Act 1983. He was charged with attempted murder. In June 1997 he was found unfit to plead and sent to Rampton Hospital.

(Published by: Nottingham Health Authority, 1998)

Report of the Independent Inquiry into the Care and Treatment of Adrian Jones and Douglas Heathwaite

Taylor, A., Baugh, S., McGinnis, P. and Tuckwell, M.

Adrian Jones, aged 30, killed Douglas Heathwaite, aged 47, following an incident at a bus stop in June 1995.

(Published by: County Durham Health Authority, 1998)

Report of the Inquiry into the Care and Treatment of Naresh Bavabhai

Lingham, R. and Khoosal, D.

Naresh Bavabhai, aged 27, pleaded guilty to the manslaughter of Kenneth Horrocks, aged 68, in November 1996 and was sentenced to 11 years imprisonment.

(Published by: Wigan and Bolton Health Authority, 1998)

The Report of the Luke Warm Luke Mental Health Inquiry

Baroness Scotland of Asthal, Kelly, H. and Devaux, M.

Luke Warm Luke (formerly Michael Folkes) stabbed to death Susan Milner, aged 33, in October 1994. He was convicted of manslaughter and made the subject of a hospital order with restrictions (ss.37/41) in April 1995.

(Published (two volumes and a summary) by:
Lambeth, Southwark and Lewisham Health Authority, 1998)

Independent Review of the Review Process into 8 Untoward Incidents of Patients who were Receiving Mental Health Services from the North Hertfordshire NHS Trust between January 1998 and June 1998

Hollis, G., Dick, D., Heatley, C., Archibald, A. and Mackay, J.

North Hertfordshire NHS Trust experienced an unusually high number of 'serious untoward incidents' over the period January to June 1998. Three of the 'incidents' involved in-patients who had died. A further five 'incidents' occurred whilst the patients were living at home, of whom four died.

(Published by: East and North Hertfordshire Health Authority, 1998)

Report of the Independent Inquiry into the Care and Treatment of Guiseppi Nacci

Price, C., Dick, D., Milne, I. and Mackay, J.

Guiseppi Nacci, aged 43, killed Barbara Coleman, aged 60, in October 1997 whilst they were living in a group home. He was convicted of manslaughter and made the subject of a hospital order with restrictions (ss.37/41) in April 1998.

(Published by: Bedfordshire Health Authority, 1998)

A Difficult Engagement – A Report of the Independent Inquiry into the Care and Treatment of Alfina Magdalena Gabriel

Double, V., Bielby, C., Rugg, T. and Wilk, R.

Alfina Gabriel, aged 28, was made the subject of a hospital order with restrictions (ss.37/41) in December 1996 after she admitted the manslaughter of Milton Lawrence, aged 73, in January 1996.

(Published by: Calderdale and Kirklees Health Authority, 1998)

The Report of the Committee of Inquiry into the Personality Disorder Unit, Ashworth Special Hospital

Fallon, P., Bluglass, R., Edwards, B. and Daniels, G.

The inquiry was established following a series of complaints concerning the Personality Disorder Unit at Ashworth by a patient who had absconded from the hospital while on a shopping trip. He returned voluntarily and made a number of allegations including the suggestion that children had been allowed to visit the unit and had had contact with convicted paedophiles.

(Published in two volumes by: The Stationery Office, 1999)

The Care and Treatment of Daniel Holden

Greenwood, W., Campbell, A., Hayward, T. and Tallentire, P.

Daniel Holden, aged 35, killed David Spencer, aged 42, in March 1996. In August 1997, he was convicted of murder and sentenced to life imprisonment.
(Published by: East Lancashire Health Authority, 1999)

Report of the Independent Inquiry into the Care and Treatment of Mr KK

Gulliver, A., Buchanan, A., Mason, L. and Mackay, J.

KK, aged 44, killed his wife, Janet, in the street. She had left her husband three months before, after years of abuse and threats to kill her.
(Published by: Enfield and Haringey Health Authority, 1999)

Report of the Independent Inquiry into the Treatment and Care of Bradley Sears-Prince

Gunn, M., Daniels, G., Foster, T. and Middleton, H.

Bradley Sears-Prince killed Adil Butt in June 1996. He was sentenced to life imprisonment at Nottingham Crown Court in July 1997.
(Published by: Leicestershire Health Authority, 1999)

Report of the Inquiry into the Care and Treatment of Micheal Donnelly

Herbert, P., Ghosh, C. and Walters, J.

Micheal Donnelly, aged 29, was made the subject of a hospital order with restrictions (ss.37/41) in December 1996 after he admitted setting fire to his mother's house, killing her lodger, Matthew Bowyer, aged 22, in March 1996.
(Published by: North Essex Health Authority, 1999)

The Dixon Team Inquiry Report

Dixon, K., Herbert, P., Marshall, S. and Pinto, R.

Magdi Elgizouli, aged 30, was made the subject of a hospital order with restrictions (ss.37/41) in April 1998 after he admitted the manslaughter of WPC Nina Mackay, aged 25, in October 1997. She was stabbed as she accompanied colleagues to arrest him for breach of bail conditions.
(Published (full report and/or summary) by: Kensington and Chelsea and Westminster Health Authority, 1999)

Report of the Inquiry into the Treatment and Care of Matthew Hooper

Curwen, M., Tennant, G. and Devaux, M.

Matthew Hooper, aged 30, was made the subject of a hospital order with restrictions (ss.37/41) in November 1996 after he admitted the manslaughter of John Trinder, aged 55, in December 1995.
(Published by: Lambeth, Southwark and Lewisham Health Authority, 1999)

Report of the Inquiry into the Care and Treatment of Lee Powell and Paul Masters

Halliday, G., Mendelson, E. and Warburg, R.

Lee Powell, aged 26, pleaded guilty in July 1997 to the murder of Paul Masters, aged 27, a fellow resident, following a fire in December 1996 at Lyme House, a rehabilitation facility near Wigan. The home is run by Transitional Rehabilitation Unit, a company specialising in the rehabilitation of people with brain injuries.
(Published by: South Cheshire Health Authority, 1999)

Report of the Independent Inquiry into the Care and Treatment of Wayne Licorish

Holwill, D., Oyebode, O., Mason, L. and Mackay, J.

Wayne Licorish, aged 32, was made the subject of a hospital order with restrictions (ss.37/41) in June 1998 after he was convicted of the manslaughter of Caroline Burningham, aged 29, who was killed in January 1997.
(Published by: Northamptonshire Health Authority, 1999)

Report of the Inquiry into the Care and Treatment of Ann Murrie

Williams, R.

Ann Murrie, aged 38, killed her daughter, Louise, aged 9, in February 1994.
(Published by: Berkshire Health Authority, 1999)

The KB Inquiry Report

Moyo, E., Read, P.H. and Coleman, K.

KB, aged 27, was made the subject of a hospital order with restrictions (ss.37/41) in November 1998 following the killing in May 1998 of his friend Vicenzo Gianni, aged 29.
(Published by: Kensington and Chelsea and Westminster Health Authority, 1999)

Bridging the Gaps – Independent Inquiry into the Care and Treatment of Naseer Aslam

Bhatoa, J., Collins, P., McNichol, E. and Whittle, K.

Naseer Aslam, aged 26, killed his sister-in-law, Mahroof Bibi, in the presence of her three young children and his mother in April 1996. He was made the subject of a hospital order with restrictions (ss.37/41) in January 1998 and detained in Rampton Hospital.

(Published by: Bradford Health Authority, 1999)

Report to Tees Health Authority of the Independent Inquiry Team into the Care and Treatment of Jonathan Crisp

Brown, T., Fraser, K., Morley, A. and Swapp, G.

Jonathan Crisp, aged 22, was sentenced to life imprisonment in May 1998 after he admitted murdering his girlfriend's ex-husband, Peter McNamee, aged 38, in June 1997.

(Published by: Tees Health Authority, 1999)

Report of the Independent Inquiry Panel into the Management of Andrew John Douglas

Robinson, N., Morgan, B. and Walsh, A.

Andrew Douglas, aged 25, was convicted in December 1998 of the murder of James Byrne in March 1998.

(Published by: Sunderland Health Authority, 1999)

Not a Real Patient? Report of the Independent Inquiry into the Care and Treatment of David Edward Roberts

Halliday, G., Daniels, O., Mackay, J. and Read, G.

In December 1998, David Edward Roberts pleaded guilty to the manslaughter of Joseph Osmond, guilty also to inflicting grievous bodily harm with intent on David Compton, and guilty of a further charge of aggravated burglary. He was made subject to detention under ss.37/41 of the Mental Health Act, and sent to a special hospital.

(Published by: Wiltshire Health Authority, 1999)

Report of the Independent Inquiry into the Treatment and Care of Richard Allott

Branthwaite, M., Fisher, N., Milne, I. and Mackay, J.

Richard Allott, aged 48, was made the subject of a hospital order with restrictions (ss.37/41) in February 1999 after he admitted killing Richard Aston, aged 20, and Richard Chandler, aged 26, in May 1998.

(Published by: Warwickshire Health Authority, 2000)

Independent Inquiry into the Care and Treatment of Feza M

Dimond, B., Carter, P., Jolley, A. and Watts, T.

Feza M, aged 36, killed Caroline Coates, aged 34, in September 1997.
(Published by: East London and the City Health Authority and the London Borough of Hackney, 2000)

Report of the Independent Inquiry into the Care and Treatment of Patient T

Galbraith, A., Humphries, S., Shewan, M. and Southall, C.

Patient T was placed on probation for two years in December 1998 for the manslaughter, in May 1997, of her former lover, Eric Kirby, aged 52.

(Published by: County Durham Health Authority, 2000)

Report of the Independent Inquiry into the Care and Treatment of Ms Justine Cummings

Laming, H., Claydon, D., Davies, C. and Womack, J.

Justine Cummings, aged 27, was made the subject of a 'hospital direction' alongside a life sentence following the manslaughter of her fiancé Peter Lewis, aged 27, in October 1997. She had been receiving psychiatric treatment since she was 15, having been beaten by both her parents. She had twice been the victim of rape and had been preyed on sexually by a police officer and a male nurse who were supposed to be caring for her.

(Published by: Somerset Health Authority and Somerset Social Services, 2000)

Report of the Independent Inquiry Panel into the Care and Treatment of TK

Etherton, T., Freeman, H. and Hennessey, M.

TK, aged 20, was made the subject of a hospital order with restrictions (ss.37/41) in December 1997 after he admitted the manslaughter of Nicholas Boyd, aged 42, in April 1997.

(Published by: Camden and Islington Health Authority, 2000)

Report of the Independent Inquiry Panel into the Care and Treatment of Stephen Allum

Eldergill, A., Bowden, P., Murdoch, C. and Sheppard, D.

Stephen Allum, aged 37, was made the subject of a hospital order with restrictions (ss.37/41) in July 1998 after he admitted the manslaughter of his wife Thelma, aged 36, in October 1997.

(Published by: Berkshire Health Authority, 2000)

Report of the Independent Inquiry into the Care and Treatment of Mrs Marie Alawode

Taylor, J., Longhurst, N., Oldridge, P. and Brown, T.

Marie Alawode, aged 45, killed her daughter Joanne, aged 3, in August 1998. She pleaded guilty to a charge of manslaughter on the grounds of diminished responsibility in January 1999 and was made the subject of a hospital order with restrictions (ss.37/41).

(Published by: Cambridgeshire Health Authority, 2000)

Report of the Inquiry into the Death of Mr David Phillips

Bell, J., Campbell, A. and Turner, T.

Andre da Conceicao, aged 31, killed David Phillips in September 1998. He was found guilty of manslaughter on the grounds of diminished responsibility in April 1999 and was made the subject of a hospital order with restrictions (ss.37/41).

(Published by: Kensington and Chelsea and Westminster Health Authority, 2000)

Report of the Independent Inquiry into the Care and Treatment of Garry Lythgoe

Dick, D. and Cartwright, I.

Garry Lythgoe, aged 25, was made the subject of a hospital order with restrictions (ss.37/41) in April 1999 after he was convicted of the manslaughter of his mother, Irene, and the attempted murder of his father, Nigel, in October 1998.

(Published by: Wigan and Bolton Health Authority, 2000)

Report of the Independent Inquiry into the Treatment and Care of Barry Halewood

Chapman, H. and Dick, D.

Barry Halewood, aged 33, was made the subject of a hospital order with restrictions (ss.37/41) in March 1999 after he admitted the manslaughter of his mother, Eileen, in October 1998.

(Published by: Liverpool Health Authority, 2000)

Report of the Independent Inquiry into the Care and Treatment of Lorna Thomas and Nicholas Arnold

Rubenstein, V., Smith, M.L., Lindsey, M., Richardson, D. and Roy, A.

Nicholas Arnold, aged 41, killed his girlfriend, Lorna Thomas, aged 21, in December 1995. He was convicted of murder in October 1996 and sentenced to life imprisonment. He unsuccessfully appealed in July 1998.

(Published by: Buckinghamshire Health Authority, 2000)

Report of the Independent Inquiry into the Care and Treatment of WM

Dimond, B., Dixon, K. and Seifert, R.

WM, aged 35, killed Beatrice Hughes, aged 91, in March 1997 after she was punched, kicked and stamped to death. He was a burglar who preyed on the old and vulnerable. He pleaded guilty to murder in January 1998 and sentenced to life imprisonment.

(Published by: Brent and Harrow Health Authority, 2000)

Report of the Independent Inquiry into the Care and Treatment of Shane Bath

Weereratne, A., Hunter, C. and Newland, A.

Shane Bath was sentenced to life imprisonment in May 1998 after pleading guilty to the murder in November 1997 of his girlfriend, Aiyse Sullivan, aged 18.

(Published by: Dorset Health Authority, 2000)

Report of the Independent Inquiry Team into the Care and Treatment of Daniel Joseph

Mishcon, J., Sensky, T., Lindsey, M. and Cook, S.

Daniel Joseph, aged 19, was made the subject of a hospital order with restrictions (ss.37/41) in July 1998 after he admitted the manslaughter of Carla Thompson, aged 57, in January 1998.
(Published by: Lambeth, Southwark and Lewisham Health Authority, 2000)

Report of the Independent Inquiry into the Care and Treatment of Alexander Cameron

Eldergill, A., Kelly, H. and Sheppard, D.

Alexander Cameron, aged 32, was made the subject of a hospital order with restrictions (ss.37/41) after he admitted killing his mother, Eileen, aged 70 in April 1997.

(Published by: Berkshire Health Authority, 2000)

Report of the Independent Inquiry into the Treatment and Care of Phillip John Craigie

Chapman, H., Davis, C. and Brand, D.

Phillip Craigie, aged 23, was made the subject of a hospital order with restrictions (ss.37/41) after he killed David Close, aged 67, in March 1999. He had pleaded guilty to causing death by dangerous driving.
(Published by: Portsmouth and SE Hampshire Health Authority, 2000)

Report of the Independent Inquiry into the Treatment and Care of Anthony Joseph

Herbert, P., Brand, D. and Bird, A.

Anthony Joseph, aged 27, was found guilty in July 1999 of the manslaughter of Jenny Morrison, aged 51, a social worker from Wandsworth Council, who was killed in November 1998 during a planned visit to a 'care in the community' hostel in Balham.

(Published by: Merton, Sutton and Wandsworth Health Authority, 2000)

Report of the Independent Inquiry into the Care and Treatment of Patient R and Patient Y

Galbraith, A., Simpson, C., Childs, A. and Parkin, D.

Patient R was sentenced to three years probation in January 1999 after she pleaded guilty to the manslaughter of Patient Y in December 1997.

(Published by: County Durham and Darlington Health Authority, 2000)

Report of the Independent Inquiry into the Treatment and Care of Paul Hundleby

Nolan, D., Payne, S., Brennan, P. and Sashidharan, S.

Paul Hundleby was made the subject of a hospital order with restrictions (ss.37/41) in May 1999 after he pleaded guilty to the manslaughter of his wife Catherine in October 1998.

(Published by: Leicestershire Health Authority, 2001)

Report of the Independent Inquiry into the Treatment and Care of Paul Horrocks

Mackay, J., Poole, R. and Sinclair, S.

Paul Horrocks was made the subject of a hospital order with restrictions (ss.37/41) in June 1999 after he was found guilty of the manslaughter of Carol Houghton in December 1998.

(Published by: Wirral Health Authority, 2001)

Report of the Independent Inquiry into the Care and Treatment of JB

Chapman, H., James, D. and Unsworth, T.

JB, aged 52, killed his wife in August 1997. He was convicted of manslaughter and sentenced to five years imprisonment.

(Published by: Brent and Harrow Health Authority, 2001)

Report of the Independent Inquiry into the Care and Treatment of John Piccolo

Bowron, M., Clarke, M. and Ledbury, B.

John Piccolo, aged 51, shot his son Darren, aged 26, at their home before shooting dead Martin Cass, aged 23, the boyfriend of his ex-lover. He then shot and wounded his former partner, Jane Smith, aged 36. John Piccolo shot himself in the head with a hand gun after he was traced and surrounded by armed police.

(Published by: North Essex Health Authority, 2001)

Report of the Independent Inquiry into the Care and Treatment of David Johnson

McGowran, T., Mackay, J., Mason, L. and Oyebode, O.

David Johnson, aged 48, threw Geraldine Simpson, aged 44, to her death from his 12th floor flat in August 1997. He was convicted of murder and sentenced to life imprisonment in May 1998.

(Published by: Birmingham Health Authority, 2001)

Independent Inquiry into the Care and Treatment of a Mental Health Client

Roy, S., Rhys, M., Brand, D. and Craig, K.

A man, aged 29, killed his older brother in April 1999. There was no evidence of animosity between them. The panel concluded that the act was strongly affected both by the paranoid and suspicious reactions caused by his mental illness and by the effects of the amount of beer and rum he had drunk.

(Published by: Barking and Havering Health Authority, 2001)

Independent Inquiry Report into the Circumstances Leading to the Death of Daniel Coleman

Armstrong, W., Humas, N. and Scofield, T.

Darryll James, aged 30, killed Daniel Coleman, aged 83, in July 1996. He admitted manslaughter and was made the subject of a hospital order with restrictions (ss.37/41) in May 1997.

(Published by: Norfolk Health Authority, 2001)

Independent Review of Services and Support Provided to Robert and Richard Turnbull and their parents on the Isle of Wight

Community Care Development Centre

In June 2000, Mrs Janquil Turnbull pleaded guilty to the manslaughter of her two sons, Robert (aged 23) and Richard (aged 20), both of whom had profound learning disabilities.

(Published by: Isle of Wight Council Social Services and Housing Directorate, Health Authority and Healthcare NHS Trust, 2001)

Complex Needs – Report of the Independent Inquiry into the Care and Treatment of Daniel Williams

Bhatoa, J.S., Davenport, S., Duffy, D. and Manby, M.

Daniel Williams, aged 28, was sentenced to life imprisonment after he admitted the manslaughter of Adrian Pawson, aged 24, whilst both were in-patients in Fieldhead Hospital, Wakefield.

(Published by: Wakefield Health Authority, 2001)

Report of the Independent Inquiry into the Care and Treatment of Kevin Hewitt

Rassaby, E., Bull, D., McCollin, D. and Murray, K.

Kevin Hewitt, aged 31, killed Wilfred Marchant, aged 72 and stabbed Brian Geeson and his son, Daniel, aged 12, in a Leicester street in August 1999. He was convicted of manslaughter on the grounds of diminished responsibility and two counts of attempted murder and was made the subject of a hospital order with restrictions (ss.37/41) in January 2000.

(Published by: Leicestershire Health Authority, 2001)

Independent Inquiry into the Care and Treatment of Mark Longman, Paul Huntingford and Christopher Moffatt

Eldergill, A., Bowden, P., Murdoch, C., Walker, J. and Welch, N.

Mark Longman, aged 27, was made the subject of a hospital order with restrictions (ss.37/41) in May 1998 after he admitted the manslaughter of his father Kenneth, aged 63, who was killed in June 1996. Paul Huntingford was made the subject of a hospital order with restrictions (ss.37/41) in November 1998 after he was found not guilty by reason of insanity following the killing of his mother, aged 84, in December 1997. Christopher Moffatt, aged 27, was made the subject of a hospital order with restrictions (ss.37/41) in December 1998 after he admitted the manslaughter on the grounds of diminished responsibility of Anthony Harrison, aged 64, and the attempted murder of his wife Jennifer, aged 61, in April 1998. Six days after the hospital order he was found hanged in Broadmoor.

(Summary report published by: North & Mid Hampshire Health Authority, 2001)

Report of an Independent Inquiry into the Care and Treatment of Paul Leane

Curwen, M., Daniels, O. and Mason, L.

Paul Leane, aged 34, killed his mother, Henrietta, aged 63, in May 1997, after he poured petrol over the living room of their home and struck a match. He admitted manslaughter and was made the subject of a hospital order with restrictions (ss.37/41) in May 1998.

(Published by: Brent and Harrow Health Authority, 2001)

Report of the Independent Inquiry into the Care and Treatment of Kevin Keogh

Mackay, J., Dent, S., Hughes, A., Radford, M. and Windle, B.

Kevin Keogh, aged 32, killed Heath Rowson in November 1998. He pleaded guilty to manslaughter on the grounds of diminished responsibility and was made the subject of a hospital order with restrictions (ss.37/41) in September 1999.

(Published by: Manchester Health Authority, 2001)

Report of the Independent Inquiry into the Care and Treatment of Christopher and Eunice Watts

Dick, D. and Hargreaves, R.

Christopher Watts, aged 57, killed his wife, Eunice, aged 55, in December 1999 and then took his own life.

(Published by: North Cheshire Health Authority, 2001)

Report of an Independent Inquiry into the Care and Treatment of Michael Abram

Roberts, G., Ferguson, B., Gorry, A., Hargreaves, R. and Pilkington, B.

Michael Abram, aged 34, was made the subject of hospital order with restrictions on discharge (ss.37/41) in November 2000 after he was cleared of the attempted murder of George and Olivia Harrison in December 1999.

(Published by: St Helens and Knowsley Health Authority, 2001)

Report of the Independent Inquiry into the Care and Treatment of Richard Gray

Downham, G., Kelly, H., Newland, A. and Webster, N.

Richard Gray, aged 38, was made the subject of hospital order with restrictions on discharge (ss.37/41) in March 1999 after he was found guilty of the manslaughter of Virginia Sivil, aged 26, in February 1998. She was attacked while walking to relieve labour pains on the day she was due to give birth to her third child, who also died. He had been the subject of a second conditional discharge following his recall to hospital in 1993.

(Summary report published by: Wiltshire Health Authority, 2001)

Report of the Independent Inquiry into the Care and Treatment of Benjamin Rathbone

Mackay, R., Badger, G., Damle, A. and Long, K.

Benjamin Rathbone was made the subject of hospital order with restrictions on discharge (ss.37/41) in June 1999 after he pleaded guilty to the attempted murder of a stranger, Will Hickin, in February 1999. Mr Hickin was pushed onto the track at Loughborough Station by Mr Rathbone who then leaped after him.

(Published by: Leicestershire Health Authority, 2001)

Report of the Independent Inquiry into the Health Care and Treatment of Dominic McKilligan

Winter, D., Preston, M. and Manby, M.

Dominic McKilligan, aged 18, killed Wesley Neailey, aged 11, in June 1998. He had been discharged from Aycliffe Young People's Centre in September 1997. He pleaded guilty to murder and was sentenced to life imprisonment in July 1999.

(Published by: Newcastle and North Tyneside Health Authority, 2001)

Report of the Inquiry into the Treatment and Care of Wayne Hutchinson

Coonan, K., Tidmarsh, D. and Hayward, P.

Wayne Hutchinson, aged 21, was convicted in January 1996 of two counts of manslaughter on the grounds of diminished responsibility, attempted murder and wounding with intent. He received six life sentences but successfully appealed against sentence in November 1996 when a hospital order with restrictions was substituted. He had been admitted to South Western Hospital in October 1994 but was allowed to leave the hospital the following month 'by mistake'.

(Published by: Lambeth, Southwark and Lewisham Health Authority, 2001)

Report of the Independent Inquiry into the Care and Treatment of Richard Smart

Mackay, J., Radford, M. and Read, G.

Richard Smart was sent to prison for five years after he admitted the manslaughter of his wife, Donna.

(Published by: Somerset Health Authority and Somerset County Council, 2001)

Report of the Inquiry into the Care and Treatment of Andrew Ackroyd

Gunn, M., Birchall, E., Lowe, J. and Vines, C.

Andrew Ackroyd, aged 37, was made the subject of a hospital order with restrictions (ss.37/41) in October 2000 after he admitted the manslaughter of his father George Ackroyd, aged 67, in October 1999.

(Published by: North Derbyshire Health Authority, 2002)

Report of the Independent Inquiry into the Care and Treatment of Alan Kippax

Gilham, C., Junaid, O. and McKeever, S.

Alan Kippax was sentenced to life imprisonment in November 1999 following the killing of Garry Warburton in November 1998.

(Published by: North West Lancashire Health Authority, 2002)

Report of the Independent Inquiry into the Care and Treatment of Matthew Hotston

Price, C., Coffey, T., Standen, R. and Wright, C.

Matthew Hotston, aged 26, was sentenced to life imprisonment in October 1998 following the killing in April 1998 of Peter Williams.

(Published by: East London and the City Health Authority, 2002)

A Part 8 Review and Homicide Inquiry Relating to A & FD

Arkley, R. and Ramsay, R.

Edward Crowley stabbed Diego Pineiro, aged 12, 30 times in front of on-lookers in Covent Garden, central London, in May 2000.
(Published by: the Camden Area Child Protection Committee and Camden and Islington Health Authority, 2002)

Report of the Independent Inquiry into the Care and Treatment of Jonathan Neale

Bradley, J., Ledbury, B. and Lindsey, M.

Jonathan Neale, aged 21, killed his mother, Rosemary, aged 52, in September 1999. He admitted manslaughter on the grounds of diminished responsibility and was made the subject of a hospital order with restrictions (ss.37/41) in February 2000.
(Published by: North Essex Health Authority, 2002)

Report of the Independent Inquiry into the Care and Treatment of Winston Williams

Johns, G., Bowden, P. and Sheppard, D.

Winston Williams, aged 52, was made the subject of a hospital order with restrictions (ss.37/41) after he admitted killing Katie Kazmi, aged 25.
(Published by: Thames Valley Health Authority, 2002)

Missed Opportunities – Report of the Independent Inquiry into the Care and Treatment of Saheeda Kapde

Smoult-Hawtree, K., McKenzie, A., Sircar, I. and Easton, A.

Saheeda Kapde, aged 30, killed her son Nihaal, aged 6, in June 2000. She admitted manslaughter and was made the subject of a hospital order with restrictions (ss.37/41) in November 2000.
(Published by: Calderdale and Kirklees Health Authority, 2002)

Report of an Independent Inquiry into the Care and Treatment of SH

Holwill, D., Cameron, A., Ghosh, C. and Lindsey, M.

SH, aged 31, killed his wife AK, aged 24, in Newham in June 2000. He was convicted of manslaughter and made the subject of a hospital order with restrictions (ss.37/41) in October 2000.

(Published by: North East London Health Authority, 2002)

Report of an Independent Inquiry into the Care and Treatment of Raymond Wills

Winter, D., Berry, A., Whittle, K. and Smith, H.

Raymond Wills, aged 29, killed his sister Caroline Wills, 26, and her son Ashley, aged 5, in March 2000. He was made the subject of a hospital order with restrictions (ss.37/41) in February 2001 after he admitted their manslaughter on the grounds of diminished responsibility.

(Published by: Northumberland and Tyne and Wear Health Authority, 2002)

Report of an Independent Inquiry into the Care and Treatment of Simon James Coombe and David Gary McMahon

Weereratne, A., Newland, A. and Hunter, C.

Simon Coombe was jailed in 1999 for murdering Michelle Lock in Kinson, Bournemouth. Police believed he stalked and raped his victim before he killed her in April 1998. David McMahon was jailed for life at Winchester Crown Court in February 1999 for the murder of William Bodle in Bournemouth in June 1998. McMahon punched and kicked Mr Bodle with whom he was living in a squat and then hit him with a bottle.

(Published by: Somerset and Dorset Health Authority, 2002)

Report of an Independent Inquiry into the Care and Treatment of DN

Mishcon, J., Snowden, P., Proctor, A., Fluxman, J. and Ward, M.

DN, aged 30, killed his paternal grandmother at her flat in Tower Hamlets in June 1998. A sentence of life imprisonment was imposed on him in March 1999 following his plea of guilty to manslaughter on the ground of diminished responsibility. He was transferred to Rampton Hospital from Belmarsh Prison in 2000 under ss.47/49 Mental Health Act 1983.

(Published by: North-East London Health Authority, 2002)

Report of the Independent Inquiry into the Care and Treatment of Matthew Martin

Downham, G., Procter, A., Campbell, A. and Clark, C.

Matthew Martin, aged 25, killed Michael Martin, aged 56, with a pickaxe at his home in Almondsbury three months after his release from Exeter Prison in 1999. He was made the subject of a hospital order with restrictions (ss.37/41) in February 2000 after he admitted manslaughter on the grounds of diminished responsibility.

(Published by: Avon, Gloucestershire and Wiltshire Strategic Health Authority, Jenner House, Langley Park Estate, Chippenham, Wiltshire SN15 1GG (Tel: 01249-858500; Fax: 01249-858501), 2003)

Report of the Independent Inquiry into the Care and Treatment of Patient Q and Patient G

Galbraith, A., Murray, K., Rippon, S. and Isherwood, J.

Patient G killed Patient Q in October 1999. They had both been in-patients at the County Hospital in Durham the previous month for detoxification. Patient G was sentenced to five years imprisonment in July 2000 after he admitted manslaughter.

(Published by: County Durham and Tees Valley Strategic Health Authority, Teesdale House, Westpoint Road, Thornaby, Stockton on Tees TS17 6BL (Tel: 01642-666700; Fax: 01642-666701), 2003)

Report of the Independent Inquiry into the Care and Treatment of H

Weereratne, A., Exworthy, T. and Flynn, C.

H, aged 37, killed his ex-partner T.L., aged 36, in November 2000. He was made the subject of a hospital order with restrictions (ss.37/41) in July 2001 after he admitted manslaughter on the grounds of diminished responsibility.

(Published by: South West Peninsula Strategic Health Authority, Lescaze Offices, Shinners Bridge, Dartington, Totnes, Devon TQ9 6JE (Tel: 01803-861874), 2003)

Report of the Independent Inquiry into the Care and Treatment of S

Weereratne, A., Exworthy, T. and Flynn, C.

S killed his wife in April 2000. He was sentenced to three years probation in December 2000, a condition of which was that he accepted treatment as determined by a consultant psychiatrist after he admitted manslaughter on the grounds of diminished responsibility.

> (Published by: South West Peninsula Strategic Health Authority, Lescaze Offices, Shinners Bridge, Dartington, Totnes, Devon TQ9 6JE (Tel: 01803-861874), 2003)

Report of the Independent Inquiry into the Care and Treatment of Matthew Steel

Greenwood, W., Campbell, A., Sloss, S. and Tallentire, P.

Matthew Steel, aged 19, stabbed Phillip Beardmore, aged 35, to death in March 2000. He was convicted at Lincoln Crown Court of murder in December 2000.

> (Published by: West Lincolnshire Primary Care Trust, Cross O'Cliff, Bracebridge Health, Lincoln LN4 2HN (Tel: 01522-513355), 2003)

A Summary of an Independent Inquiry Report into the Care and Treatment of X

Manby, M. and Subotsky, F.

X, aged 16, stabbed a woman, aged 35, to death in February 2000. She was convicted at Manchester Crown Court of manslaughter in July 2001.

> (Published by: Greater Manchester Strategic Health Authority, Gateway House, Piccadilly South, Manchester M60 7LP (Tel: 0161-236-9456), 2003)

Report of the Independent Inquiry into the Care and Treatment of Gregory Marden

Holwill, D., Mackay, J. and Radford, M.

Gregory Marden, aged 26, killed his father, Richard, aged 69, in May 1999. He was convicted of manslaughter on the grounds of diminished responsibility in August 1999.

> (Published by: Leicestershire, Northamptonshire and Rutland Strategic Health Authority, Lakeside House, 4 Smith Way, Grove Park, Enderby, Leicester LE19 1SS (Tel: 0116-295-7500), 2003)

Report of the Independent Inquiry into the Care and Treatment of GE

Taylor, J., Freeman, R. and Oldridge, P.

In October 1999 George Eckersley, 52, battered his wife Denise to death. He was jailed for life at Leeds Crown Court in 2000.

> (Published by: West Yorkshire Strategic Health Authority, 2003)

Report of the Independent Inquiry into the Care and Treatment of AB

Sedgman, J., Allen, B. and Davies, C.

AB killed her lover, Hugh McCaffrey in March 1998. She was convicted of manslaughter and sentenced to three years imprisonment in October 1998.

(Published by: North West London Strategic Health Authority, Victory House, 170 Tottenham Court Road, London W1T 7HA (Tel: 020-7756-2500), 2003)

Report of the Independent Inquiry into the Care and Treatment of Mr A

Bhatoa, J. S., Brabbins, C., Davis, H. and Hargreaves, R.

Mr A, aged 25, killed Mr B in September 2000. He was sent to Rampton Hospital in May 2001 after Bradford Crown Court found he had killed but was not guilty by reason of insanity.

(Published by Bradford Health Authority, 2003)

Report of the Independent Inquiry into the Care and Treatment of KB

KB killed his wife, DB in January 1998.

(Report accepted by the Norfolk, Suffolk and Cambridgeshire Strategic Health Authority in April 2003 but not published)

Report of the Independent Inquiry into the Care and Treatment of Kevin Littlewood

Robinson, N., Anderson, T., Day, K., Morgan, W. and Wressell, S.

Kevin Littlewood was a patient of Child and Adolescent Mental Health Services from 1997 until he was arrested and subsequently found guilty of killing John Paul Jeffries, an 18-year-old student, with a hammer in December 2001.

(Published by: County Durham and Tees Valley Strategic Health Authority, Teesdale House, Westpoint Road, Thornaby, Stockton on Tees TS17 6BL (Tel: 01642-666700), 2003)

Report of the Independent Inquiry into the Care and Treatment of Mark Harrington

Greenwood, B., Anderson, T., Campbell, A., Curtis D. and Tallentire, P.

Mark Harrington, 21, pleaded guilty to the manslaughter of his friend Anthony Rigby, 18, who died in January 2002 after he was shot in the back of the head. He was made the subject of a hospital order with restrictions on discharge (ss.37/41) Mental Health Act 1983 after he admitted manslaughter on the grounds of diminished responsibility at Preston Crown Court in September 2002. He had been receiving care at the psychiatric unit at Blackburn's Queen's Park Hospital.

(Published by: Blackburn with Darwen PCT, Guide Business Centre, School Lane, Blackburn, Lancashire BB1 2QH (Tel: 01254-267000), 2003)

Report of the Independent Inquiry into the Care and Treatment of Mr A

Curwen, M., Holloway, F. and Tarbuck, P.

In May 1999, A pushed Stelios Economou, aged 20, a man unknown to him, in front of an oncoming train, causing his death. He pleaded guilty to manslaughter on the grounds of diminished responsibility and was made the subject of a hospital order with restrictions on discharge (ss.37/41).

(Published by: North West London Strategic Health Authority, Victory House, 170 Tottenham Court Road, London W1T 7HA (Tel: 020-7756-2500), 2003)

Report of an Independent Inquiry into the Care and Treatment of Dr Daksha Emson and her daughter Freya

Joyce, L., Hale, R., Jones, A. and Moodley, P.

Dr Daksha Emson, a psychiatrist, aged 34, who suffered from bipolar affective disorder, killed her 3 month old daughter Freya and then herself in October 2000.

(Published by: North-East London Strategic Health Authority, Aneurin Bevan House, 81–91 Commercial Road, London E1 1RD (Tel: 020-7655-6600), 2003)

Report of the Independent Inquiry into Suicides, Attempted Suicides and Related Serious Untoward Events relating to In-patients of the Mental Health Unit, Blackpool, Wyre and Fylde Community Health NHS Trust

Gilham, C., Hargreaves, R., Junaid, O. and McKever, S.

(Published by: Cumbria and Lancashire Strategic Health Authority, Preston Business Centre, Watling Street Road, Fulwood, Preston PR2 8DY (Tel: 01772-647000), 2003)

Part IV

Inquiries into the abuse of people with learning disabilities

Chapter 10

Learning disability, abuse and inquiry

Rachel Fyson, Deborah Kitson and Alan Corbett

Introduction

In comparison with the other client groups covered in this book, there have been relatively few recent inquiries relating to people with learning disabilities, and even fewer that have received widespread media attention. The reasons for this are varied, but certainly include the fact that people with learning disabilities are not generally perceived as being of interest to the public at large. Unlike children, adults with learning disabilities do not offer photogenic images of innocence; unlike people with mental health problems, they seldom pose a threat to public safety.

It has proved extremely difficult to gain an accurate picture of the number or types of inquiry which have taken place in the field of learning disability in recent years, largely because so few inquiries are reported nationally. However, it also appears to be the case that abuse of people with learning disabilities is not very likely to be inquired about. This may be because the victims are unable to effectively instigate complaints themselves; because police and regulatory authorities are unlikely to see the protection of people with learning disabilities from abuse as a priority; and because, moreover, low-level abuse merges so seamlessly with 'mere' poor practice that victims may be unaware that they can either expect better standards of care or do anything to improve their situation.

The few inquiries that have broken through the inertia of press and public disinterest, however, provide examples of appalling lack of care which in some cases had continued over years before being investigated and halted. We succeeded in identifying only seven inquiries into the abuse of people with learning disabilities since the 1990s. Clearly, this is unlikely to be an accurate picture of the number of inquiries that have actually taken place, and it is certainly not a true reflection of the frequency with which people with learning disabilities are seriously abused. What it does reflect, however, is the fact that there is no systematic, official collation of inquiry findings in relation to this group of people. The only attempt to gather together information of this

Table 10.1 Details of inquiries into the abuse of people with learning disabilities

Author, date and place of publication	Inquiry details
Bell *et al.* October 1992 Staffordshire	Report of the Committee of Inquiry into the Death of Freda Latham at Stallington Hospital. Freda Latham died after having been left tied by a bib to a toilet cistern. She choked on her own vomit after inhaling the medication which had been administered 40 minutes prior to her death.
Warner *et al.* May 1994 Thameside	Report of the Inquiry into aspects of Learning Disabilities Services managed by Thameside Community Healthcare NHS Trust. A report by the local Community Health Council, following complaints made by relatives about inadequate investigations of complaints through the Trust's complaints procedure and poor communication with relatives of six patients.
Myers *et al.* October 1996 York	Report to City of York Council following the death of Zoe Fairley. Zoe Fairley died of suffocation whilst being restrained by four workers in a local authority respite care home.
Brockington and McDonough June 1997 Durham	Report of an investigation into the Learning Disability Service at Earl's House and recommendations for action. Allegations of abuse were made against 16 staff, resulting in two further investigations by the staff's professional body and three written warnings.
Buckinghamshire County Council June 1998 Buckinghamshire	*Independent* Longcare Inquiry. An investigation of the roles of statutory authorities following the criminal conviction of staff for abusing residents at two large, privately owned residential care homes. Residents had suffered years of physical, sexual, emotional and financial abuse and neglect.
Community Care Development Centre, King's College London June 2000 Isle of Wight	*Independent* Review of Services and Support provided to Robert and Richard Turnbull and their parents on the Isle of Wight. Mrs Turnbull pleaded guilty in June 2000 of the manslaughter of her two severely learning disabled sons, following the failure of health and social services to provide adequate support to meet their care needs.
Commission for Health Improvement March 2003 Bedfordshire	Investigation into Learning Disability Services provided by the Bedfordshire and Luton Community NHS Trust. After two (unrelated) deaths in 1997 and 1999 and ongoing reports of alleged abuse, a Commission for Health Improvement report identified commonplace practices which infringed the human rights of service users with a learning disability – notably choices and freedoms being restricted by poor planning which meant that daily life was not much different to being in a long-stay hospital.

nature is on an independent website (IMHL 2003, see Chapter 9) but it cannot be assumed that this provides comprehensive coverage.

Brief details of the inquiries are identified in Table 10.1. These are undoubtedly not the only inquiries to have taken place into the abuse of people with learning disabilities within the past decade.

Of the inquiries in the table, all but one are cases of institutional abuse, where staff paid to provide care and support had instead used their position of trust to inflict emotional, physical and sexual abuse upon those in their care. As organisations working to protect people with learning disabilities from abuse and ameliorate its devastating effects, *The Ann Craft Trust* and *Respond* are aware that abuse in such settings occurs with distressing frequency. Indeed, the terms of reference of the inquiry in Bedfordshire (Commission for Health Improvement 2003) makes reference to no less than five previous inquiries having taken place within the same service over a period of only six years, although it was not possible to track down further details of these. The fact that only seven inquiries have resulted in findings which are available to the wider public says much about the value – or rather lack of it – that society places on the quality of life of people with learning disabilities. More worryingly, it could give an impression that abuse of people with learning disabilities is a relatively rare occurrence, when research proves time and again that this is not the case.

People with learning disabilities are at significantly greater risk of abuse than the general population for a number of reasons. This includes the facts that they are more likely to be in situations where other people have power over them because of their need for help in various aspects of life ranging from personal care to finances; that they may have difficulties with verbal communication and so find it harder to disclose abuse that has happened to them; that they may not understand either that they have been abused or that they have a right to complain; and that they may not be believed or listened to when abuse is disclosed. Studies (Beail and Warden 1995; Brown *et al.* 1995; Brown and Stein 1997) clearly demonstrate that abuse – and in particular sexual abuse – is a common occurrence in the lives of people with learning disabilities and that it is most likely to occur in their homes, perpetrated by people known to them.

The inquiries listed above, although limited in number, do give some insight into the types of incident which may instigate an inquiry being set up. With the exception of the Isle of Wight inquiry (Community Care Development Centre 2000) following the manslaughter of Robert and Richard Turnbull, the inquiries all concerned acts of abuse which had occurred within residential care settings. Furthermore, in each case it appeared that cultures of poor and abusive practice had been allowed to develop unhindered within services, had not been identified by statutory inspections, and had only ceased following either the death of an individual, *repeated* complaints by relatives, or whistleblowing by concerned members of staff. Moreover, it is similarly noteworthy that only two of the inquiries listed were independent of the services in which the abuse had occurred, and in both of these cases the independent inquiry had been instigated in the wake of criminal proceedings. Since it is known that very few cases of abuse of people with learning disabilities ever reach court, this suggests that independent inquiries may be as much about services wishing to appear responsive *post hoc* as about any widespread desire to use inquiries to promote better working practice. More positively, however, independent inquiries do at least result in greater publicity – both the Bedfordshire and Isle of Wight inquiries were reported in the mainstream UK press – and their resultant findings, unlike those of internal inquiries, are available in perpetuity through the British Library.

It is also interesting to note that all but one of these episodes of abuse took place within settings which were created as a result of the reprovision *in the community* of services for people who might in other times have been resident in long-stay 'mental handicap' hospitals. This begs the question as to whether current services have adequately learned the lessons from earlier inquiries into learning disability services. In the past, it would seem that inquiries into the abuse of people with learning disabilities have been a driving force behind radical service developments. More recently, however, service change has been driven more clearly by an agenda of rights and independence – in which people with learning disabilities themselves are playing a central role. During this time, inquiries (notably the Longcare inquiry, Buckinghamshire County Council 1998) have been one of several important factors which have fed into the development of adult protection initiatives, but they have played a much less significant part in shaping the provision of general support services for people with learning disabilities.

To summarise, it can be argued that, within learning disability services, scandal and inquiry historically played a major role in determining the overall shape of service provision; more recently the discovery of abusive practices has resulted in inquiries which, while resulting in calls for changes in working practice, have had a lesser role in determining the overall shape of service provision.

Learning disability, scandal and inquiry: a brief history

The lives of people with learning disabilities (and mental health problems) first became the subject of widespread public debate during the first half of the nineteenth century. A Royal Commission was established to examine issues of inheritance and infringement of personal freedom relating to individuals locked in asylums. The resulting Lunatics Act of 1845 introduced measures aimed at preventing miscarriages of justice and abuse of power, with regard to both public and private asylums (Jones 1960). However, as the century wore on, witnessing both the growth of government and an increasing scientific interest in eugenics, such people began to be perceived as not only economically unproductive – a burden on their families and society as a whole – but also as a potential threat to the health of the country's genetic stock (Ryan with Thomas 1987; Means and Smith 1994; Felce 1996). Public demand grew for intervention to curb the perceived dangerous increase in 'idiocy'.

The government of the day was pressured into action and in 1913 the Mental Deficiency Act was passed, introducing compulsory certification for people admitted to institutions and labelled as 'mentally defective' (a classification which included the mentally ill and the morally feckless as well as the learning disabled). This legislation established for the first time a separate and unified service for people with learning disabilities, a service, moreover, which excluded them from other welfare and mainstream educational facilities. A combination of scandal, inquiry and public approbation had laid the foundations for the large-scale institutional services which were to be the mainstay of learning disability services for over half a century, and the remnants of which still exist today in some parts of the UK.

The next significant shift in attitudes towards people with learning disabilities arose largely as a by-product of the Second World War: as a result of the atrocities committed in its name by the Nazi regime, the eugenics movement lost support dramatically (Leighton 1988), leading some to question the policy of separation and asylum. Accordingly, in 1954, a Royal Commission was again established to examine issues concerning the care of the learning disabled and mentally ill. The Commission's findings formed the basis of the 1959 and 1960 Mental Health Acts. This legislation provided the framework for the first mandatory provision of services to 'mentally disordered' people living in the community. The underlying aims of the Acts were anti-institutional, with a strong emphasis on training and employment for people with learning disabilities, to enable them to participate as far as possible in ordinary social and economic life. However, despite the high ideals of both the inquiry and the ensuing legislation, few people left institutional care at this time.

In fact, the status quo remained largely undisturbed until the 1967 Ely Hospital scandal. The *News of the World* reported in graphic detail the appalling living conditions and lack of adequate care being provided in Ely Hospital, Cardiff – a large but typical institution for people with learning disabilities. More revelations followed. In 1968, the *Guardian* conducted investigations into the condition of residents at Harperbury Hospital and discovered similar, unacceptably poor, service provision. These discoveries, and subsequently a number of official inquiries, led to public outcry. Change was demanded and the government responded by publishing the White Paper, *Better Services for the Mentally Handicapped* (Department of Health 1971). This was the first explicit government recognition that hospitals and the 'medical model' might be inappropriate ways of providing care for people with learning disabilities. Targets were set for reducing the number of people living in such institutions.

In the aftermath of the 1971 White Paper, a slow but steady shift from large-scale, hospital-based provision of care towards a model of smaller, community-based services began to take place. This trend was boosted significantly by the publication in 1979 of *The Report of the Committee of Inquiry into Mental Handicap Nursing and Care* (the 'Jay Report') (Jay 1979). The Jay Report was notable for being the first government-backed investigative report into services for people with learning disabilities which was not conducted either in the wake of public scandal concerning standards of care, nor with ulterior aims, such as reducing expenditure. Its proposed model of services still exceeds, in scope and vision, the pattern of provision prevalent in some parts of the country today. The report broadly restated the case for adopting the principles outlined in the 1971 White Paper but was also strongly influenced by the emerging theory of 'normalisation' (Wolfensberger 1972), and specifically recommended that community residential provision should take the form of small, socially integrated, group homes. However, these proposals were never fully endorsed by the government, in part due to cost implications.

Following the Jay Report, although learning disability services continued to strive towards provision which gave individuals more choice and greater independence, little attention was paid to the issues involved by central government. Changes that occurred within services were influenced more by local factors, and pioneering individuals, than they were by concerted pressure being brought to bear upon statutory services. During this period, professionals who worked with people with learning disabilities were increasingly aware of, and influenced by, Wolfensberger's theories of normalisation (1972) and in the early 1980s, O'Brien and Tyne published their 'five accomplishments' (O'Brien and Tyne 1981), which in essence provided a blueprint against which services in the UK could measure their progress towards the provision of learning disability services which broadly met the pre-requisites for achieving the aim of normalisation. Indeed, these criteria were still relevant enough to form the value base of the most recent learning disability White Paper, *Valuing People* (Department of Health 2001).

In 1993 the community care element of the 1990 National Health Service and Community Care Act came into operation. This legislation was promoted as enabling all adults who required social care, whether learning disabled, physically impaired, elderly or mentally ill, to have greater choice in the services they received, more individualised packages of care and (again) services which were based on support within the community rather than in institutional settings. As such, it may have been influenced to some extent by the ongoing legacy of institutional abuse, but the immediate cause for government action was at least as much to do with a desire to reduce public expenditure in this area and encourage private sector provision of care services (Lewis and Glennerster 1996). As a consequence of this focus, the issue of abuse prevention received relatively little attention within this legislation, although individual care plans, which were meant to follow all social service assessments of need, should include an individual 'safety plan' in cases where someone was known to have been abused or where they were considered to be at risk.

Recent government guidance on learning disability services

In the intervening years, particularly during the late 1990s, numerous pieces of government guidance have been produced to encourage the provision of better services for people with learning disabilities. These publications, however, have not come about as a result of public inquiries, indeed, none makes any reference to the occurrence of any inquiries or the existence of the ensuing reports. Rather, these documents have been part of the wider government agendas of promoting efficiency and accountability in public services and of reducing social exclusion. More worryingly, these reports and guidance have paid relatively little attention to issues of abuse prevention, as if the reprovision of services in the community will act as an automatic barrier to the development of abusive practices of the type which have in the past led to scandal and inquiry in older, larger institutions.

The 'abuse awareness' demonstrated in major government reports and guidance produced in the run-up to the *Valuing People* learning disability White Paper (Department of Health 2001) was at best limited and at worst non-existent. *Signposts for Success* (Department of Health 1998a) describes itself as good practice guidance for commissioners and providers of learning disability services. It mentions in one of its many 'checklists for action' the need to: 'Ensure that there are systems in place for preventing, detecting and responding to abuse and exploitation' (Department of Health 1998a: 11). However, the guidance fails to explain what this might entail in practice and provides no details about where to find out more about this topic in its extensive section on further sources of information. Likewise, the suggestion that commissioners should: 'Encourage non-statutory counselling services to develop their skills in working with people with learning disabilities' (op. cit. p. 11) is not backed up by any further detail.

Moving into the Mainstream (Department of Health 1998b), the report of a national inspection of services for adults with learning disabilities performs even less well. Services were measured against a total of 41 separate criteria: of these, two refer to the need for complaints procedures to be in place, but none mentions abuse prevention *per se* or what should occur when complaints are raised. *Facing the Facts* (Department of Health 1999), a policy impact study of social care and health services for people with learning disabilities, fares slightly better than its two predecessors. It not only specifically talks about the fact that: 'Protecting people from abuse and otherwise helping to keep them safe is an absolute priority for services' (Department of Health 1999: 21) but also provides some useful examples of good practice in protecting service users from potential abuse.

The *Valuing People* (Department of Health 2001) White Paper, like the reports and recommendations which preceded it, paid little more than lip service to issues of abuse prevention: one 'sub-objective' of quality services is declared to be: 'Ensuring that local adult protection policies and procedures are in place and fully complied with' (Department of Health 2001: Annex A). However, unlike many of the other objectives and sub-objectives outlined, there is no corresponding performance indicator for this measure of service quality.

All in all, these recent reports and guidelines appear to have been little influenced by either previous inquiries or the possibility of inquiries arising in the future. The reasons for this may be many, but one issue stands out as being of prime importance: the value base upon which these publications were – implicitly or explicitly – premised. *Valuing People* provides the clearest exposition of the 'key principles' upon which it is based, namely: rights, independence, choice and inclusion. These principles have not been plucked from thin air, but reflect both the growing involvement of people with learning disabilities in the planning and control of their services and the continuing influence of Wolfensberger and O'Brien. The fact that people with learning disabilities were actively involved in writing *Valuing People*, and continue to be actively involved in its implementation, represents an important and positive step in their fight for control of their own lives and lifestyles. However, it would probably be true to say that those people with learning disabilities who have been most active in this process have been those with less severe impairments and who are, as such, less vulnerable to abuse than people with multiple and profound disabilities. In this context, words such as 'protection' may be felt to have negative connotations, which hearken back to the asylums, and this may have contributed to the low profile of abuse prevention in policy statements.

That said, it is not the case that abuse prevention has had no champions in recent years, indeed there is a small but growing literature which unambiguously describes the need for safety and abuse prevention matters to be a central element in the planning and provision of services to people with learning disabilities (Sobsey 1994; McCarthy and Thompson 1996; ARC/NAPSAC 1996; White *et al.* 2003). There are also published materials to assist managers in the aftermath of abuse allegations being made (Bailey and Kitson 2001) and which demonstrate the profound need for therapeutic responses to abuse (Corbett *et al.* 1996). However, there has to date not been a sufficient connection made between those on the one hand who champion rights and independence for people with learning disabilities and those on the other hand who work to prevent abuse and to ameliorate its potentially devastating effects.

Developments in adult protection: another world?

In the decade since the enactment of the NHS and Community Care there have been no further major legislative changes that have radically altered the types and scope of public provision of learning disability services. While *Valuing People* (Department of Health 2001) sets out a new vision for learning disability services, as a White Paper it does not create any new statutory powers nor command significant extra monies. There has, however, been a significant number of steps taken towards the protection of people with learning disabilities from abuse. Progress in this area has not been specific to learning disability, but has instead been part of a wider adult protection agenda, incorporating matters relating to both abuse prevention and protection of vulnerable witnesses. Progress to date is outlined in Table 10.2.

It is in this field, of abuse prevention and vulnerable witness protection, that inquiries – in particular *Longcare* (Buckinghamshire County Council 1998) – can be seen to have played a significant role in the development of new statutory frameworks and policy guidance. However, inquiries have been only one of the major influences which have been brought to bear upon this area of work. Ongoing research, lobbying and publications emanating from voluntary sector organisations (ARC/NAPSAC 1996 and 1997; Mencap, Respond and Voice UK 2001) have also been an important factor in the development of adult protection policies and the commensurate legislative frameworks. This work has been driven by a knowledge of, and desire to eliminate, the abuses suffered by people with learning disabilities, but also a belief that it is time for the successes of child protection initiatives to be replicated across services for adults. In this respect, developments in the protection of vulnerable adults can be seen as an attempt to build an adult protection framework which mirrors the structures and procedures that already exist for the protection of children. In many senses the inquiries and lobbying which are currently occurring in relation to adult protection mimic similar events that took place several decades ago in the field of child protection. The battle is still, essentially, to get the abuse of vulnerable adults recognised by public and politicians alike as being both commonplace and completely unacceptable. In this respect the media have a significant role to play, and arguably programmes such as BBC1's *MacIntyre Investigates* (BBC 1999), where undercover filming revealed the violent ill-treatment of learning disabled residents in a private care home in Kent, have done as much as many more formal inquiries to raise public awareness of the abuses which may occur even in community-based residential support services.

Table 10.2 Progress towards the protection of people with learning disabilities

Legislation/guidance	What it says	Provenance
Human Rights Act (Home Office 1998)	Applies equally to all UK citizens, including those with a learning disability. Includes the right not to be discriminated against.	Election pledge, to bring UK in line with European legislation.
Speaking Up for Justice (Home Office 1998)	78 recommendations to ensure a fairer hearing and better access to criminal justice for vulnerable adults. This included 'special measures' in court (e.g. removal of gowns and wigs; use of screens and video links; communication aids; supporters; unsworn evidence). All 78 recommendations were accepted, with those requiring legislation being incorporated in the Youth Justice and Criminal Evidence Act.	Report of inquiry following concerns raised at the number of abuse cases not reaching court because victims and/or key witnesses were deemed 'unreliable'. Ties in with other initiatives to ensure that vulnerable and intimidated witnesses are given access to justice.
Working Together to Safeguard Children (Department of Health 1999)	Government guidance on inter-agency co-operation in relation to promoting children's welfare and protecting them from abuse and neglect. It is addressed to those who work in the health and education services, the police, social services, the probation service, and others whose work brings them into contact with children and families. It is relevant to the statutory, voluntary and independent sectors.	A response to inquiries into child abuse, which have repeatedly highlighted the need for better communication and co-ordination between the various agencies involved in child protection.
Youth Justice and Criminal Evidence Act (Home Office 1999)	Legislation required to realise the recommendations of 'Speaking Up For Justice'. Implementation began in February 2002.	A necessary legislative response to the Speaking Up for Justice report.

No Secrets (Department of Health 2000)	All local authorities are required to have policy and procedures relating to the protection of vulnerable adults in place by October 2001. The setting up of Adult Protection Committees is recommended, but not made mandatory.	A result of pressure from previous inquiries and voluntary sector campaigns. These policies were required in order to ensure consistency of approach towards issues of adult protection.
Care Standards Act (Department of Health 2000)	Creates a national inspection services for social care. Amongst other things, introduces a register (POVA: Protection of Vulnerable Adults) of individuals deemed unfit to work with vulnerable adults, against which all employees must be checked prior to commencing work. Phased implementation, due to start 2004.	Heavily influenced by the need for *national* standards, as identified by the report of the *Longcare* inquiry.
Learning Disability White Paper (Department of Health 2001)	Sets out a new framework for the provision of services for people with learning disabilities in England, based on an agenda of rights, independence, choice and inclusion.	Impetus from one interested Minister, with strong input from self-advocates and other learning disability organisations.
Achieving Best Evidence (Home Office 2002)	Good practice guidance on interviewing children and vulnerable adults and preparing them for court. Aimed at all those in the criminal justice system (police, CPS, solicitors, judiciary, etc). Replaces previous memorandum of good practice, which only applied to children.	Following on from, and adding practical detail to, the recommendations of *Speaking Up for Justice*.
Protecting the Public (Home Office 2002)	Proposals for a Bill to pass through parliament in this session. It strengthens the existing protection against sex offenders and reforms the law on sex offences. It includes particular measures relating sexual crimes perpetrated against both children and vulnerable adults (e.g. capacity to consent)	Revision of sexual offences bill considered to be long overdue, following high profile paedophile cases; lobbying by women's groups re: rape laws; and pressures from voluntary sector adult protection special interest groups.

Moving forward after abuse inquiries

The importance of inquiries, of course, lies not in their frequency or in their findings *per se*, but in the impact they have on the future pattern of service development and delivery. The hope is that they act as a kind of punctuation mark – a full stop to abusive practices and failures of regulatory practice. The reality appears to be that they act instead as a comma, a brief pause before the next scandal, a scandal that tends to possess striking similarities to those preceding it. Thus the inquiry reports themselves tend to have a 'Groundhog Day' feel to them – the same concerns raised, leading to the same recommendations made. The publication of *No Secrets* (Department of Health 2000) has attempted to provide the full stop, containing as it does a distillation of the recommendations which have been repeated in various reports over the past 15 years, but it remains dispiriting that key recommendations have yet to be implemented.

When inquiries report, but no action follows, there is a sense in which they may add to rather than diminish public and professional outrage about the continuing vulnerability of people with learning disabilities and the terrible abuses which some suffer. Part of the reason for the lack of impact, and a reason why inquiries are often so rapidly forgotten, is the format in which they are presented and their choice of emphasis. Abuse inquiries are seldom easy to read, but not for the reason one might expect: *Longcare* is actually rather coy about stating what abuses occurred. The difficulty in reading arises simply from the use of dry, repetitive official language. The inquiry's findings are presented in a language devoid of humanity – as if by exorcising emotion from its lexicon it could similarly excise its effect upon the victims. Would it were so.

The *Longcare* report (Buckinghamshire County Council 1998) produced a range of excellent recommendations designed to ensure greater transparency, stronger legal powers for Registration and Inspection Units, and a more rigorous process of investigating complaints. All of this was essential and overdue. What was absent was a meaningful examination of the emotional world of the victims of *Longcare*. It was stated both that: 'Inspection should be more focussed on the mental, physical and social well-being of the residents and the care they receive' (op. cit. p. 10) and that: 'Inspectors should seek the views of residents, their families and their social workers as to the standard of care residents are receiving' (op. cit. p. 11). This is not enough.

What is missing is an understanding of the deeper emotional needs of those traumatised within the *Longcare* homes. This is an omission that has been replicated in most inquiry reports examining the abuse of people with learning disabilities. This oversight cannot be attributed solely to the understandable preference for a format for reports that focuses on practical change rather than accommodating a more therapeutic perspective. An important question to pose about inquiries into the abuse of people with learning disabilities is:

Why is so little space given to examining the long-lasting effects of abuse? The space currently given to such issues is patently lacking, but is undoubtedly connected with a societal denial of the emotional needs of people with learning disabilities. The fact that having a learning disability places a person at greater risk of abuse than other sections of society is an unpalatable reality that is studiously avoided by most inquiries. The fact that the emotional consequences of trauma can be long-lasting and require specialist intervention is similarly overlooked.

It is interesting to note that this failure to consider fully the emotional needs of people with learning disabilities is mirrored in other settings. The world of mainstream psychotherapy and counselling, for example, has assiduously ignored the needs of people with disabilities. Most training bodies do not permit their students to take on people with learning disabilities as training patients, and offer little or nothing in the way of theoretical or practical input into working with this client group. The results of this are of extreme concern, because it has led to a scarcity of psychotherapeutic provision that can be accessed by people with learning disabilities. There remain too few therapists prepared to work with too many survivors of abuse. This situation, sadly, makes something of a mockery of the calls in *Signposts for Success* (Department of Health 1998a) for commissioners to promote the development of therapeutic services for the learning disabled.

It is essential that future inquiries learn new ways of including the voice of the service user in their method of investigation and reporting. Progress has been made in opening up the policy making process and the same now needs to be done with inquiries and inquiry reports. People with learning disabilities (at all ends of the spectrum of ability) need access to the kind of information generated by inquiries, so that they are able to effectively advocate for themselves to prevent further abuse.

Conclusion

In attempting to assess the impact which recent inquiries have had upon services for people with learning disabilities three points must be emphasised. First, that recent inquiries have been a response to abuse or death, rather than more open-ended and outward-looking systemic reviews. Second, that very few inquiries concerning people with learning disabilities ever receive widespread public attention, nor even a great deal of attention from policy makers in the field of learning disability. And third, that if levels of abuse are to be reduced, future policy makers and service planners must pay a great deal more attention to this subject than they appear to do at present.

Abuse occurs because of both organisational and individual failures to provide support and protection to vulnerable members of society. Whilst it may not always be possible to prevent the actions of a determined individual, organisational failures cannot be allowed to continue unchecked. Abuse inquiries must not be left to gather dust; their findings should become a vital tool in furthering our understanding of why abuse occurs and how to prevent it recurring. Recent service developments within the field of learning disability have focused on the need to promote rights and independence. These core values ought never again to be lost, but a way does need to be found of successfully incorporating the very real issues of protection from abuse into service development without limiting the opportunities of people with learning disabilities to lead fulfilling lives. Human rights and protection from abuse are *not* antithetical; rather each is implicit in the other. Rights can only be fully realised when people are free from the threat of abuse in their daily lives, and when those who have already suffered are given ready access to the counselling and support services which they will need to rebuild their shattered emotional landscape. Once this happens, perhaps the underlying need for inquiries will begin to lessen.

References

ARC/NAPSAC (1996) *It Could Never Happen Here! The Prevention and Treatment of Sexual Abuse of Adults with Learning Disabilities in Residential Settings*, Chesterfield/Nottingham: ARC/NAPSAC.

ARC/NAPSAC (1997) *There Are No Easy Answers: The Provision of Continuing Care and Treatment to Adults with Learning Disabilities Who Sexually Abuse Others*, Chesterfield/Nottingham: ARC/NAPSAC.

Bailey, G. and Kitson, D. (2001) *Facing the Possibility: Supporting Service Managers in Handling Allegations Against Staff*, Chesterfield: ARC.

Beail, N. and Warden, S. (1995) 'Sexual abuse of adults with learning disabilities', *Journal of Intellectual Disability Research*, 39: 382–7.

British Broadcasting Corporation (BBC) (16 November 1999) *McIntyre Investigates*.

Brown, H. and Stein, J. (1997) 'Sexual abuse perpetrated by men with intellectual disabilities: a comparative study', *Journal of Intellectual Disability Research*, 41: 215–24.

Brown, H., Stein, J. and Turk, V. (1995) 'Report of a second two-year incidence survey on the reported sexual abuse of adults with learning disabilities: 1991 and 1992', *Mental Handicap Research*, 8: 3–24.

Buckinghamshire County Council (1998) *Independent Longcare Inquiry*, Buckingham: Buckinghamshire County Council.

Care Standards Act 2000, London: The Stationery Office.

Corbett, A., Cottis, T. and Morris, S. (1996) *Witnessing, Nurturing, Protesting: Therapeutic Responses to Sexual Abuse of People with Learning Disabilities*, London: David Fulton Publishers.

Department of Health (1971) *Better Services for the Mentally Handicapped*, Cmnd. 4683 London: HMSO.

Department of Health (1979) *Report of the Committee of Enquiry into Mental Handicap Nursing and Care*, Cmnd. 7468 (Jay Report) London: HMSO.

Department of Health (1998a) *Signposts for Success in Commissioning and Providing Health Services for People with Learning Disabilities*, London: Department of Health.

Department of Health (1998b) *Moving into the Mainstream: The Report of a National Audit of Services for Adults with Learning Disabilities*, London: Department of Health.

Department of Health (1999) *Facing the Facts: Services for People with Learning Disabilities: A Policy Impact Study of Social Care and Health Services*, London: Department of Health.

Department of Health (2000) *No Secrets: Guidance on Developing and Implementing Multi-Agency Policies and Procedures to Protect Vulnerable Adults from Abuse*, London: Department of Health.

Department of Health (2001) *Valuing People: A New Strategy for Learning Disability for the 21st Century*, Cm 5086, London: Department of Health.

Department of Health, Home Office and Department for Education and Employment (1999) *Working Together to Safeguard Children: A Guide to Inter-Agency Working to Safeguard and Promote the Welfare of Children*, London: Department of Health.

Felce, D. (1996) 'Changing residential services: From institutions to ordinary living', in P. Mittler and V. Sinason (eds), *Changing Policy and Practice for People with Learning Disabilities*, London: Cassell.

Human Rights Act 1998, London: The Stationery Office.

IMHL (2003) www.davesheppard.co.uk

Independent Review of Services and Support Provided to Robert and Richard Turnbull and their parents on the Isle of Wight (2000) London: Community Care Development Centre.

Investigation into Learning Disability Services provided by the Bedfordshire and Luton Community NHS Trust (2003) London: Commission for Health Improvement (http://www.chi.nhs.uk)

Jay, P. (1979) *The Report of the Committee of Inquiry into Mental Health Handicap Nursing and Care*, London: HMSO.

Jones, K. (1960) *Mental Health and Social Policy*, London: Routledge & Kegan Paul.

Leighton, A. (1988) *Mental Handicap in the Community*, Cambridge: Woodhead-Faulkner.

Lewis, J. and Glennerster, H. (1996) *Implementing the New Community Care*, Buckingham: Open University Press.

McCarthy, M. and Thompson, D. (1996) 'Sexual abuse by design: an examination of the issues in learning disability services', *Disability and Society*, 11: 205–18.

Means, R. and Smith, R. (1994) *Community Care: Policy and Practice*, London: Macmillan.

Mencap, Respond and Voice UK (2001) *Behind Closed Doors: Preventing Sexual Abuse Against Adults with a Learning Disability*, London: Mencap.

O'Brien, J. and Tyne, A. (1981) *The Principle of Normalisation: A Foundation for Effective Services*, London: Campaign for People with Mental Handicaps.

Ryan, J. with Thomas, F. (1987) *The Politics of Mental Handicap*, London: Free Association Books.

Sobsey, D. (1994) *Violence and Abuse in the Lives of People with Disabilities: The End of Silent Acceptance?*, Baltimore, MD: Paul H. Brooks Publishing.

Thompson, D. (2000) 'Vulnerability, dangerousness and risk: the case of men with learning disabilities who sexually abuse', *Health, Risk and Society*, 2: 33–46.

White, C., Holland, E., Marsland, D. and Oakes, P. (2003) 'The identification of environments and cultures that promote the abuse of people with intellectual disabilities', *Journal of Applied Research in Intellectual Disabilities*, 16: 1–9.

Wolfensberger, W. (1972) *The Principle of Normalisation in Human Services*, Toronto: National Institute of Mental Retardation.

Youth Justice and Criminal Evidence Act 1999, London: The Stationery Office.

Chapter 11

Abuse inquiries as learning tools for social care organisations

Paul Cambridge

Introduction

As learning tools for organisations and indeed for wider society – in relation to how social care services are funded and organised, and how we value difference and disability – abuse inquiries expose limits and present opportunities. The purpose of this chapter is to explore how abuse inquiries at both local and national levels can be as productive as possible in relation to learning, while remaining functional. In undertaking this task, a focus is provided on services for people with learning disabilities. A major aim of most inquiries will be learning, but it is observed that there are limits to the extent that learning from individual inquiries can be transferred to services in general. However, some observations are evident for adult protection in general and services for people with learning disabilities in particular.

Such an analysis needs to explore the different purposes of abuse inquiries, which are established for a variety of reasons (other than organisational learning). Considerations of inquiry construction, design, and process are also relevant – sound inquiries and robust methodologies have the capacity to generate reliable and transferable findings and associated learning opportunities. Part of the task is also to consider the wider and sometimes multiple demands experienced by social care organisations – political pressures and resource constraints can distort inquiry design and process and the interpretation of evidence.

Little attention has been given to lines and hierarchies between local and national inquiries, local inquiries and investigations of individual cases and the potential connections between these different hierarchies and levels of inquiry. In-house alerts may lead to investigations, which may lead to broader inquiries, depending on respective outcomes and visibility. These will involve the police if criminal acts are alleged or suspected. Sometimes, situations may be so confused, complicated or disastrous, that national inquiries are needed, encompassing any local actions, findings or interventions. The respective learning from different levels of inquiry therefore needs to be carefully targeted.

Box 11.1   The Inquiry process – a case study

- Established by local commissioner, in response to disclosures of abuse and service collapse
- Service provided in small group home for two people with learning disabilities and challenging behaviours
- Terms of reference and background information provided
- Ran in parallel to police investigations
- Small local team established to lead inquiry including health, social services and independent representatives
- Undertook interviews with staff and managers
- Additional information and chronologies developed
- New disclosures of abuse emerged
- Issues of race and culture surfaced
- Users unable to be interviewed
- Parents declined interview due to legal action
- Developed analysis of culture of abuse
- Provided recommendations in key areas of organisation and policy
- Developed action points for commissioners, providers and services
- Reported to joint public body

(Cambridge 1999a)

In addressing the above tasks, reference will be made to my own experience as a member of a local inquiry team, and the individual and collective learning, as well as the local and general findings from this inquiry (Cambridge 1999a). Often there is little linkage between the management of abuse inquiries and practice, let alone an attempt to link such work into broader knowledge or use it to inform academic work and research. Box 11.1 profiles the case study inquiry into abuse in a small learning disability residential service which is referred to at various points in this chapter.

What we know already

Scrutiny and exposure of poor quality or abusive services have clearly led to improvements in the lives of people with learning disabilities through new philosophies of support and service models and better management and practice. Critical analyses of institutionalised care (Townsend 1962; Morris 1969; Robb 1967) and a chain of abuse scandals, exposés and inquiries (e.g. Department of Health and Social Security 1969, 1971 and 1974), contributed to the closure of the long-stay institutions and the development of community care. These helped to address fundamental questions of segregation, isolation and neglect, which were themselves characteristics of abusive regimes. However, we have since learned that deinstitutionalisation *per se* does not protect against the abuse and neglect of people with learning disabilities.

Inquiries into the abuse of people with learning disabilities in community based residential services such as Longcare (Buckinghamshire County Council 1998) or less structured exposés (Macintyre 1999) also influenced government and public opinion, with adult protection being made visible in efforts to improve value and performance management in social care (Department of Health 1998, 1999). Indeed, it could be argued that accumulated evidence and heightened national awareness and guilt stemming from such exposés have been instrumental in ensuring the prominence and implementation of national policy and strategy in generic adult protection as exemplified in *No Secrets* (Department of Health 2000).

Adult protection policy and practice had previously tended to develop *ad hoc*, through a growing body of research evidence, mainly in services for people with learning disabilities and particularly in relation to sexual abuse (e.g. Brown *et al.* 1995). Logic and understanding progressed through a series of reports and texts building on clinical, management and practice experience, outside a strategic national policy framework (see, for example, Brown 1996; Brown *et al.* 1996; ARC/NAPSAC 1993 and 1997; AIMS 1998, 1999).

Most inquiries, together with the raft of historical evidence on abuse in institutions, have tended to identify common factors associated with abusive cultures and regimes. Whilst such factors have the potential to be used as indicators or predictors of potentially abusive service environments or dependency relationships, they are also frequently characteristic of poor quality services *per se* (Cambridge 2002), suggesting conceptual links between abuse and service quality and between competence and resources. Such links, however, also dilute their usefulness as learning points for organisations or potential triggers for intervention in relation to adult protection.

The Longcare Inquiry (Buckinghamshire County Council 1998) into abuse in a private residential service for people with learning disabilities, starkly illustrated how the institutionalised abuse of people with learning disabilities can emerge in community based provisions, with residents systematically sexually and physically abused and subjected to humiliation and neglect. The inquiry found that social services had continued to purchase care despite various allegations of abuse and that the inspection service had failed to spot or act on the appalling conditions prevailing. Such observations point to how fractures in accountability across contracts and functions in community care markets can lead to isolation and increased risks for service users (Cambridge and Brown 1997).

Martin (1984), reviewing the findings of abuse inquiries in institutional (hospital) care, summarised the ingredients of institutionalised abuse as individual callousness and brutality, low standards and morale, weak and ineffective leadership, pilfering by staff, vindictiveness towards complainants and the failure of management to concern itself with abuse, characteristics also theorised by other observers (Goffman 1961; Foucault 1977).

The combined evidence from a range of studies and commentaries on abuse in the community describes the primary characteristics of abusive cultures. These include isolation, ineffective supervision and management distance, intimidation, institutionalised practice, inexperience and anti-professionalism (Cambridge 1999a). Also significant is the neutralisation of normal moral concerns, particular models of work, inward looking organisations and the nature of certain client groups (Wardhaugh and Wilding 1993). Isolation, coupled with routinised personal care work and control of private spaces by staff have been referenced as related factors (Lee-Treweek 1994), along with invisibility in high dependency care situations (Williams 1995), such as the vulnerability of clients in private and intimate care situations (Cambridge and Carnaby 2000a, 2000b).

Other formulations theorise risk factors and their location, highlighting the boundaries and relationships between abuse, neglect and mistreatment. These include carer stress leading to abusive or neglectful care (Sobsey 1994), which is increasingly an issue in unpaid care and in services with a poorly qualified workforce where increased pressures on performance and regulation impact on management time.

Wolfensberger (1975) described the production of sub-human language and images associated with infantilisation, depersonalisation, dehumanisation and victimisation and Sobsey (1994) identifying the use of euphemisms to decriminalise crimes committed against people with learning disabilities, highlighting the social learning of abuse by staff and service users as witnesses and victims. The various interpretations and meanings of dependency which can distort the caring relationship have also been described in relation to the risks of abuse (Hollins 1994), as have the construction and management of private and collective care spaces in services (Biggs *et al.* 1995). Other observations include the lack of competence in critical areas of practice such as physical interventions (Harris 1996; Harris *et al.* 1996) and intimate care (Cambridge and Carnaby 2000a).

The purpose of abuse inquiries

Inquiries into the abuse of people with learning disabilities and other vulnerable adults and children will not succeed in ensuring that abuse *'never happens again or never happens to someone else'*, despite such aims frequently being voiced. Individual circumstances and characteristics relating to service users, staff, social and physical environments and wider organisational and resource systems provide unique combinations of factors, making it difficult to construct transferable lessons. However, the construction and organisation of services also have much in common and if general lessons are to be drawn, then they need careful targeting and interpretation in relation to the specific service or care domains in which they occur. Learning for local organisations is easier, as recommendations tend automatically to reflect local conditions, assuming that such considerations are properly addressed.

Rowlings (1995) and Clough (1999) focus on the interplay of 'structural' and 'environmental' factors with the 'individual characteristics' of staff and residents as a means to understand how abuse is caused. Systems of regulation and management along with the nature of communal and private spaces can therefore be related to how individuals in care situations interact, how and where abuse might surface, whether, where and when it is recognised and what measures are taken to detect or respond to abuse. Building on such systems approaches, it has been possible to identify a series of levels within a service system to assess and manage risk (Cambridge 2003) and to interpret and locate the findings of an abuse inquiry (Cambridge 1999a).

In addition to providing lessons, abuse inquiries have a number of other potential roles that need to be considered when developing learning points (Cambridge 2001). These include demonstrating openness and a recognition of responsibilities among commissioners or providers, acceptance of public and management accountability, signalling a willingness to address failures in service management or organisation, and making a commitment to user-centred services, quality and value.

National inquiries such as Longcare (Buckingham County Council 1998) have the additional function of demonstrating wider political recognition of the needs of vulnerable adults and socially excluded groups such as people with learning disabilities. In addition, they signify the importance of responding to particularly serious disclosures of abuse and recognising some level of political accountability in higher tiers of government. Therefore, they reflect situations where national guidelines or standards have been disregarded, the severity or scale of abuse is such that local inquiries are likely to be inadequate or public sector agencies have transparently failed to meet their statutory responsibilities. Issues of public interest or wider public good may also determine the level of any inquiry as well as press for wider coverage or concern in the media. Also impacting on the profile of inquiries will be the perceived failure of regular quality monitoring or review arrangements, or where there has been a deliberate attempt to cover up disclosures or failures to act (Cambridge 2001).

Most inquiries, rightly or wrongly, also seek to establish some level of individual responsibility or blame. However, caution needs to be maintained when interpreting evidence of abuse in relation to individuals, with some important caveats evident for interpreting the findings of such inquiries and the consequent development of organisational learning.

General limits to learning

'Failings in care' cases of abuse are easy to attribute to an individual or group of people and their particular actions or inactions, suggesting a degree of individual culpability. However, such conclusions are potentially naive and even dangerous, in that they can distract attention away from more fundamental learning points for organisations. Blaming someone can be used as an excuse for not making broader systems level improvements, for example, in relation to inter-professional working or care management.

The focus on individual perpetrators or blame also constrains the interpretation of abuse as a product of wider social determinants (Sobsey 1994). More relevant are service level factors and explanations for abuse within the economic or socio-political context of service provision and labour relations, or as a product of disorganised capitalism (Harvey 1989). Cambridge and Brown (1997) identified the influence of the market shift in service provision in the UK in the 1990s on service production, leading to de-professionalisation and casualisation of the workforce and business styles of management. Such shifts have distorted user-centred provisions, fractured accountability and distanced service users from decision-making, raising additional risk management and duty of care concerns for adult protection.

The scrutiny of practice and management in abuse inquiries will usually be undertaken through a general trawling exercise of available information and evidence. However well such exercises are designed and undertaken (Cambridge 2001), there are potentially serious methodological and interpretative pitfalls to be acknowledged and avoided.

These include interactions between staff and users or particular interventions such as physical restraint. Abuse can be attributed to them in a simple cause and effect relationship, yet correlation is not the same as causation. Implicated behaviours may have been happening previously without abuse as a hypothesised outcome and such behaviours may be established elsewhere in services without attracting attention or even be sanctioned. Even if a cause and effect relationship between individuals, staff or client behaviours and abuse can be established, this may fail to acknowledge the complexities apparent from a deeper analysis of intent or experience on the part of the abuser and abused.

When interpreting evidence on prevalence and incidence from statistics or when constructing chronologies of events or actions, local policies and guidelines may provide useful baselines. However, multiple abuse may be better recognised with generic policies and procedures (Brown and Stein 1998) and reports may mainly concern service users already known to the organisations involved, diverting attention from risks in private and unregulated care settings.

A worrying aspect of high profile abuse inquiries is that they risk distracting attention away from home circumstances and at worst, providing a sort of voyeuristic gratification that such terrible things could 'never happen here'. It is important that we acknowledge the limits of inquiries and investigations in relation to prevention, but also understand how to disseminate most effectively the lessons transferable to general practice. Although admitting to mistakes or failures can be a positive learning experience and help make services more open and less defensive and arguably safer, errors of professional or management judgement which can be linked to abuse need to be placed in an operationally and organisationally appropriate context to be valid. Conversely, if lessons are culturally inappropriate, counter-intuitive or ignore the reality of management or practice experience, then they will be of little use to care staff, families or practitioners.

Graphic descriptions of individual cases of abuse can undoubtedly help increase our understanding of how a culture of abuse can develop, the risk factors and characteristics associated with the perpetration of abuse and the reasons abuse sometimes remains unchallenged or informally sanctioned. There are many complex reasons why colleagues who witness abuse, managers in service providing organisations and senior managers in public sector purchasing agencies, sometimes fail to recognise abuse or are reluctant to disclose it. Only by making such situations stark, is it possible to increase our awareness of risk, remain alert and develop interventions designed to minimise opportunities for abuse or maximise the chances of early detection.

In fighting abuse we also need to recognise the importance of empowering service users, advocates, front line staff and managers in relation to best care practices. For example, ways to address the low levels of self-advocacy in services for people with learning disabilities, coupled with a reluctance to discuss certain aspects of sexuality, the difficulties in organising quality intimate and personal care and the problems associated with developing safe physical interventions for challenging behaviour, all suggest the need for a paradigm shift from receiving services to promoting user and staff rights.

In relation to managing the consequences of disclosures of abuse, we also arguably need a parallel shift from punitive responses, which scapegoat individual managers and staff, to facilitative and emancipatory responses, which empower and encourage positive changes in behaviour and attitudes. Such responses could also help confront the need to address power relations within social care organisations and between professionals and service users. Non-punitive approaches to tackling abuse – as opposed to a serious sexual or physical assault, where there are legal responsibilities and where the criminal justice system actually stands some chance of success – maximise opportunities for individual learning. They also create chances for professionals, teams and organisations to productively learn from and apply the findings of abuse inquiries or local case investigations in grounded ways.

Part of the answer is clearly systemic, lying in valuing users, staff and managers and investing in human capital in ways which avoid institutionalising that investment in the propagation of power and powerlessness. The White

Paper, *Valuing People* (Department of Health 2001) and the raft of changes in relation to best value, inspection, care standards, quality and workforce development in social care initiated by New Labour represent opportunities for landmark steps in the right direction. However, implementation and delivering the outcomes expected will be a huge challenge for all working in and living in services for people with learning disabilities.

Extending the boundaries to interpretation and understanding

The impact of abuse on people with learning disabilities can be severe and prolonged. Their particular vulnerabilities outlined earlier mean that abusive experiences can be particularly difficult for people with learning disabilities to understand outside an individual context of self-blame and negative self-image. There are also limited opportunities for people with learning disabilities to disclose abusive experiences, such as through sex education. Disclosure is further restricted by the poor development of self-advocacy in many localities, the continued exclusion of people with more profound and multiple learning disabilities and the difficulties often experienced in accessing psychological therapies. This is despite evidence that most cases of sexual abuse, for example, are detected through self-disclosure (Brown *et al.* 1995).

Table 11.1 summarises a formulation for defining suspected abuse which, unlike some approaches, acknowledges that there are sometimes no clear lines between intent and experience and that many cases of suspected abuse will be very difficult if not impossible to be sure about. Boundaries also vary immensely between the different types of abuse perpetrated and the levels and extent of abuse.

Table 11.1 Deconstructing the boundaries between intent and experience

Categories of intent and experience	Intended as abusive	Not intended as abusive	Difficult or impossible to ascertain intent
Experienced as abusive	Clearly abuse	Probably abuse	Should be initially treated as abuse
Not experienced as abusive	Generally considered as abuse	Clearly not abuse	Probably not abuse
Difficult or impossible to ascertain how experienced	Should be initially assumed and treated as abuse	Probably not abuse	Impossible to tell whether or not abuse

Developed from McCarthy and Thompson (1994)

Examples include the direct sexual abuse of a person with a learning disability by a non-learning disabled person, compared with the failure to keep to agreed care guidelines because of pressure of work. Non-consenting sex may not always be experienced as abusive. There may sometimes simply not be the information required to ascertain whether a particular act was or was not abuse. People with a severe and multiple learning disability might be unable to relate their experience of an act or interaction because they have not learned effective ways to communicate non-verbally.

Before we learn how to respond to abuse and learn from our experiences recognising and managing individual abuse investigations or wider inquiries, we need to acknowledge the limits imposed on our individual and collective understanding and interpretation.

Accepting the variability and continuum of uncertainty inherent in the above framework, it is also evident that we require a range of flexible responses and robust rationales. Investigations and inquiries generally have the capacity to develop these. At the individual level, for example, adult protection investigations, through planning meetings and case conferences, should develop rationales for action, intervention and worker responsibility, or indeed inaction. Internal inquiries, navigating a variety of sometimes conflicting or contradictory evidence should have the capacity to distil critical information and interpret evidence, in making effective and useful recommendations. In short, we need to think about how we can respond most productively to abuse when it is recognised, and this will often require creative and lateral thinking.

Some responses to proven or suspected abuse may be similar or identical therefore, to interventions to improve poor quality care or low management or practice standards. We will need the capacity and resilience to adjust thresholds and tolerance in relation to individual circumstances unless we are to sink into a conceptual trap and moral quagmire. The same requirements apply to effectively transferring lessons to management and practice.

Brown and Stein (1998) identified the tension between formal and informal responses in relation to thresholds for responding and other workload considerations. The former included 'draconian' and 'all or nothing' approaches and the latter 'tea and sympathy' and 'blind-eye' approaches, the ability to differentiate being seen as a key to coherent reporting and effective intervention. This approach recognises the need to ground responses in an understanding of local pressures and demands while trying to maintain notions of fairness, equity and justice in adult protection practice. Most importantly, responses should be both informed and value led, with the consequences for users, services and organisations fully considered. Only by facilitating a shift from defensive management and practice to openness and honesty can we begin to learn real lessons about providing good quality support and care for people with learning disabilities.

In the context of adult protection it is also helpful to consider the idea of risk management at the macro-level (Cambridge 2002). Such approaches are particularly important for organisations because of their conceptual links to cost–benefit analysis (Eby 2000) and the high profile of development of functions and processes such as performance management and best value in social care (Cambridge 2000 and Cambridge 2002 – developed from Carson 1990). The construction and application of effective learning points for organisations will be an essential part of such an approach. Effectiveness will be determined by a range of considerations, including identifying action that can be taken to reduce uncertainty.

It is important to support the agency or worker in informed decision-making, to define the steps which need to be taken to make the benefits or advantages more likely to occur for the organisation, client, service and staff involved and reference the long-term gains and risks of particular actions against the short-term ones. Identifying action points and priorities for implementation, suggesting mechanisms and devices for facilitating consultation and change and linking these to agencies and organisations within the local service system are helpful ways of mapping the desired state and the organisational and individual responses and actions needed to achieve it.

Developing wider frameworks for understanding and learning

It is useful to differentiate the immediate circumstances and individual players surrounding instances of abuse from wider factors within service systems that potentially influence the recognition, conduct or management of abuse. In the inquiry described in this chapter (Cambridge 1999a), the characteristics of a particular culture of abuse were identified and described at four different levels within the service and service system: the individual (user); house (service); professional (team) and organisational (provider). However, a broader hierarchical framework can be constructed for risk assessment and management in services for people with learning disabilities, building on the original four levels (Cambridge 2003).

Such analyses help focus attention beyond simplistic 'bad apple' interpretations of abuse, such as the actual abuse perpetrated over a period of time by the proprietor in the Longcare example (Buckinghamshire County Council 1998). They help structure more systemic action and meaningful learning, for example, how the abuse developed, why it was tolerated for so long and what interventions might have prevented it. This encourages inquiries to look beyond the immediate and obvious to the dynamics of the establishment and its hierarchy and relationship with the outside world (Brown 1999), allowing conflicts such as those between the development and policing roles of commissioners and regulators to be taken into account.

The argument has been made in the first part of this chapter that abuse can be linked conceptually to poor quality services and it is possible to identify common failings in services and service systems which directly or indirectly contribute to opportunities to abuse or to abuse remaining hidden or unreported. Quality in services does not simply relate to the direct support of service users, although this is a fundamentally important dimension – demonstrated by the dominance of normalisation and social role valorisation, an ordinary life and the five accomplishments in services for people with learning disabilities (Wolfensberger 1980, 1984; King's Fund 1980; O'Brien 1987), supported by research evidence on levels of engagement and staff user interaction (Jones *et al.* 1999; Felce *et al.* 1998).

Quality is also concerned with management and support systems for staff, team-working and reflective practice, the implementation of policies and guidelines in critical areas such as physical interventions and intimate care, care management arrangements (Cambridge 1999b). As implied earlier, it is also critically dependent on the effective implementation of contractualism and market management, joint commissioning (Cambridge 1999c), best value and performance management (Cambridge 2000). The management, policy and interventions required to implement such instruments need to keep dimensions of user and policy outcome, such as adult protection, in sight. These include user-centred arrangements such as person-centred planning and direct payments, for example, and how users are protected from abuse or exploitation within them.

Hierarchical models can also be utilised to construct and target learning for organisations from abuse inquiries. The seven levels outlined below provide a framework for reviewing the robustness of services in relation to critical factors for adult protection and for the navigation of adult protection inquiries and the conduct of investigations.

1. Individual client level

Individual service users, their lives, characteristics, behaviours and experiences form a natural baseline for constructing lessons from an abuse inquiry. Information will include individual planning, behavioural programmes, activity records, engagement, individual guidelines and so on.

2. Staff level

The qualifications, experience, backgrounds and attitudes of individual support staff are central to relationships with service users, interactions, activities and consequently the quality and the appropriateness of care. Information for any inquiry may include training records, job applications, job and person specifications, supervision and appraisal records, observational data on interaction and so on.

3. Service level

The direct service supports and resources provided for service users and the staff team, staff and management cultures, line management and supervision will usually require scrutiny and action in abuse inquiries. Such information will include operational policies and guidelines, planning and staff records, systems for recording and sharing information, group activities, induction systems and so on.

4. Professional and specialist level

The organisation of human resources provided for or directed to service users, including team working in residential or day support settings and the management of specialist outside inputs, provide the basis for effective trans-disciplinary working. Information in this area will include assessment records and notes from different professionals and specialists, training records, care management systems and records, risk assessment and risk management information and so on.

5. Organisational level

The visibility of adult protection policy and procedures in organisational systems and cultures and guidelines for using physical interventions is a necessary prerequisite to effective adult protection practice. Information will include contracts and inter-agency agreements, responsibilities defined in policies, agency mission and value statements, appointment and supervision procedures, best value reviews and so on.

6. Systems level

Considerations of process and organisation within the lead agencies for adult protection, particularly in relation to policy development and training, are required for effective policy implementation. Information will include commissioning strategies and community care plans, service planning and care management arrangements, inspection and registration records, service audit, training strategies and so on.

7. Policy level

The influence of *No Secrets* and other relevant central policy initiatives and the use of research to develop evidence-based practice provide a baseline for assessing local adult protection practice. Information will include policy reports and documents, academic and research literature, training initiatives and inquiry reports.

Methodology, process and outcome

Investigative methodologies are an essential part of the inquiry process and relevant to the subsequent reliability, validity and usefulness of any lessons and recommendations. A number of methodological considerations are evident, mirroring approaches to utilisation focused evaluation (Patton 1997). In the particular inquiry referred to in this chapter (Cambridge 1999a, 2001) questions were asked from the start, about the accountability and autonomy of the inquiry, the type and level of information required, how best to collect a range of supporting evidence and how findings would be used.

An essential starting point is to identify and define the terms of reference. It may also be helpful to say what the inquiry should *not* include or is *not* about, for example, not interviewing people about whom allegations have been made or who are being investigated by the police. More practical considerations include expectations for reporting and delivery, for example, to whom the report will be going, when it will be required and what it will be used for. Such an approach will assist the inquiry panel plan and timetable its work, target the report and recommendations and address considerations of confidentiality (Cambridge 2001). It will also help answer the basic question 'what is the most effective way to deliver the information required by the brief in relation to the various limits evident?' and map the broader demand and response system in which the inquiry will operate (Beckhard and Harris 1987).

Internal management and accountability for inquiries need to be transparent in order to maintain credibility within the organisation(s) involved. Clear leadership will be required in order to undertake key tasks effectively (Cambridge 1999a, 2001). Relevant concerns include:

- handling and processing inquiries from any advisory body, with the help of a co-ordinator or lead link. The Chair is often best placed to perform this function;
- co-ordinating the work of the panel with various outside interests. The Chair should oversee co-ordination, but individual members may be best placed to liaise with their respective parent organisations or hold the skills or identity to work most effectively with families, carers, advocates or other interested parties, with advice from and feedback to the inquiry team;
- chairing meetings of panel members. Status, experience and respect are important attributes for this task and this usually means a senior manager from health or social services may be best placed to chair the inquiry panel or team;

- managing lines of accountability within the inquiry panel itself. The Chair, with the support of an administrator, would usually hold this responsibility;
- helping make strategic decisions about the conduct of the inquiry. Ideally, this should be a collective decision by consensus in the core team, but the Chair may on occasions need to direct the team on the basis of legal advice or operational expediency, depending on the critical nature or urgency of making a decision;
- liaising with and updating the commissioners of the panel. Regular written or verbal reports should be passed through the Chair to the commissioners, following circulation and consultation amongst the team. It will help if one person takes the lead in drafting reports or updates;
- leading contact with the police or liaison with other investigations. The Chair will usually undertake this responsibility with effective administrative support and feedback and updating for the wider team;
- managing the reporting and dissemination process. Again, an individual team member with good writing, reporting and communication skills can be delegated this task following drafting, circulation and consultation amongst the team.

Abuse inquiries should also consider the benefits of involving someone on the inquiry panel without local interests or connections, thus providing an element of objectivity and a capacity to compare circumstances with those elsewhere. Ideally, such individuals should have broad perspective or experience of the management and practice issues in social care, the specialist needs of the user group in question and an understanding of the nature and characteristics of abuse.

Someone in such a position might be an adult protection co-ordinator from another local authority, a specialist senior practitioner in learning disability, an experienced care manager in adult protection or an academic involved in applied research in adult protection, learning disability, challenging behaviour or any area of expertise relevant to the particular case or investigation. Such involvement can help maintain the wider credibility of the inquiry and relate local evidence to wider management or practice experience or research evidence.

In services for people with learning disabilities, it is virtually unheard of for a user representative to be directly involved in an inquiry, but there is no valid reason why a user representative or someone from a self-advocacy group should not be directly involved in interpreting the evidence, helping make recommendations or safeguarding the interests of those who may have been victims.

In cases of abuse which include oppression on the basis of race, culture or ethnicity or where gender or sexuality have played a particularly visible part, best practice would also suggest equivalent representation on the inquiry.

This will help ensure that investigations are grounded in the experience of structural or institutionalised oppression, questions are appropriately and sensitively formulated and recommendations are relevant to wider issues of social exclusion or discrimination. Advice might also be sought from community or self-help groups on appropriate arrangements and representation. In the inquiry referred to in this chapter, a black practitioner was asked to join the team due to the prominence of race and culture as intervening variables in the service in question and the allegation of abuse.

As noted earlier, important sources of information will be various staff, user, management, planning and intervention records, as well as wider policies and procedures. These can help provide contextual and supporting evidence on care standards and processes, service quality and management inputs and guidance and make the location of learning points relevant to the organisation. It is therefore important for inquiries to agree principles for accessing such information. In the inquiry discussed in this chapter (Cambridge 1999a), the commissioner, as the agency responsible for jointly purchasing services for people with learning disabilities in the local area, compiled sets of records and reports relating to the allegations of abuse and the management of the service itself, for the inquiry panel to scrutinise. In addition, information was collated from a range of other sources, including the provider agency and local authority policies, guidelines and procedures on risk management, control and restraint and adult protection, recruitment and selection arrangements, staff supervision systems, complaints procedures and service audit. At the same time, it needs to be recognised that records have obvious limits. Abusers will avoid recording abusive acts and some aspects of service provision, such as intimate care, will remain unobserved for reasons of privacy and respect. Complete pictures are rarely available from such sources.

It is evident that co-operation from both purchasers and providers is essential for establishing comprehensive baseline information for abuse inquiries. However, in some instances it may be risky to rely on an interested party to obtain information for and on behalf of inquiry panels, as the objectivity of the inquiry or the information provided may be compromised by potential conflicts of roles or interests. Conversely, a co-operative culture is likely to prove an essential part of a successful and productive inquiry, requiring two-way trust.

In relation to interviewing as a source of intelligence, it makes moral and intellectual sense to interview the victims or possible victims of abuse (when checking the possibility of more widespread abuse). However, there are particular considerations regarding supporting people with learning disabilities to participate productively and safely in such a process. These include support from a keyworker or advocate, help with communication through translation of speech or signing and the possibility of psychological therapy or a support group following disclosures of abuse. In addition, there needs to be a clear rationale with expert advice if there is a chance of criminal proceedings against the perpetrator, as poor interviewing procedures could open the inquiry to allegations of suggestibility (see various papers in Churchill *et al.* 1997).

Witness evidence is also an important source of information for abuse, and is a particularly important form of evidence in criminal cases (Brown *et al.* 1995; AIMS 1999). It is therefore probable that inquiries will seek to interview potential witnesses and those who might have access to relevant information about users or the staff and professionals in contact with them. Such people are also in a good position to provide impressions about the culture within services, the attitudes of key players and make observations about the signs and signals that usually surround abuse. Inquiries will of course need to be aware of the probability that interviewees who suspected or witnessed abuse may be reluctant to disclose this, as this might be perceived to reflect poorly on their professional capability or possibly be interpreted as negligent.

However, the experience with the case study described in this chapter suggests that, without criminal investigations and the power to require potential witnesses or informants to attend police interviews and disclose information, key players in abuse inquiries are likely to be unavailable or decline participation. This invariably limits the pool of available intelligence and therefore the thoroughness of inquiries. This will often apply to the most important source of information and intelligence, namely people with learning disabilities themselves. In the case study, both were unable to be interviewed by either the police or the panel due to their difficulties with all forms of expressive or receptive communication.

In the case study inquiry, careful planning was invested in the conduct and content of interviews, in order to maintain consistency and fairness, as well as to maximise effective and productive interviewing (Cambridge 2001). A standard interview schedule, with sub-questions reflecting the roles of the key interviewees, was developed for the inquiry. These also reflected the terms of reference. A set of rules for participation, representation and interviewing was also constructed, with participants briefed prior to the interview. They included:

- having two interviewers present;
- having an interviewee representative if desired (although not to become involved in the discussion);
- an introductory letter explaining the inquiry brief (e.g. to examine policies, procedures and systems, but not to attribute blame);
- not permitting interviewees to see the questions before the interview;
- ensuring the initial questions asked are taken from the interview schedule;
- only asking additional questions for clarification or to explore particular issues or lines of inquiry;

- selecting questions which are relevant to the role and responsibilities of the interviewee;
- treating interview notes as confidential to the inquiry panel;
- recording interviewer observations and interpretations following each interview;
- prior briefing of interviewees about the scope and limits of confidentiality;
- explaining the necessity to pass on any additional disclosures of abuse.

Such protocols help make for a balanced and considered approach and can provide useful protection for both interviewees and interviewers, the latter usually being members of the inquiry team. Many of those who have witnessed and/or disclosed abuse will also have been disempowered by the experience, especially in the absence of policies aimed at protecting whistle-blowers. It will therefore be important to try to ensure that interviews are not experienced as aversive.

An essential task of most inquiries will be to examine the robustness and comprehensiveness of adult protection policies and procedures used and referenced by commissioners and providers (Brown and Stein 1998) and any other relevant guidelines, such as those on physical interventions (Harris 1996; Harris *et al.* 1996) sexuality and personal relationships (Cambridge and McCarthy 1997) and intimate care (Cambridge and Carnaby 2000b). Often failure to implement policies and related guidelines contributes to the late detection of abuse or to the neglect of service users. Such analyses will invariably generate learning points for organisations.

To make their findings as relevant and powerful as possible, inquiries should seek to develop partnership models of working. For example, providers should be involved in inquiries initiated by commissioners, and family members consulted and interviewed if their relatives have been abused, and so on, depending on considerations of confidentiality and appropriateness. Options include the service or provider agency in question being given an opportunity to comment on draft reports or seeing the final report in advance of wider circulation to enable a response to be prepared.

Where there are a large number of potential stakeholders involved, such as parents, user/advocates, a residential or day service provider organisation, peripatetic team, professionals, national voluntary organisation as well as purchasers from health and social services, consideration could be given to developing an advisory group for the inquiry. Although this was not appropriate for the case study inquiry due to the polarised interests between the commissioner, provider service and relatives, such a group has the potential function of defining the terms of reference, identifying the lines of inquiry or defining the questions for the investigation. It can also help develop the co-operation of individuals from the organisations or interests represented for implementing recommendations and lead to more meaningful learning on the part of the different stakeholders.

Structuring the analysis and describing the abuse

It will usually prove helpful for the inquiry team to map the chronology and morphology of the abuse itself, in order to make what has happened transparent and to reduce any resistance to acting on evidence or recommendations. The nature, patterns and wider characteristics of any additional abuse uncovered by the inquiry will also need to be described, as this will help target the findings and facilitate learning points for organisations and individuals within them. Attention will, of course, need to be given to issues surrounding confidentiality for individual staff and service users.

At a broader level, inquiries will undoubtedly point to inherent weaknesses in our care systems. These exist at all levels, as mapped above, but most worrying are likely to be those between staff and users, different professionals involved with individuals or services and between commissioners and providers of services. These are the critical junctures at which practice, interagency working, inspection and regulation and care markets break down. Inter-disciplinary working is often fractured by accountability to different agencies and different lines of management and professional accountability (Cambridge and Brown 1997).

Comparing experience between different user groups (see Stanley *et al.* 1999), can also help widen our understanding of abuse and its economic and social determinants, particularly in relation to the formal dependency relationships constructed through the use of paid labour in social care and the contractual relationships between purchasers and providers. For example, the market in residential and social care for older people carries risks of isolation, neglect and physical abuse which might be relevant to informing the regulation and inspection of private sector residential care for people with learning disabilities. In fighting abuse in services for people with learning disabilities we therefore need to consider the wider context of abuse, as much as the individual characteristics of abusive acts or interactions between staff and residents.

Yet it will be unusual for there not to be a number of facets to individual cases of abuse, especially considering the particular vulnerabilities of people with learning disabilities and characteristics of offenders or perpetrators. Emotional abuse in the form of threats and intimidation is commonly associated with sexual abuse and physical abuse may be perpetrated alongside financial abuse and exploitation of individuals or within services (Brown *et al.* 1995), making it necessary to employ some categorisation of abuse (this is best done by referring to those specified in local vulnerable adults or abuse policies) and exploring connections between different types of abuse.

The attributes of abusive cultures can themselves also be distilled and summarised in the findings of inquiries, as in the case study inquiry which analysed the underlying culture of abuse and identified its key characteristics.

This can add conceptual depth to a report and make for a grounded story; one that local players and interests can identify with and act on.

Reporting and making recommendations

The findings of inquiry panels will generally be delivered through a formal written report with recommendations, but this is not mutually exclusive of other modes of reporting and dissemination. Such devices can include regular interim reports, summary updates on progress, verbal briefings for commissioners and briefing or issue papers identifying the emerging themes or findings. The targeting of the findings and recommendations can also be achieved through separate dissemination for particular audiences, including executive summaries (for commissioners) or action papers (for providers and professionals).

Having summary versions of the main findings or recommendations can help make for effective dissemination and reporting, as one large report is often difficult to interpret and time-consuming to read. Professionals and user groups need easy and ready information to act on. A feedback sheet for care staff could summarise the main findings relevant to direct support or one for managers setting the lessons relating to supervision or staff training. A user leaflet in plain English or using local symbols could inform service users of their rights and who to disclose abuse to.

It will generally prove unhelpful to circulate reports widely for comments before general release, apart possibly to the commissioners of the inquiry or the organisation, service or professionals in question (the latter could provide for problems which are unlikely to be resolved and hold up wider reporting). Moreover, there may not necessarily be an obligation on the part of the inquiry or organisation concerned to circulate the findings more widely. Any advantages of having sole access to a report will need to be balanced against wider expectations about openness and the need to target and implement action and learning, as well as relevant questions of anonymity and confidentiality.

Much will hinge on the actual findings and recommendations, making some reciprocal criticism about accuracy or interpretation almost inevitable. Such criticism should be constructively addressed by the inquiry and it will be critically important to differentiate between facts on the one hand and impressions and views on the other in the findings in order to maintain robust critiques and interpretations.

Managerially and operationally relevant recommendations are an essential product of an abuse inquiry and one way to help meet this objective is to identify the aspects and components of the service, system or policy which failed to perform adequately in relation to the abuse and why this was the case. For example, the case study inquiry profiled earlier (Cambridge 1999a) used a series of headings for reporting the findings and recommendations which related to service operation and management. These included staff supervision arrangements, training and staff development, service audit and challenging behaviour, inter-professional working arrangements, clarity over care management responsibilities and individual service co-ordination, market management, relationships between the commissioner and provider organisations and information exchange and accountability within and between provider services.

Areas where adult protection policies and procedures could be improved were also identified, including policy development in whistle-blowing, supporting witnesses, managing disclosure and policy implementation and leadership in adult protection. Related action points referenced the responsibilities of the various parties and interests involved for facilitating change and improvement.

Action point 1, for example, detailed how the development of new inter-agency policy on whistle-blowing could be progressed, linking with adult protection and through consultation with the various stakeholders. Action point 2 detailed measures for improving inter-agency co-ordination in adult protection, including liaison with the police. Action point 3 detailed the development of adult protection competence in provider services, through induction training and basic skills in recognition and reporting. Action point 4 profiled the establishment of a small task force to help move forward multi-disciplinary and inter-professional liaison and co-ordination on individual cases. Action point 5 detailed how all purchasers in the local area could clarify care management arrangements and responsibilities. Agencies and individuals responsible for implementing the recommendations of abuse inquiries need to be given the tools, resources and authority to manage and negotiate change effectively. More often they are left powerless.

Conclusion

The resource implications of taking adult protection forward in services for people with learning disabilities are potentially very significant and include expenditure on policy development and review, staff training, the pump-priming of specialist services such as advocacy and individualised communication, workload management across community teams and caseload management for care managers and senior practitioners.

The costs attached to an individual investigation or inquiry can also be considerable in terms of administrative support and professional time. Moreover, the implementation of any action or recommendations invariably carries costs. These may range across the various levels and include developing individual guidelines, programmes and plans, risk management, briefing professionals, reviewing and amending policies and procedures, changing contracting processes, commissioning new services such as advocacy or communication support, specifying training interventions, initiating new lines of accountability or models of supervision or establishing educational groups or workshops for service users.

However, the short-term costs associated with implementing the findings of abuse inquiries bear no comparison to the costs of failing to act on abuse or the recommendations of abuse inquiries. The latter can impact massively in terms of damage to the credibility or reputation of organisations, staff, managers, or professionals and to the self-respect of service users and their families. Too often the hidden costs to individual staff and service users of inaction, costs that cannot be priced, are never brought into the equation. At the same time, abuse will never be eradicated in a society in which structural inequalities remain stark. We continue to institutionalise capital in services, dependency relationships are an important means of economic production, many staff remain undervalued or poorly supported and oppression on the basis of gender, race and sexuality often remains acute.

Focused work in learning disability on risk (Manthorpe *et al.* 1997) and sexual abuse (Brown *et al.* 1995; McCarthy and Thompson 1996) has provided essential insights into the patterns and circumstances surrounding the abuse of people with learning disabilities, but there remains a need to strengthen generic comparisons and perspectives (Decalmer and Glendenning 1997). The exchange of experience in the detection and management of abuse and the development and implementation of learning between user groups, services and organisations should therefore also receive priority.

References

AIMS (1998) *The Alerter's Guide*, The Aims Project, Brighton: Pavilion.

AIMS (1999) *The Investigator's Training Manual*, The Aims Project, Brighton: Pavilion.

ARC/NAPSAC (1993) *It Could Never Happen Here!*, Association for Residential Care/ National Association for the Protection from Sexual Abuse of Adults and Children with Learning Disabilities, London: Department of Health.

ARC/NAPSAC (1997) *There Are No Easy Answers*, Association for Residential Care/ National Association for the Protection from Sexual Abuse of Adults and Children with Learning Disabilities, London: Department of Health.

Beckhard, R. and Harris, R. (1987) *Organizational Transitions*, Wokingham: Addison Wesley.

Biggs, S., Phillipson, C. and Kingston, P. (1995) *Elder Abuse in Perspective*, Buckingham: Open University Press.

Brown, H. (1996) *Towards Safer Commissioning: A Handbook for Purchasers and Commissioners*, Nottingham: NAPSAC.

Brown, H. (1999) 'Abuse of people with learning disabilities: layers of concern and analysis', in N. Stanley, J. Manthorpe and B. Penhale (eds), *Institutional Abuse: Perspectives Across the Life Course*, London: Routledge.

Brown, H. and Stein, J. (1998) 'Implementing adult protection policies in Kent and East Sussex', *Journal of Social Policy*, 27(3): 371–96.

Brown, H., Stein, J. and Turk, V. (1995) 'The sexual abuse of adults with learning disabilities: report of a second two year incidence survey', *Mental Handicap Research*, 8(1): 1–22.

Brown, H., Brammer, A., Craft, A. and McKay, C. (1996) *Towards Better Safeguards: A Handbook for Inspectors and Registration Officers*, Nottingham: National Association for the Protection from Sexual Abuse of Adults and Children with Learning Disabilities.

Buckinghamshire County Council (1998) *Independent Longcare Inquiry*, Buckingham: Buckinghamshire County Council.

Cambridge, P. (1999a) 'The first hit: A case study of the physical abuse of people with learning disabilities and challenging behaviours in a residential service', *Disability and Society*, 14(3): 285–308.

Cambridge, P. (1999b) 'Building care management competence in services for people with learning disabilities', *British Journal of Social Work*, 29: 393–415.

Cambridge, P. (1999c) 'More than just a quick fix? The potential of joint commissioning in services for people with learning disabilities', *Research, Policy and Planning*, 17(2): 12–22.

Cambridge, P. (2000) 'Using "best value" in purchasing and providing services for people with learning disabilities', *British Journal of Learning Disabilities* 28: 31–7.

Cambridge, P. (2001) 'Managing abuse inquiries: Methodology, organisation, process and politics', *Journal of Adult Protection*, 3(3): 6–20.

Cambridge, P. (2002) 'Assessing and managing risk', in S. Carnaby (ed.), *Learning Disability Today (learning disability certificate reader)*, Brighton: Pavilion Publishing and Tizard Centre.

Cambridge, P. (2003) 'The Risk of Getting it Wrong: Systems Failure and the Impact of Abuse', in D. Allen (ed.), *Ethical Approaches to Physical Interventions: Responding to Challenging Behaviour in People with Intellectual Disabilities*, Kidderminster: British Institute of Learning Disabilities.

Cambridge, P. and Brown, H. (1997) 'Making the market work for people with learning disabilities: An argument for principled contracting', *Critical Social Policy*, 17(2): 27–52.

Cambridge, P. and McCarthy, M. (1997) 'Developing and implementing sexuality policy for a learning disability provider service', *Health and Social Care in the Community*, 5(4): 227–36.

Cambridge, P. and Carnaby, S. (2000a) *Making it Personal: Providing Intimate and Personal Care for People with Learning Disabilities*, Brighton: Pavilion.

Cambridge, P. and Carnaby, S. (2000b) 'A personal touch: managing the risks of abuse during intimate and personal care', *Journal of Adult Protection*, 2(4): 4–16.

Carson, D. (1990) 'Taking risks with patients – your assessment strategy', in *Professional Nurse, The Staff Nurse's Survival Guide*, pp. 83–7, London: Austen Cornish.

Churchill, J., Brown, H., Craft, A. and Horrocks, C. (1997) *There are No Easy Answers*, London: Association for Residential Care/National Association for the Protection from Sexual Abuse of Adults and Children with Learning Disabilities.

Clough, R. (1999) 'The abuse of older people in institutional settings: The role of management and regulation', in N. Stanley, J. Manthorpe and B. Penhale (eds), *Institutional Abuse: Perspectives Across the Life Course*, London: Routledge.

Decalmer, P. and Glendenning, F. (eds) (1997) *The Mistreatment of Elderly People*, London: Sage.

Department of Health (1998) *Partnership in Action*, London: HMSO.

Department of Health (1999) *Modernising the Social Services*, London: HMSO.

Department of Health (2000) *No Secrets: Guidance on Developing and Implementing Multi-Agency Policies and Procedures to Protect Vulnerable Adults from Abuse*, London: The Stationery Office.

Department of Health (2001) *Valuing People: A New Strategy for Learning Disability for the 21st Century*, London: Department of Health.

Department of Health and Social Security (1969) *Report of the Committee of Inquiry into Allegations of Ill-treatment of Patients and Other Irregularities at the Ely Hospital, Cardiff* (Cmnd. 3975), London: HMSO.

Department of Health and Social Security (1971) *Report of the Committee of Inquiry at Farleigh Hospital* (Cmnd. 4557), London: HMSO.

Department of Health and Social Security (1974) *Report on the Care of Patients at South Ockendon Hospital*, London: HMSO.

Eby, M. (2000) 'The challenges of being accountable', in A. Brechin, H. Brown and M. Eby (eds), *Critical Practice in Health and Social Care*, London: Sage.

Felce, D., Lowe, K., Perry, J., Jones, E., Baxter, H. and Bowley, C. (1998) *The Quality of Residential and Day Services for Adults with Learning Disabilities in Eight Local Authorities in England: Objective Data Gained in Support of a Social Services Inspectorate Inspection*, Cardiff: Welsh Centre for Learning Disabilities, University of Wales.

Foucault, M. (1977) *Discipline and Punish*, London: Allen Lane.

Goffman, E. (1961) *Asylums*, New York: Anchor.

Harris, J. (1996) 'Physical restraint procedures for managing challenging behaviours presented by mentally retarded adults and children', *Research in Developmental Disabilities*, 17: 99–134.

Harris, J., Allen, D., Cornick, M., Jefferson, A. and Mills, R. (1996) *Physical Interventions: A Policy Framework*, Kidderminster: British Institute of Learning Disabilities.

Harvey, D. (1989) *The Condition of Postmodernity*, Oxford: Blackwell.

Hollins, S. (1994) 'Relationships between perpetrators and victims of physical and sexual abuse', in J. Harris and A. Craft (eds), *People with Learning Disabilities at Risk of Physical or Sexual Abuse*, Seminar Papers No. 4, Kidderminster: British Institute of Learning Disabilities.

Jones, E., Perry, J., Lowe, K., Felce, D., Toogood, S., Dunstan, F., Allen, D. and Pagler, J. (1999) 'Opportunity and the promotion of activity among adults with severe intellectual disability living in community residences: The impact of training staff in active support', *Journal of Intellectual Disability Research*, 43(3): 164–78.

King's Fund (1980) *An Ordinary Life*, Project Paper No. 24, London: King's Fund Centre.

Lee-Treweek, G. (1994) 'Bedroom abuse: The hidden work in a nursing home', *Generations Review*, 4(1): 2–4.

Macintyre, D. (1999) *Macintyre Undercover*, BBC1, 16 November.

Manthorpe, J., Walsh, M., Alaszewski, A. and Harrison, L. (1997) 'Issues of risk practice and welfare in learning disability services', *Disability and Society*, 12(1): 69–82.

Martin, J. (1984) *Hospitals in Trouble*, Blackwell: Oxford.

McCarthy, M. and Thompson, D. (1996) 'Sexual abuse by design: an examination of the issues in learning disability services', *Disability and Society*, 11(2): 205–17.

Morris, P. (1969) *Put Away*, London: Routledge.

O'Brien, J. (1987) 'A Guide to Lifestyle Planning', in B. Willcox and G. Bellamy (eds), *The Activities Catalogue*, Baltimore: Brookes.

Patton, M. (1997) *Utilization Focused Evaluation*, London: Sage.

Robb, B. (1967) *Sans Everything: a Case to Answer*, London: Nelson.

Rowlings, C. (1995) 'Elder abuse in context', in R. Clough (ed.), *Elder Abuse and the Law*, London: Action on Elder Abuse.

Sobsey, D. (1994) *Violence and Abuse in the Lives of People with Learning Disabilities*, Baltimore: Brookes.

Stanley, N., Manthorpe, J. and Penhale, B. (eds) (1999) *Institutional Abuse: Perspectives Across the Life Course*, London: Routledge.

Townsend, P. (1962) *The Last Refuge*, London: Routledge.

Wardhaugh, J. and Wilding, P. (1993) 'Towards an explanation of the corruption of care', *Critical Social Policy*, 37: 4–31.

Williams, C. (1995) *Invisible Victims: Crime and Abuse against People with Learning Difficulties*, London: Jessica Kingsley.

Wolfensberger, W. (1975) *The Origin and Nature of our Institutional Models*, Syracuse: Human Policy Press.

Wolfensberger, W. (1980) 'The definition of normalisation: update, problems, disagreements and misunderstandings', in R. Flynn and K. Nitsch (eds), *Normalisation, Social Integration and Community Services*, Baltimore: University Park Press.

Wolfensberger, W. (1984) 'A reconception of normalisation as social role valorisation', *Mental Retardation* (Canadian), 34: 22–5.

Part V

Inquiries into the abuse and neglect of older people

Chapter 12

Older people, institutional abuse and inquiries

Bridget Penhale and Jill Manthorpe

Introduction

The abuse of older people receiving care in institutions is not a new phenomenon. Reports of mistreatment and neglect appear regularly but are somewhat cursorily covered by the media. The abuse of older people who live in institutions is seemingly part of the experience of many residents in a number of different settings and such abuse may be both widespread and systematic (Glendenning 1999a). As Glendenning (1999b: 2) observed, there has been a lengthy tradition in the UK of scandals in institutional care relating to older people and, in the United States, detailed research stretches back to the early 1970s. Such scandals tend to have been investigated and treated as separate inquiries into standards of care rather than as directly concerned with abuse. Interest tends to be short-lived and rather superficial in such scandals and the infrequent inquiries that are established. There are a number of reasons for this, but the nature and impact of ageism and ambivalence concerning the care afforded to older people may be important factors.

The focus of this chapter concerns inquiries into institutions for older people that provide care, protection and sometimes treatment. In these locations, the duty of care is perhaps of paramount concern especially when it relates to those older people who are particularly frail and vulnerable and in the latter stages of life. When abuse occurs in such settings, it may be perceived as particularly at variance with the institution's stated aims and objectives. The chapter will examine and compare recent inquiries concerning three separate NHS units that provided care for older people. First we consider definitions and understandings concerning the abuse of older people that occurs within institutions.

Multiple definitions of institutional abuse, a variety of indicators of abuse and the inclusion and exclusion of neglect are evident in the UK, despite the sharper policy focus of *No Secrets* (Department of Health 2000). Public inquiries into institutions may employ differing definitions, or move between 'bad practice', 'unacceptable care', 'mistreatment' and 'abuse'. Differing definitions need not be problematic (Penhale 1993) but greater clarity could be helpful. Any investigation should draw some distinction between individual acts within institutions, abusive regimes, and examples of poor, or even bad, practice relating to both management and care. This may also help to address organisational and structural problems (Bennett *et al.* 1997).

Inquiries into institutional abuse may focus on individuals and their personality or practice; the so-called 'bad apple' approach (Biggs *et al.* 1995; Manthorpe and Stanley 1999). This means responses to abuse will focus on flushing out real or potential abusers. Developments in professional screening and regulation such as the setting up of and proposed extensions of the General Social Care Council, the extension of criminal record screening, and the proposed register for staff who are judged as not suitable to work with vulnerable adults are responses to these concerns.

Like abuse within domestic spheres, elder abuse in institutional settings involves differing types of abuse. Abuse may be physical, including sexual abuse; or it may be psychological and emotional, including bullying and intimidation. Neglect, whether intentional or not, is usually incorporated and may include such aspects as enforced isolation, lack of activities and deprivation (food or drink, clothes or personal care). The misuse of medication within care settings has also evoked concern (Chambers 1999), as has the use of physical restraints, which may result in physical injury (Bright 1999a). Financial or material abuse, the misappropriation of money, property, possessions, or exploitation, is also sometimes found in institutions although this appears common in all settings (Aitken and Griffin 1996).

Abuse may occur in institutions run by public, private and voluntary, or not-for-profit organisations. Hospitals, residential and nursing homes and day care settings are all possible locations in which abuse or neglect has been found. All vulnerable older people who use such institutions could potentially be at risk of experiencing abuse or an abusive regime. In these settings, there is an organisational context to the delivery of care in which the behaviour of a particular individual towards a resident or patient has to be set. As the numerous inquiries into deficiencies in the institutional care of older people have shown, abuse may flourish within a culture that allows it to be acceptable and where boundaries are not respected (Martin 1984; Clough 1999a; Stanley *et al.* 1999).

Interwoven aspects of abuse and poor standards of care are illustrated in the examples of abuse in the UKCC report into professional misconduct cases (UKCC 1994), a report which, it has been said, should be 'mandatory reading for all nurses' (Nolan 1994). Between 1990 and 1991 and 1993 and 1994, the number of allegations involving older people rose, both absolutely and as a proportion of all cases. The Council drew particular attention to the rise in the number of misconduct cases in nursing homes, which, by 1994, constituted the highest single group of cases:

Whilst the complaints reveal serious professional misconduct such as physical and verbal abuse, they also identify wholly inadequate systems of drug administration, ineffective management systems, lack of systematic care planning or effective record keeping and almost non-existent induction or in-service training . . . Financial controls and audit procedures designed to safeguard residents' finances appear to be woefully inadequate.

(UKCC 1994: 7)

However, this only indicates an issue, not the extent of abuse or its causes. There is 'extremely limited empirical evidence' (Gilleard 1994: 195), about the role of professionals within such situations. The limited research, much of it from the United States, concentrates on nursing home assistants, rather than qualified staff (see, for example, Fader *et al.* 1990).

In addition to different types of abuse and different settings, there may be a range of participants involved: residents; staff; relatives, friends or volunteers (see Stanley *et al.* 1999). Abuse within institutions may arise because of the regime or system operating in which residents are mistreated and their personhood denied (Bright 1999b). At the other end of the continuum, however, are individual acts of abuse that happen but are not part of the overall regime or organisational culture. Abuse may also occur between a resident and a member of care staff, initiated by the older person as protagonist, so there may be dual directionality of abuse, or abuse solely from resident towards a staff member (McCreadie 1996).

This broad arena means there is limited research and such as there is becomes thinly stretched to inform inquiries' deliberations. Although there have been numerous scandals relating to the care of older people receiving institutional care (Clough 1999b), at central level, the Department of Health's (1993) initial focus was on abuse in domestic settings. However, a more coherent and consistent approach emerged during the 1990s (Department of Health/SSI 1999). Institutional abuse is now highlighted within policy documents as an area where attention is needed (Department of Health 1998, 2000).

Indeed, the *No Secrets* document, published in 2000 (Department of Health 2000), gave a clear mandate to English Social Services Departments to take a lead role in the co-ordination of multi-agency work in relation to adult protection. This ranges from the setting up of inter-agency policies and procedures through to the development of investigations and responses to abuse and neglect. Institutional forms of abuse clearly fall within the provisions of the document, which includes institutional abuse as a distinctive form of abuse together with more 'traditional' forms of abuse. Matthew *et al.*'s (2002: 9) work on the implementation of policies and procedures shows that representatives from the local authority inspection unit were heavily consulted and that most (71 out of 110) contracts between local authorities and providers of residential and nursing homes required adherence to vulnerable adult procedures.

Inquiries into the institutional care of older people

In comparison with inquiries into the care of children, reported in earlier chapters, there has been limited attention to inquiries' role in enhancing the quality of residential care or lasting improvements. This is reflected in the short-term interest accorded to inquiries involving abuse of older people; and we argue that ageism and the marginalisation of older people are the most convincing explanations for this.

In the late 1980s, Roger Clough was commissioned to review ten inquiry reports for a government review of residential care (the Wagner Committee). Only two of the reports concerned older people, although these represented the most recent inquiries that he studied (Clough 1999b) and one concerned the full range of residential provision for older people in a London borough. This work was later complemented by further studies of abuse within residential settings, which incorporated insights developed as a result of Clough's professional involvement in inquiries (Clough 1996, and see Chapter 13 this volume). The three reports chosen for this chapter concern hospital provision not residential care, although the needs of the older people involved were evidently as much for social care as much as for health care. In the UK, the search for the 'right' place to support older people with high levels of disability, particularly if this is the result of cognitive and behavioural problems combined with illness or frailty, is an enduring tussle between health and social services. The inquiries discussed here centre on the NHS but in our view they have broad relevance to any long-term, or 'home for life' environment. As we argue, the factors identified as contributing to abuse are not restricted to the NHS but may apply to any marginalised, low priority or isolated service or sector. The first inquiry relates to an internal inquiry, the other two to external reviews, developed following initial internal inquiries. The third report relates to a review and investigation by a national organisation, the Commission for Health Improvement (renamed the Healthcare Commission in 2004). These reports were published later than Clough's unpublished review for the Wagner Committee or his work relating to inquiries (1999b). The issues they raise, however, have some distinct similarities.

The three inquiries cover events in long-term units for older people provided by the NHS in three very different areas of England. One was in London, at St Pancras Hospital, serving an inner city community (Camden and Islington Community Health Services NHS Trust 1999); another in the North-West in a predominantly rural area, although the hospital was located on the edge of a regional centre, Carlisle (North Lakeland Trust 2000). The final report concerned a mental health unit run by Manchester Mental Health and Social Care Trust (Commission for Health Improvement

2003). These were all units that were well established, self-contained and separate from the main hospital provision, although sited within the main hospital campus. As a result of the events that took place, including the inquiries, in London and Carlisle the units were closed and the remaining patients transferred to newer units. In the case of the Carlisle hospital, the hospital itself (Garlands) was closed, although this appeared to be due to service changes rather than the events that had occurred in one specific unit of the hospital. In Manchester, patients were moved from Rowan Ward to a temporary ward location in another hospital prior to their movement to accommodation run by Anchor Trust, a not-for profit Housing Association (Commission for Health Improvement 2003: 3.46). For the purpose of clarity, the units considered here will be referred to by name: Beech House (St Pancras), Kielder House (North Lakeland Trust), and Rowan Ward (Manchester) for the remainder of this account.

The reports

The similarities between the three reports are striking. All three units provided care for older people with enduring mental health problems. Kielder House had been opened in 1997 and provided for 30 older people with mental health difficulties. The unit had been formed by the amalgamation of staff and patients from three continuing care wards at the hospital. The reports of mistreatment were therefore made at most two years after the opening of the unit (in December 1998). A decision was taken for the initial investigation to only consider the allegations made at the particular time that the report was made.

Beech House unit had been established in 1993 to house 12 older people who had been transferred following the closure of a psychiatric hospital covered by the same health authority. The reports concerning this unit were made in April 1996, after the unit had been open for three years. During the investigations that took place, a decision was taken to consider the entire period that the unit had been open, as evidenced by the title: *Beech House Inquiry: report of the internal inquiry relating to the mistreatment of patients residing at Beech House, St. Pancras Hospital during the period March 1993–April 1996*. Both these units had therefore been established relatively recently.

According to staff and the local Community Health Council, Rowan Ward had become a 'forgotten service' (Commission for Health Improvement 2003: 3.11) after other wards and services moved from the Withington Hospital site in 2001. Indeed some staff referred to Rowan Ward as the 'naughty ward' where staff were sent as punishment (Commission for Health Improvement 2003: 3.15). The ward had been due to move to a new facility, run by Anchor Trust in 1999, but this was delayed. The 16 patients were described as individuals needing continuing care; most had dementia, others had conditions such as depression, schizophrenia or 'challenging behaviour'.

Initial reporting of incidents

In two units, some of the initial concerns about practice were raised by individuals often considered to be the most powerless and disenfranchised within this type of work: healthcare or nursing assistants (Pillemer 1988 and Pillemer and Moore 1990 make similar points about low status in the US context). These concerns did not refer solely to single incidents, but consisted of a catalogue of events. At Kielder Ward, matters were raised by temporary (bank) healthcare staff who were working on the ward. The manager of the unit had already raised issues with the hospital management relating to the physical environment of the ward, under-staffing and injuries to existing staff. This happened at least a month before the reports of mistreatment were made. This had resulted in temporary staff being drafted into the unit to assist who became extremely concerned about the staff's treatment of patients. Two healthcare assistants made allegations concerning abuse of patients by a number of staff within a short period of time (several weeks only) of arriving on the ward; the incidents that were reported therefore covered a relatively limited period. Following these reports, a number of staff on the ward were suspended from duty and an investigation was initiated.

However, it emerged during the external review process that a previous investigation into the conditions and actions by staff on one of the predecessor wards at Garlands Hospital had taken place in 1996. The issues had been reported by several student nurses on placement on the ward who had raised concerns with one of their tutors, which were then more formally reported to the Trust. A number of the reports by the student nurses were similar to those made later about Kielder House. Following the 1996 internal investigation, many of the staff concerned had been transferred to Kielder House when this had opened. However, the existence and findings of this earlier report had not been made known to those investigating the subsequent situation at Kielder House and this only came to light at a later stage of the external review. In addition, three of the staff, including the ward manager, who had been subject to the investigation in 1996, were subsequently implicated in the investigation concerning Kielder House.

At Beech House, the initial report was instigated by one healthcare assistant on the ward, with the support of a junior manager, who had encouraged her to raise her concerns to the Co-Director of Nursing (Sarah Andrews) at the hospital. This report also referred to patient abuse on the ward by a number of members of staff. As Andrews recalled: 'This was one individual and these were issues of having seen individual patients hit. To begin with it was about issues of hitting and not letting patients go back to bed if they were tired' (Andrews 2003). As a result, the staff who were alleged to have been involved were suspended from the ward and an investigation was set up. Initially, three members of staff were suspended from the unit; a fourth person, who was working a period of notice before leaving the hospital, was instructed not to return to work. A fifth member of staff was suspended on his return to work following a period of annual leave.

Andrews recalled: '. . . as the investigation flowed forward and other witnesses were enabled to feel safe enough to speak out, we uncovered a range of other issues, which on the face of it and taken individually, didn't appear to mean an awful lot by themselves' (Andrews 2003). It emerged that a broader review of the circumstances relating to the unit was needed. However, because the matter was principally being dealt with as relating to disciplinary concerns about staff members, there was a significant delay in achieving the broader review. Andrews described this unfolding: 'So it was over many months that I was hearing some material for individuals that I could not deal with by simply looking at individual cases, so I then needed to go to the then Chief Executive and say that there was unfinished business and say that I wanted a Serious Incident Enquiry' (Andrews 2003).

In Rowan Ward, initial concerns were raised through the Trust senior staff; as a result, a Nurse Development Plan was put in place. During this process, further concerns were raised by the ward staff and one nurse in particular used the Trust's whistle-blowing procedure to expose possible long-term abuse of patients. These allegations were later supported by a number of the nurse's colleagues. They led to suspensions of five unqualified and two qualified staff. A police investigation followed but no prosecution ensued. During this time, both the Trust and the local Strategic Health Authority (Commissioner) decided an external review was necessary, the patients' relatives group also supported this (Commission for Health Improvement 2003: 2.20).

In all three locations, the existence of situations of abuse, neglect and abusive regimes, not to mention poor care practices and management, appeared to be of quite long duration. The reports from each setting reveal that the investigations instigated as a result of the formal reports were established through the use of the hospital disciplinary procedures for staff, rather than under policies relating to Serious (or Untoward) Incidents. As we shall see, this appears to have had major consequences for the outcome of the inquiries.

The incidents reported

Clough's review of inquiry reports referred to the following instances of mistreatment: neglect of care (including personal hygiene); punishment of residents who complained; inappropriate use of the bar by staff and non-residents of the homes; institutionalised (and inhumane) practices (Clough 1988, cited in Clough 1999). In his later work, Clough categorised the general range of abuse and neglect detailed in inquiry reports as follows:

- Physical cruelty
- Indifference towards and neglect of residents
- Institutionalised practices (including treating residents 'en masse')

- Humiliation
- Too authoritarian a lifestyle
- A dull and depressing lifestyle
- Overcrowded and rundown environments
- Disharmony amongst the staff team
- Inappropriate use of resident money or goods by staff (including theft and other forms of misappropriation)

(Clough 1999b)

This combination of abuse, neglect and institutional malpractices appear to be subtly intertwined and may lead to a situation which becomes seen as institutional abuse, since it involves the regime or whole system of the care institution.

In the hospital units considered here, similar practices to some of those raised by Clough were uncovered that exposed the physical mistreatment of some patients by some staff. At Kielder House, allegations, substantiated by the subsequent investigation, included: rough handling of patients; swearing and verbal abuse; lack of personal care (including personal hygiene); brusque and uncaring attitudes; physical abuse (some serious); withholding of normal diet; feeding of liquidised diet (when not specifically recommended); deliberate withholding of adequate clothing and blankets; irregularities relating to medication; physical restraint of a patient (tied to a commode) and feeding of patients whilst on the commode or toilet.

At Beech House, the initial reports by the healthcare assistant referred to physical mistreatment (hitting) of patients by staff. Following disciplinary and other investigations relating to the internal inquiry, it was established that all five members of staff had either: 'directly harmed patients or knowingly supported their physical mistreatment' (Camden and Islington Community Health Services NHS Trust 1999: 5). The types of incidents that were substantiated included: physical abuse (hitting); inappropriate use of restraint; verbal abuse and threats; inappropriate attitudes towards patients and patient care; bathing of a patient in cold water; withholding of fluids from a patient.

In addition to these, however, were issues such as the failure of staff to protect patients or to act to stop abuse; to adequately supervise staff or to take appropriate action (for example, failure to discipline a member of staff who had caused distress to a patient); creation of an environment of intimidation on the unit; and staff sleeping whilst on night duty. These factors seem to relate in more general terms to significant failures in management practices. Several of these management issues, in particular, those relating to supervision and management at ward level, were also apparent at Kielder House.

A preliminary draft of the internal inquiry report together with an analysis of patient records by Sarah Andrews was reviewed by Bennett (a geriatrician and expert on elder abuse). This occurred following the disciplinary hearings but prior to the internal inquiry. From the review and analysis of patient records, a number of issues became apparent. Andrews' review of records revealed:

- Indicators of very poor clinical standards (possibly constituting neglect)
- Inappropriate responses following the reporting of falls or injuries
- Acceptance of physical decline evidenced through pressure ulcers and weight loss
- Evidence of dishonest reporting by nurses
- Evidence of unauthorised absences of staff from the unit
- Inadequate, possibly falsified, nursing records
- Inappropriate reliance by medical staff on nursing reports
- Limited understanding about care requirements
  (Camden and Islington Community Health Services NHS Trust 1999)

The factors that Bennett recalled included: slapping and punching of patients; verbal threats; withholding of liquids on a regular basis; theft of ward supplies and intimidation of witnesses to the inquiry by those suspended staff members who were under investigation (Bennett 2003).

Those features that related to theft and intimidation were considered to be of particular concern (Bennett 2002) because of their effects on the nature of the environment. Theft of essential items can lead to a very impoverished setting, whilst a culture of intimidation is likely to be experienced by vulnerable patients as well as more junior members of staff. The fear of intimidation appears to have permeated Beech House. Thus the inquiry report refers to the existence of an 'intimidatory environment on the ward' (Camden and Islington Community Health Services NHS Trust 1999), which related to patient care as much as to staff matters. Further, in connection with the investigation and subsequent inquiry process, Andrews also recalled: '. . . at the same time we'd had threats made against some of the witnesses and the original whistle-blower we had to give protection to' (Andrews 2003). This led to difficulties in acquiring information and evidence, as individuals were understandably reluctant to be involved.

The silencing and secrecy about what had happened in Beech House and in Kielder House and during the inquiries resulted in additional problems. At Kielder House, for instance, although most of the staff on the unit were interviewed about the situation, the report details that: '. . . current Kielder House ward staff did not give any evidence to support the allegations and what corroboration there was came from staff who no longer worked on the ward' (North Lakeland Healthcare 2000: 10). Prior to the investigation, the unit was perceived as providing a 'model of good healthcare' (North Lakeland Healthcare 2000: 8). This is at odds with an early finding of the internal review that there appeared to be an unacceptable regime operating at ward level, created and maintained by 'strong-willed individuals' (North Lakeland Healthcare 2000: 12). However, the internal report was apparently clear that:

> . . . these behaviours were not consistently displayed by all staff towards all patients. It appears that this type of behaviour appears to have been directed by a few staff towards a small number of particular patients.
>
> (North Lakeland Healthcare 2000: 12)

This does not seem to have been as evident to those concerned with the external review. In addition, some elements of the hospital management during the internal inquiry considered that '. . . there is a still a culture that believes that the staff who were disciplined were unfairly and injustly (*sic*) dealt with' (North Lakeland Healthcare 2000: 11).

At Beech House, there were similar findings in relation to the investigation and inquiry. The internal inquiry report stated that:

> Many of those interviewed were extremely anxious and reluctant to have their concerns put in writing, fearing reprisals. . . . One member of staff was not prepared to give a statement or attend any hearing. Another attended an investigatory meeting but refused to allow any notes to be taken. A further member of staff made repeated appointments to be inter- viewed but failed to attend any of them. Another nurse went off sick as soon as the investigation began. He only returned once the disciplinary process was completed, when the five suspended members of staff had been dismissed or otherwise left the Trust and the closure of Beech House had been completed. Several witnesses revealed more details at the initial investigatory meetings than they were subsequently prepared to commit to statements.
>
> (Camden and Islington Community Health Services NHS Trust 1999: 15)

Additionally, Andrews recalled that, as the investigation progressed, '. . . it was quite difficult to get more information than we had already had, but we did thoroughly interview a whole raft of people. A lot of them we sought out – previous employees, doctors, nurses and managers to interview them and find out about their memories and what their experiences of Beech House had been at that time' (Andrews 2003). Yet, even following the investigation and inquiry and the findings that abuse and mistreatment of older patients had probably occurred at Beech House over a substantial period of time, Andrews observed:

But there are still some who say that we got it all wrong; some who still work in the system who say that it didn't happen. They can't believe it happened; who claim that it didn't.

(Andrews 2003)

On Rowan Ward, care was too institutionalised and regimented (Commission for Health Improvement 2003: 3.12) and although the inquiry report focused on the old age service in the Trust, not the allegations of psychical and emotional abuse, the inquiry (it termed itself an 'investigation') acknowledged the vulnerability of the patients and the risk factors on the ward that enhanced the patients' vulnerability. These included a poor and institutional environment, low staff levels, high turnover, temporary staff, limited training, lack of supervision, weak management and confused reporting and accountability. Abuse at this unit was said to have included 'hitting, stamping on feet, intimidating language, withholding food and playing on patients' anxieties' (Kmietowicz 2003).

The involvement of residents and relatives

One of the key differences between the investigations and inquiries concerns the extent of involvement of residents (or patients) and their relatives in the processes. In Kielder House it does not appear that either patients/residents or their relatives were involved in the investigations that took place. In contrast throughout the Beech House report, there is a focus on residents. Indeed, a number of residents and their relatives were involved in the process of the investigation. As part of the initial investigation, a group of ten residents were interviewed by a consultant old-age psychiatrist, together with a ward manager and a union representative. The consultant then provided a written report for the investigation. Additionally, a number of relatives were interviewed in person or by telephone and four letters received from relatives (of three residents) were also considered. In overall terms, neither relatives nor residents expressed misgivings about the care received. Indeed, relatives in particular voiced praise for the staff of the unit.

This appears to have complicated matters, as Andrews indicated:

. . . as part of the individual interviews for the disciplinary hearings, which is when thorough interviews with residents and some of their relatives were undertaken, all appeared from the viewpoint of residents and relatives to be well. No issues were raised. And then when we did the Serious Incident Enquiry, we took a decision, which with hindsight was the wrong one, and because of the evidence we had from the relatives and our knowledge about the ability of residents to give helpful accounts, we decided not to re-interview them.

It later emerged that a number of relatives, in particular, did have concerns about the unit. Andrews reported:

> It was only after the inquiry was released publicly that we then went to see the relatives of all the residents who had been involved . . . and that which has never been published are the accounts . . . of what the relatives were then, and only then . . . prepared to tell us. . . . And some of the most interesting material came out of being with those relatives, who were very angry, but were also then prepared to say: 'Well of course, we always knew that all was not well'; but it was a fairly familiar account of 'well we didn't like to say anything because we were fearful of retribution'.
> (Andrews 2003)

This highlights one of the major difficulties relating to this area of work. If, during an investigation or inquiry, an individual or a relative is reluctant to discuss a situation, their reluctance or anxiety can be ascribed to fear or intimidation and an inquiry may decide to explore this further with the person. However, if an individual, or a relative, or groups of respondents answer without apparent hesitation or reluctance, how can one be sure that the information given is accurate and not similarly affected by fear of reprisal? This is of particular relevance to the situation of relatives, who may not be concerned about their own safety or possible direct reprisals, but may be very anxious about the well-being of their relative. It may be easier for relatives to deny that there is any problem. This may present those charged with rectifying a situation and implementing changes with a particular set of challenges, as Andrews revealed: 'So how could we be sure, as far as we could be, that this time we had taken the right action to really hear what we were being told by relatives and really act on what we found as a result of the inquiry to improve the quality of life patients, but also to improve the possibility for the staff to do a good job?' (Andrews 2003).

In Rowan Ward, the inquiry interviewed five sets of relatives and its members attended relatives' group meetings, with 15 relatives. Appendix D of the report summarises the relatives' views and those of the 'public' (community and voluntary groups) contacted by posters, letters, leaflets, and the press. Relatives were concerned about the isolation, and environment of the ward, and anxious about the future care of their relatives. However, the inquiry reports that 'most relatives were generally satisfied with care provided' (p. 55), although there were mixed views and experiences. It is evident from this inquiry that the relatives felt that communication with them had at times been insensitive, inconsistent and upsetting. This potential for investigations of any type to add to distress is one key message in our view from the Rowan Ward report: it has much to suggest about ongoing communication with relatives and the need for this to be well handled in any care setting.

Messages from the inquiries

The three reports considered here are concerned with long-term care in the NHS, but although such units continue to be moved to the independent social care sector, the lessons from these detailed inquiries are transferable. In our view, the move to a fragmented social care system of care of some of the most vulnerable people in society (often without family or friends to advocate for them) will compound the risk factors in some instances. The NHS may not seem to have much to be proud of when these inquiries are considered, but it opened its doors to review and in some cases 'volunteered' for the harsh spotlight of an inquiry. Commercial and not for profit care providers may fear and avoid this level of scrutiny.

In our view, there are three main sets of messages from the reports considered here. These build on the previous reports into residential care for older people in the UK and resonate with research from other contexts (see the collection assembled by Glendenning and Kingston 1999). They also have much in common with care services for other marginalised groups, as Chapter 10 in this volume illustrates. However, common messages from inquiries should not mean that inquiries simply repeat each other. Local contexts are important. We have been surprised to see word-for-word repetition of the Beech House report in the Kielder House report (North Lakeland Healthcare 2000) and suggest that this is particularly inappropriate in sections where some reassurance is being given.

Vulnerable residents/risky environments

There is uncertainty about whether an impairment or disability such as dementia is a risk factor for abuse and, if so, what is the nature of any relationship (Penhale 2003). What is less disputed is that people with dementia are vulnerable and that providing care for them is demanding and distressing at times (as is much social care work, Department of Health 1998: 5.2). The inquiry reports recognise this but it is clear that the services under scrutiny consistently failed to see this area of their responsibility as the most difficult area in which to work. Indicators of vulnerability among residents were rarely addressed. Patients/residents lived in enclosed, isolated environments, with advocates, volunteers and other professionals, generally absent. The medical profession, for example, is particularly shadowy in all the reports, despite the hospital locations.

Those familiar with older people's services may recognise this as another example of an 'inverse care law': that those who are most vulnerable are less supported and protected than others who pose danger or evoke fear. Positive developments in dementia care may need to identify the issue of risk of abuse for service users rather more conspicuously and consistently.

The reports discussed in this chapter do just this but they also raise the potential for the creation of a new category of a 'risky environment', characterised by an accepted checklist of factors, such as temporary staff, poor environment, organisational neglect, and so on. The Commission for Health Improvement (2003) report on Rowan Ward is most developed in this respect. Risk factors are helpful but risk assessment is not a science. Judging any environment by whether it contains such factors and then making decisions on the basis of these along is likely to lead to false positives (Munro 1999). We do not have evidence of how such risk factors operate, or their interaction. Hindsight, as the introduction to this book argues, needs to be used with caution.

The second message distilled from the three reports discussed here is that the inquiry process is often one of a number of reviews and investigations. Beneath the water-line, a series of interviews, records, disciplinary and human resources investigations and meetings have taken place. Lengthy investigations may compromise the ability to deal with abuse and its impact. In contrast to inquiries into mental health homicides, the inquiries into care provision and care for larger numbers of individuals are more diffuse and harder to follow. In the absence of a criminal trial, or hearing by a professional regulatory organisation, the inquiry often represents a partial view. We are less able to hear the 'voices' of those involved.

Our third point relates to the 'aftermath' of institutional inquiries. In all three discussed here, the 'units' were dissolved. We have no evidence of the long-term impact on patients/residents, on families, the wider community or on services. Pritchard's (2003) work on support for older people who have been the subject of domestic/family abuse has the potential to assist in developing thinking here. It is important to know more about good practice in re-building trust and restoring goodwill, motivation and confidence.

Acknowledgements

The authors wish to acknowledge the invaluable assistance of Professor Sarah Andrews and the late Professor Gerry Bennett who were interviewed concerning the Beech House Inquiry and gave freely of their time in relation to this chapter.

References

Aitken, L. and Griffin, G. (1996) *Gender Issues on Elder Abuse*, London: Sage.
Andrews, S. (2003) Personal communication.
Bennett, G. (2002) *Institutional Abuse*. Presentation to the Valencia Research Forum (unpublished), Valencia: Spain.
Bennett, G. (2003) Personal communication.

Bennett, G., Kingston, P. and Penhale, B. (1997) *The Dimensions of Elder Abuse*, Basingstoke: Macmillan.

Biggs, S., Phillipson, C. and Kingston, P. (1995) *Elder Abuse in Perspective*, Basingstoke: Macmillan.

Bright, L. (1999a) 'Restraint: cause for continuing concern?', *Journal of Adult Protection*, 3(2): 42–7.

Bright, L. (1999b) 'The abuse of older people in residential settings: residents' and carers' stories', in N. Stanley, J. Manthorpe and B. Penhale (eds), *Institutional Abuse: Perspectives Across the Lifecourse*, London: Routledge.

Camden and Islington Community Health Services NHS Trust (1999) *Beech House Inquiry: Report of the Internal Inquiry Relating to the Mistreatment of Patients Residing at Beech House, St. Pancras Hospital During the Period March 1993–April 1996*, London: Camden and Islington Community Health Services NHS Trust.

Chambers, R. (1999) 'Potential for the abuse of medication for the elderly in Residential and Nursing Homes in the UK', *Journal of Elder Abuse and Neglect*, 10(1/2): 79–90.

Clough, R. (1988) 'Scandals in Residential Centres: A report to the Wagner Committee', unpublished, cited in Clough, R. (1999) 'Scandalous Care: Interpreting Public Enquiry reports of Scandals in Residential Care', *Journal of Elder Abuse and Neglect*, 10(1/2): 13–26.

Clough, R. (ed.) (1996) *The Abuse of Care in Residential Institutions*, London: Whiting and Birch.

Clough, R. (1999a) 'The abuse of older people in residential settings: The role of management and inspection', in N. Stanley, J. Manthorpe and B. Penhale (eds), *Institutional Abuse: Perspectives Across the Lifecourse*, London: Routledge.

Clough, R. (1999b) 'Scandalous care: Interpreting public enquiry reports of scandals in residential care', *Journal of Elder Abuse and Neglect*, 10(1/2): 13–26.

Commission for Health Improvement (2000) *Investigation into the North Lakeland NHS Trust*, London: Commission for Health Improvement.

Commission for Health Improvement (2003) *Investigation into Matters Arising from Care on Rowan Ward, Manchester Health and Social Care Trust*, London: Commission for Health Improvement.

Department of Health (1993) *No Longer Afraid: the Safeguard of Older People in Domestic Settings*, London: HMSO.

Department of Health/Social Services Inspectorate (1996) *Responding to Residents*, London: HMSO.

Department of Health (1998) *Modernising Social Services*, London: HMSO.

Department of Health/Social Services Inspectorate (1999) *No Secrets: the Protection of Vulnerable Adults-Guidance on the Development and Implementation of Multi-Agency Policies and Procedures* (consultation document), London: Stationery Office.

Department of Health (2000) *No Secrets: Guidance on Developing and Implementing of Multi-Agency Policies and Procedures to Protect Vulnerable Adults from Abuse*, London: Department of Health.

Fader, A., Koge, N., Gupta, G.L. and Gambert, S.R. (1990) 'Perceptions of elder abuse by health care workers in a long-term care setting', *Clinical Gerontologist*, 10(2): 292–8.

Gilleard, C. (1994) 'Physical abuse in homes and hospitals', in M. Eastman (ed.), *Old Age Abuse*, 2nd edn, London: Age Concern England/Chapman & Hall.

Glendenning, F. (1999a) 'The abuse of older people in institutional settings: An overview', in N. Stanley, J. Manthorpe and B. Penhale (eds), *Institutional Abuse: Perspectives Across the Life Course*, London: Routledge.

Glendenning, F. (1999b) 'Elder abuse and neglect in residential settings: The need for inclusiveness in elder abuse', in F. Glendenning and P. Kingston (eds), *Elder Abuse and Neglect in Residential Settings: Different National Backgrounds and Similar Responses*, New York: Haworth Press.

Glendenning, F. and Kingston, P. (eds) (1999) *Elder Abuse and Neglect in Residential Settings: Different National Backgrounds and Similar Responses*, New York: Haworth Press.

Kmietowicz, Z. (2003) Bullying and harassment rife in Manchester Unit, reports say, *British Medical Journal*, 327: 697.

McCreadie, C. (1996) *Elder Abuse: An Update on Research*, London: HMSO.

Martin, J. (1984) *Hospitals in Trouble*, Oxford: Blackwell.

Manthorpe, J. and Stanley, N. (1999) 'Conclusion: Shifting the focus from bad apples to users' rights', in N. Stanley, J. Manthorpe and B. Penhale (eds), *Institutional Abuse: Perspectives Across the Lifecourse*, London: Routledge.

Matthew, D., Brown, H., Kingston, P., McCreadie, C. and Askham, J. (2002) 'The response to *No Secrets*', *Journal of Adult Protection*, 4(1): 4–14.

Munro, E. (1999) 'Protecting children in an anxious society', *Health Risk and Society*', 1: 117–27.

Nolan, M. (1994) 'Deregulation of nursing homes: a disaster waiting to happen?' *British Journal of Nursing*, 3(12): 595.

North Lakeland Healthcare (2000) *External Review Report*, NHSE: Carlisle: North Lakeland Healthcare and North Cumbria Health Authority.

Penhale, B. (1993) 'The abuse of elderly people: Considerations for practice', *British Journal of Social Work*, 23(2): 95–112.

Penhale, B. (2003) 'Elder abuse and people with dementia', in T. Adams and J. Manthorpe (eds), *Dementia Care*, London: Arnold.

Pillemer, K.A. (1988) 'Maltreatment of patients in nursing homes', *Journal of Health and Social Behaviour*, 29(3): 227–38.

Pillemer, K.A. and Moore, D.W. (1990) 'Highlights from a study of abuse in nursing homes', *Journal of Elder Abuse and Neglect*, 2(1/2): 5–29.

Pritchard, J. (2003) *Support Groups for Older People Who Have Been Abused*, London: Jessica Kingsley.

Stanley, N., Manthorpe, J. and Penhale, B. (eds) (1999) *Institutional Abuse: Perspectives Across the Lifecourse*, London: Routledge.

United Kingdom Central Council for Nursing, Midwifery and Health Visiting (UKCC) (1994) *Professional Conduct – Occasional Report on Standards of Nursing in Nursing Homes*, London: UKCC.

Chapter 13

Inspections and inquiries

Roger Clough and Jill Manthorpe

Inquiries are brought into being when an event is judged to be of sufficient magnitude and of sufficient concern to warrant investigation. The reasons for holding an inquiry in such circumstances rather than an internal, organisational review are numerous but include the following:

- to ensure that people outside the organisation examine the event(s);
- to show the public or government that the events are viewed as of a serious nature and demand serious study;
- a threshold has been crossed;
- to involve people with expertise to make judgements both about what happened and about the consequent actions that the organisation should take;
- to provide additional powers for those investigating, for example, to require the attendance of witnesses.

As is apparent throughout this book, a serious event almost inevitably is followed by calls from different sources for an inquiry. At times, organisations may set up inquiries to ensure that they are seen to act properly rather than because of their belief that an inquiry is appropriate to the seriousness of the event and the risk of repetition. Sometimes an organisation holds its own inquiry in parallel with that from outside experts. Faced with a serious event, the senior staff of an organisation and of their management body will consider how to address the best way to investigate an event, the remit of any investigation, and who should head the investigation.

It is intriguing that inspectorates, whether local, regional or national, may not be viewed as appropriate for the task. This chapter considers that conundrum. Are inspectorates disregarded because they are not thought to be impartial or because they are not considered to be sufficiently competent?

We start the chapter by setting out some scenarios from inspection activity that we hope will allow us to consider the roles of inspectorates in inquiries. Our focus is on older people, but we will draw on our experiences conducting inquiries (RC), in inspection services (RC), in commissioning a local inquiry

(JM), and in appearing as a witness in front of an unpublished mental health homicide inquiry (JM). We have also read and considered a large number of inquiries, spanning a wide range of settings and user groups and use some of these to illustrate certain points.

The tasks of inspection

Most regulatory activities contain elements of setting standards, monitoring, enforcement and development. From these it is possible to set up outcomes that should be expected, such as:

- required standards will become accepted by stakeholders;
- overall standards within inspected facilities improve;
- enforcement action is taken;
- people feel confident in the quality of the work of inspectorate staff.

There is no point in having inspectorates if they do not have an impact on practice. Their influence should be more than cosmetic. For their work to be of value, there should be evidence of better practice in that higher standards have been set and achieved. Such improvements may come about by developmental work or sanctions.

The regulatory task is not straightforward: firm standards, applied even handedly, are needed but flexibility may be required. In addition, there may be intended or unintended side effects from the setting of standards. For example, imposing health and safety regulations has resulted in most residents of homes for older people being excluded from kitchens. This removes older people, most of whom will be women, from tasks and environments that may hold particular pleasure, memory and meaning for them, as well as emphasising that they are no longer in their own homes.

The nature of evidence

To take action, regulators need firm evidence. As with the police, it is not always easy to demonstrate what others claim or inspectors suspect. It is tempting to ignore concerns if the evidence does not seem of the right type: it is easier to take action on what is most obvious and demonstrable, whether the room size meets minimum requirements or the temperature of the hot water does not exceed safe levels. As Sinclair (2002: 435) observes, in relation to residential care: 'There is some evidence that things go a good deal better if staff are given considerable autonomy rather than being hemmed in with rules and regulations.'

The evaluation of an event such as a meal can be by *components or indicators*. For example, the following could be assessed: inputs, shown by the quality of the food used; the environment in which the cooking takes place (for example, hygiene, health and safety); choice for residents and their involvement; outputs in terms of the quality of food produced; quality of service by staff. An indicator by its nature is selective: it has the potential to capture some elements, to ignore others and to miss out on the total experience, in this case the ambience or pleasure of a meal.

Lewis (2002), considering the nature of evidence, a central feature of both inspection and inquiries, stresses the importance of professional judgement. She defines this as: 'Knowledge + evidence + practice wisdom + user experience'. It is important to introduce the notion of 'professional judgement' as something that is distinct from the narrower frame of 'evidence'. The key point is that evidence has to be interpreted and it is both naive and inaccurate to think that evidence on its own determines action. The view that inspectorates should be firm, consistent and flexible makes more sense when seen in the context of professional judgement.

However, whether inspectorates take action depends also on how decisions are made as to whether in the particular circumstances it is appropriate to intervene. This has similarities with the police passing its evidence to the Crown Prosecution Service for a decision about prosecution. Similar tests ought to apply for inspectorates. First, on the available evidence, how likely is a prosecution to be successful? Secondly, importantly and often neglected, even if a successful prosecution looks unlikely, is there a public interest in which the inspectorate should be seen to act against bad practice?

Freedom to act impartially

Inspectorates have to be subject to regulation themselves but free from interference with decisions concerning the competence of individual organisations. Whatever the reality, one of the criticisms of inspectorates when located within and even when at arm's length from local authority social services departments was that they did not seem to be at arm's length from social services operations and its management or politicians. So a key test, whether for an inspectorate or an inquiry, is whether the system and the individuals involved allow judgements to be reached without fear or favour.

There are different sorts of pressures. In an audit of practices in the Social Services Inspectorate Wales, one of us (RC) had the experience of examining the quality of practice and integrity of an inspector who had been charged with assaults against children in an earlier job (Clough and McCoy 2000). A leading councillor had claimed on television that the Social Services Inspectorate Wales was not taking the concerns seriously enough and that all of that inspector's work must be tainted. The consequence of such comments was that it felt as if the integrity of the investigation team would be best maintained if we were to find faults in the work of the individual. The team found only minor problems and held to that position.

Whether involved in inspections or inquiries, people should be aware of the pressures that are exerted. The notion that an independent inspection or inquiry takes place outside a social, political and legal context is naive, and Prins, in Chapter 2 of this volume, has added considerably to our knowledge of the processes involved in the initial phases of inquiries.

The impact and outcome of inspections

The experience of being inspected, while a real pressure, may provide an opportunity for people to address some key questions regarding their work and their concerns. The same questions arise in respect of inquiries:

- are they worth their expense?
- do they produce change?
- if so, what are the means by which they achieve change?
- which, if any, of the participants or stakeholders find the experience valuable?

Inspectorates must be able to justify their existence – and in particular the standards they are demanding – to everybody with an interest in their work. Frequently, inspectorates are attacked for focusing on inessentials. It may be that they are highlighting areas where they know they can collect evidence, that they are demanding performance in relation to an indicator (rather than the activity which the indicator was designed to assess), or that others have failed to understand the importance of a particular standard.

The competence of inspectorates can be judged against each of the activities listed earlier: setting standards, monitoring, enforcement and development. However, the competence should be measured also against the extent to which all the activities are advanced at the same time.

Examples of the sorts of questions that can be used to assess the competence of inspectorates are:

- is there evidence for the importance of the standards which are set? and
- does the achievement of a particular indicator (or performance target) matter – or is it more important to assess whether the bigger goal is being achieved, for example, whether people are being treated with respect?

This is an important balancing act. Commentators such as Richard Clough (1998) allude to the need to enhance public confidence in residential care but also identify the necessity for staff morale to be improved and for care workers not to feel under continuous scrutiny. Thus, too great a burden of inspection may be counter-productive. It is obvious that standards of service should rise as a consequence of regulation and inspection, but as with the negative impacts of inquiries, there are costs as well as benefits of systems of inspection. Authors such as Fook (2000) and Froggett (2002) indicate the importance of attending to the feelings of ambivalence evoked by institutions. Practitioners' doubts concerning the institutional enterprise, together with defensiveness in response to scrutiny may make apparently rational processes, such as inspection, fraught and risky. Additionally, the area is replete with conflicts of interest. It is worth remembering that if reliance had been placed on hearsay evidence concerning whether older people wanted to have single rooms in residential homes, the majority of residents would still be living in shared accommodation.

Inspectorate codes of practice

Most inspectorates have published objectives and standards of practice. They provide interesting evidence of what are judged to be the important objectives and attributes of inspections. We will consider later their relevance as benchmarks for inquiries. The former National Care Standards Commission (recently re-organised into the Commission for Social Care Inspection) claimed to embrace the following standards: fairness and even-handedness; transparency and accountability; willingness to listen and learn; honesty and integrity; responsibility and accountability; valuing diversity. It stated that it would seek to be:

> a learning organisation, open and accountable for its actions, striving for continuous improvement . . . giving a central role to the views of service users in *all* its regulatory work.
>
> (NCSC website 2003)

The Audit Commission (2003) has set out what it terms the principles of inspection:

1 *Inform the public about the performance of local services now and their likely performance in the future, and so enhance local accountability.* Importantly, the authors argue, that there are multiple audiences, not just the public.
2 *Focus on public services as users experience them.* The objective here is to report 'how well and efficiently public services meet needs'.
3 *Take into account the use of money, people and assets and promote economy, efficiency and effectiveness.*
4 *Act as a catalyst to help public bodies to improve*: this involves seeking 'to secure the ownership of findings by the body under inspection'.
5 *Identify what works, to inform policy nationally and practice locally.*
6 *The scale of inspection should be proportionate to risk.*

7   *The methodology and criteria on which judgements are based should be explicit
    and based on evidence of what works in improving services.*
8   *Inspection should be carried out without fear or favour.*

These are less general and provide a framework within which to establish
the merits of regular inspection, 'one off' inspections and inquiries. Rather
than avoiding resources issues they make it clear that these need to be
addressed, for the good reason perhaps, that with finite resources (both financial, but also time and energy), expenditure may come at the cost of direct
services.

Inquiries: task and competence

Taking examples from regulation about principles and values allows us to
pose questions about the nature and effectiveness of inquiries. The first of
these relates to terminology: how does an inquiry differ from inspection,
audit or other regulatory activity? An inquiry is likely to examine a discrete
event or series of events: it is a one-off episode, typically with special arrangements being made for that investigation.

However, inspectors could conduct an inquiry. An example of this was an
inquiry (never published) undertaken by inspectorate staff into the murder of
an older person by a person who entered a local authority managed residential
home. Of course there was a police investigation but the authority wanted to
know if there had been failings by staff. We report this not to question the
procedure that we have no reason to judge inappropriate. It is interesting
to conjecture whether, had the same thing happened to a child in a residential
home, there would have been different action.

This highlights what we have termed the threshold: an inquiry is brought
into being when the event is regarded as sufficiently serious and, possibly,
unusual. As argued in the introduction to this book, an inquiry addresses
issues that assume some moral status, the event under the spotlight is seen
to mark a specific failing in an area where social care or health services have
legitimate responsibility and accountability cannot be exercised by the
inspectorates alone.

We noted earlier that most inspectorates publish codes of practice. One of
the purposes of such codes of practice is to make clear what people should
expect from an inspection. This allows the public and witnesses to judge
the practice. They will know what to expect and, if they wish, how to
make a complaint about the conduct of the inspection. Inquiries, as single
events, rarely have such codes of practice. Against what principles are
inquiries to be judged in terms of quality of practice? Should we expect standards of openness, integrity, style of conduct, including treatment of
witnesses? Do people know what to expect of the event? Have they a means
of complaining?

In terms of the core task of the inquiry, there are parallels with any inspection: to study the evidence, to analyse the findings, to reach a judgement on the information provided. What has to be recognised, whether in inspection or inquiry work, is that such tasks may be carried out with great skill or very little skill. Just because someone undertakes an inquiry does not mean that they understand the activity into which they are inquiring sufficiently well to know what are the key questions to ask or where are the places to look; alternatively, the person may be skilled in knowing just these things, but unskilled in how to ask questions to elicit the information wanted. The quality of an inquiry is dependent, as are inspections, on the capacity of those undertaking the inquiry. At all levels these will draw on management skills (Clough 2000), whether as the inspector or member of an inquiry panel, or as a witness or employee of the organisation undergoing an inspection. This process of inquiry covers a range of skills – not simply inquisitorial but also the construction of the final product, the report and its handling or dissemination. The Commission for Health Improvement (2003), for example, on the publication of its inquiry into Rowan Ward (see Chapter 12), made it clear that this was the third in a series of such reports to comment on the dismal quality of care of older people with mental health problems, thus placing its report in a context, establishing that the events portrayed were more than isolated occurrences and pointing out that remedies will require political action rather than single system change.

Monitoring inquiries

The task of the inquiry is usually set out clearly in the invitation to the members of the inquiry. However, there may be comparatively little other guidance. Without such explicit statements, it is difficult to monitor the effectiveness of inquiries. Not all inquiries tell us about their terms of reference, although within mental health inquiries there appears to have evolved a 'skeleton' of terms of reference to which local factors are added. This makes it possible to have a sense of the shape of such inquiries and, as Prins notes in Chapter 1, this is largely based on Department of Health guidance (Department of Health NHS Executive 1994). Such guidance is worth exploring because, as the catalogue of inquiries compiled by Sheppard in Chapter 9 demonstrates, they are so numerous, and the processes are often similar.

Among these terms of reference there is evidence about the extent to which the inquiry is able to be proactive. The inquiry into the care and treatment of Peter Richard Winship from 1992 to 1996 (Chapman et al. 1997), for example, sets out in an appendix its 'remit'. This covers four main tasks, the first of which is to examine in detail Mr Winship's treatment and care, in particular: the quality of health, social care and risk assessments, the suitability of his treatment, the extent to which his care met statutory obligations and the extent to which his care plans were appropriate, known, complied with and monitored. Furthermore, this inquiry's remit was 'to consider the quality of any relevant professional judgements', to examine the adequacy of collaboration and communication, and finally to produce a report with recommendations.

However, inquiries may cast a wider net in light of the individual circumstances or history of the individual in question or in light of accumulated concerns. The inquiry into the care and treatment of Wayne Licorish (Holwill *et al.* 1999), for example, notes that their terms of reference included the context of the number and nature of his convictions. Other inquiries appear to have been given specific areas to consider, such as the inquiry into the care and treatment of Jonathan Crisp (Brown *et al.* 1999), where 'the appropriateness and adequacy of professional and in-service training of those involved in the care of Jonathan Crisp' was an area of scrutiny.

However, these are only a segment of the inquiry industry and great variation occurs within both adult services' and child protection inquiries' terms of reference. These may range from the brief but broad approach typified by the case review in respect of PM (Manby *et al.* 1998: 2) where the independent review panel was appointed:

- to review the circumstances which led to the death of PM on 6.12.97
- review the involvement of all agencies known to have had contact with PM, his family and significant others particularly in the period May to December 1997
- and to make recommendations to the APCP in relation to improving the child protection system, and 'public confidence in it' together with an action list.

These terms of reference are similar to those devised by an adult protection committee that sought to investigate the death in a nursing home of an older man, and in doing so needed to agree terms of reference for this and other possible inquiries with local agencies including the then National Care Standards Commission regional office (Manthorpe 2003).

In contrast, the report of the Bridge Consultancy into the circumstances of the death of Sukina (Bridge Consultancy 1991) set out its commission from the Department of Health in nine areas, including:

- was Sukina's death preventable?
- what services were offered to Sukina?

Such questions may in essence be the same as those set out by, or implicit in, the terms of reference for all inquiries. What seems to be important is the way in which an inquiry's terms of reference may give it permission to go beyond a forensic approach to consider wide issues and systems. It is evident that the Climbié inquiry (Laming 2003) was able to construe its role as a policy instrument – criticising the law, policy and operational issues – because it was both given but also interpreted its terms of reference proactively. Likewise, the Beech House internal inquiry (Camden and Islington Community Health Services NHS Trust 1999) (see Chapter 12) received a set of terms of reference from the Trust's chief executive but focused on four key questions that were broader than its original remit. These four comprised:

- What was discovered during the disciplinary hearings?
- What were the circumstances that led to patient harm?
- What action has the Trust taken since the discovery of the circumstances at Beech House?
- What steps should be taken to minimise the risks of a similar situation arising in future?

(Camden and Islington Community Health Services NHS Trust 1999: 13)

Internal inquiries clearly have much potential and can be set up fairly quickly at local level to speak to local systems and communities. Their drawback lies in their perceived lack of independence. It is easy to see this simplistically. Inquiries are expected to be independent, but what is the nature of that independence and what results are achieved by independence? Indeed, to whom are those who carry out inquiries accountable other than to the organisation which issued them with the contract to undertake the work?

In both inquiries and inspections, the process of the investigation is important: information is collected from records, interviews, written statements or observation; the material is reviewed and analysed; emerging questions are checked; judgements are reached. Such a process may be conducted well or badly. It is concerned with the management of relationships (Clough 1994: 167), rather than the management of paper and data. If necessary, is it possible for people to examine the conduct of an investigation? Again we can learn from inspections and we use those inquiries mentioned above to illustrate the potential directions and processes.

The Winship Inquiry (Chapman *et al.* 1997) set out its procedure in an appendix. This is a set of commitments about its communication with witnesses – how and what they will be told, what forms of representation will be permitted, the privacy of the sittings, and so on. In essence this is a procedural 'code of conduct' and is laid out as un-contentious. What we know, however, is that this code has to be negotiated in the absence of national guidance (see Chapter 1) and that to witnesses or observers this code may favour a professional perspective (see Paul and Audrey Edwards' account in Chapter 2). This inquiry does not reflect on this procedure and whether, with the benefit of hindsight, it was appropriate or beneficial. Few inquiries, to the best of our knowledge, have outlined the extent of intimidation of witnesses as chronicled by the Beech House internal inquiry (Camden and Islington Community Health Services NHS Trust 1999: Appendix F).

Clough and McCoy (2000), undertaking their audit, concluded that there was not sufficient information to track back and examine from paper or computer records the way an inspection had been managed:

> We can tell little about the management of the inspection from the files and are concerned about the limited information that is kept on files, for example, planning notes, records of observations and interview notes were rarely stored in the files. We were unable to identify questions which were raised by inspectors or lay assessors, how these were to be pursued, and, to examine the management of any difficulties during the inspection. We are not confident that there is full enough information to allow adequate management and overview by a line manager.
>
> (Clough and McCoy 2000: 7.44)

Further, they noted that, as a sizeable amount of material related to inspections is kept by individual inspectors, in particular on their computers, 'the content of work was now less available for scrutiny by management than when paper copies were kept of pieces of work'. To what extent should the conduct of an inquiry be open to similar examination?

Distinctive characteristics of inquiries

We have noted earlier that inquiries are conducted under terms different from those of inspections. Often they have a legal framework and, indeed, many are chaired by lawyers who are presumed to have skills in sifting evidence (see Chapter 1). However, those undertaking inquiries may still be boxed in by regulations that are not of their making. For example, some inquiries have been unable to report their findings in public because the insurers of the local authority have stated that they will refuse cover to the authority if the outcome were publicised. For over ten years, central government has demanded that inspection reports should be made public; the same is not guaranteed for inquiries, often to the frustration of those undertaking the work who think that their conclusions should be in the public arena.

Inspections reviewed

This chapter has explored the changing nature of inspection and commented on its potential to operate as a form of inquiry. This is counter to the view expressed in *Moving Forward* (Department of Health 1995) that inspections should focus on the basic standards necessary to fulfil legal requirements.

The notion that there can be tiers of inquiries is seductive, but the commissioning of a public inquiry may remain within the 'gift' of government ministers or local politicians in order to restore shaken public confidence. If the inquiry becomes a matter of 'routine', as has sadly become the case in inquiries into mental health homicides where conclusions are converging, then the system begins to resemble an albatross. Professional development and quality improvements are impeded when a blame culture ossifies an agency.

What is evident, however, is that inspection reaches out beyond the public sector, whereas most inquiries in health and social care have concerned public sector organisations. Few believe that this suggests there is no cause for concern outside the public sector. It may be time for the public sector to argue that the new independent inspectorate in social care should open up the doors of independent organisations to the same degree.

This chapter has identified the 'grey area' between inspection, investigation and inquiries but it is evident that the final responsibility for these overlaps lies with central government. Central government has both a permissive role, in allowing latitude and flexibility at local levels, but it has mandatory powers, for example, it is government that is 'modernising' inspection to combine aspects of the work of the National Care Standards Commission, the Social Services Inspectorate and the Audit Commission. Such reorganisation is in the name of rationalisation, to avoid duplications and to combine expertise. It also reflects a prime purpose, to achieve better and more consistent outcomes for service users. This of course will need to be judged, especially in light of the potential undermining it represents of the Social Services Inspectorate's (SSI) approach of engaging with practitioners and managers as temporary or seconded members of its staff. While the SSI reports have provided accumulations of evidence of the 'deficiencies in the quality, effectiveness and efficiency of social services' (Hill 2000: 182), the legacy of the inspectorate's service reviews has been positive, notably, in this area, its practice guidance *No Longer Afraid* (Social Services Inspectorate 1993).

As Hill notes (2000: 189), the Department of Health in England undertakes 'general surveillance' over the work of local social services departments, but this is a strategic overview. In fact, the 'peculiar position of local authorities in a centralised state' (Hill 2000: 146) leads to tensions between local autonomy and central control. Inspection stands in midst position here, with local authorities currently under greater scrutiny, both in respect of their provision of services, but also with regards to judgements on their commissioning (best value reviews) and performance. Local authorities have increasingly turned to market models of audit, surveys and quality control: all of which are replacing the language of inspection (so much so that the term inspection is hardly discernible in many social work texts and commentaries). It is curious how the positive experiences of involving the public as lay assessors (Williams 1998: 31) have not been highlighted; this at a time when citizen and user involvement is a policy goal, and when there is interest in drawing on residents' insights to develop quality standards (Raynes 1998).

The Department of Health's power to set in train an inquiry within a local authority is further evidence of its ability to prescribe action and to open the doors of local agencies. While this is used sparingly, and flexibly, the main developments in regulation and inspection were set in train following the Burgner review (Department of Health 1996) (the author being the Chair of the Longcare inquiry, Buckinghamshire County Council 1998) but also were outlined in the thinking behind the consultative document *Moving Forward* (Department of Health 1995). This forms the backcloth to the National Care Standards Commission under the Care Standards Act 2000. Independence from government is thus a matter of definition and degree since both the NCSC and its successor, the Commission for Social Care Inspection (CSCI), are heavily dependent on government. This chapter thus concludes that inspections have great potential for inquiry and they offer a degree of consistency and accountability. What they lack, however, is political ownership, and this of course is advantageous to some and not to others.

We noted earlier the Audit Commission's 'Principles of Inspection'. This chapter has argued that they are unevenly applied in inquiries but provide a sensible framework within which other stakeholders' views should be canvassed. We have mentioned the involvement of lay assessors in residential care inspections and see merit in strengthening this role in new systems, notably to include users in developing standards, monitoring and evaluation (Beresford and Croft 2003). Inspections will always be more numerous than inquiries, and if inspections can combine a 'forensic' but also a good practice approach then they may be able to avert the need for inquiries by illuminating service deficiencies at an earlier stage.

References

Audit Commission, www.audit-commission.gov.uk/reports/guidance accessed: 6 Oct 2003.

Beresford, P. and Croft, S. (2003) 'Involving service users in management: Citizenship, access and support', in J. Reynolds, J. Henderson, J. Seden, J. Charlesworth and A. Bullman (eds), *The Managing Care Reader*, London: Routledge.

Bridge Consultancy (1991) *Sukina: An Evaluation Report of the Circumstances Leading to Her Death*, London: The Bridge Child Care Consultancy Service.

Brown, T., Fraser, K., Morley, A. and Swapp, G. (1999) *Report to Tees Health Authority of the Independent Inquiry Team into the Care and Treatment of Jonathan Crisp*, Middlesbrough: Tees Health Authority.

Buckinghamshire County Council (1998) *Independent Longcare Inquiry*, Buckingham: Buckinghamshire County Council.

Camden and Islington Community Health Services NHS Trust (1999) *Beech House Inquiry: Report of the Internal Inquiry Relating to the Mistreatment of Patients Residing* at Beech House, St. Pancras Hospital During the Period March 1993–April 1996. London: NHSE: Camden and Islington Community Health Partnership NHS Trust.

Chapman, H., Higgins, J. and Sandford, T. (1997) Report of the Independent Inquiry into the Treatment and Care of Peter Richard Winship, Nottingham: Nottinghamshire Health Authority.

Clough, R. (1994) 'The context of inspection', in R. Clough (ed.), Insights into Inspection, London: Whiting & Birch.

Clough, R. (Richard) (1998) 'The future of residential care', in R. Jack (ed.), Residential Versus Community Care, London: Macmillan.

Clough, R. (2000) The Practice of Residential Work, London: Macmillan.

Clough, R. and McCoy, K. (2000) An Audit of the Working Practices of the Social Services Inspectorate, Wales, a Report Presented to the National Assembly for Wales, Cardiff: National Assembly for Wales.

Commission for Health Improvement (2003) Investigation into Matters Arising from Care on Rowan Ward, Manchester Health and Social Care Trust, London: Commission for Health Improvement.

Department of Health (1995) Moving Forward: A Consultative Document on the Registration and Inspection of Social Services, London: Department of Health.

Department of Health (1996) The Regulation and Inspection of Social Services (The Burgner Report), London: Department of Health.

Department of Health NHS Executive (1994) Guidance on the Discharge of Mentally Disordered People and their Care in the Community HSG/94/27, London: Department of Health.

Fook, J. (2000) 'Deconstructing and reconstructing professional expertise', in B. Fawcett, B. Featherstone, J. Fook and A. Rossiter (eds), Practice and Research in Social Work: Postmodern Feminist Perspectives, London: Routledge, 104–19.

Froggett, L. (2002) Love, Hate and Welfare, Bristol: The Policy Press.

Hill, M. (2000) 'The Central and Local Government Framework', in M. Hill (ed.), Local Authority Social Services, Oxford: Blackwell, 130–57.

Holwill, D., Oyebode, O., Mason, L. and Mackay, J. (1999) The Independent Inquiry into the Care and Treatment of Wayne Licorish, Northampton: Northamptonshire Health Authority and Northamptonshire Social Services.

Laming, H. (2003) The Victoria Climbié Inquiry: Report of an Inquiry by Lord Laming, London: The Stationery Office.

Lewis, J. (2002) 'The contribution of research findings to practice change', MCC: Building Knowledge for Integrated Care, 10(1): 9–12.

Manby, M., Evans, I. and Hall, S. (1998) Case Review in Respect of PM. Born 15th September 1993, Died 6th December 1997. Report of an Independent Review Panel for North East Lincolnshire Area Child Protection Committee, Grimsby: North East Lincolnshire ACPC.

Manthorpe, J. (2003) 'Informing local inquiries: developing local reviews in adult protection', Journal of Adult Protection, 5(4): 18–25.

National Care Standards Commission (2003) website http://www.carestandards. org.uk

Raynes, N. (1998) 'Involving residents in quality specifications', Ageing and Society, 18(1): 65–78.

Sinclair, I. (2002) 'A quality-control perspective', in M. Davies (ed.), *The Blackwell Companion to Social Work*, Oxford: Blackwell, 431–7.

Social Services Inspectorate (1993) *No Longer Afraid: The Safeguard of Older People in Domestic Settings*, London: HMSO.

Williams, J. (1998) 'Drawing the boundaries of risk and regulation', in I. Allen (ed.), *Best Value, Regulation and Risk*, London: Policy Studies Institute.

Index